BRING YOUR OWN BANDAGES

98% of the content in *Bring Your Own Bandages: Medicines and Supplies to Have on Hand Before Disaster Strikes* comes from the Prep School Daily blog (prepschooldaily.blogspot.com). You can read everything from the blog for free. However, keep in mind that the medical articles in *Bring Your Own Bandages* are the abridged versions. What remains here is the bare-bones content you want to prepare and care for your family.

BRING YOUR OWN

BANDAGES

MEDICINES AND SUPPLIES

TO HAVE ON HAND BEFORE DISASTER STRIKES

JENNIFER RADER

Edited by: Kristine Collier
Cover design by: Berge Design

Published by
Juniper Ridge Press

Publisher's Note: Neither the publisher nor the author is associated with any company, vendor, product, or brand listed in this volume.

While the publisher and author have been careful in the preparation of this guidebook, it does not offer professional medical advice. All information contained herein is solely for educational and entertainment purposes. It does not constitute medical advice nor the practice of medicine. The reader must seek the services of licensed and qualified medical professionals for medical care. As medical care and knowledge are constantly expanding, it is not possible for this to be an all-encompassing guide.

At the time of publication, the author and publisher have made every effort to provide accurate Internet addresses. Naturally, the author and publisher cannot assume any responsibility for errors or changes that occur after publication.

ISBN: 978-1-7348261-0-4

For Jared, Luke, Sarah, Becky, Charlotte, and Lydia,
and all the children I hope you have:

May you prepare everything necessary for your families,
and may you never need any of it.

And for Aaron, my eternal companion and best friend,
whose life as a type-1 diabetic brought the necessity of
being medically prepared to the forefront
the day we started dating.

CONTENTS

INTRODUCTION **15**

SECTION 1—BASIC HEALTH AND NUTRITION **20**

1. THE RATIONING OF MEDICAL CARE AND SUPPLIES **20**

2. THE GREATEST MEDICAL ADVANCES **24**

3. WATER **26**

BOILING 26

BLEACH 27

CALCIUM HYPOCHLORITE 28

WATER PURIFICATION TABLETS 31

SOLAR DISINFECTION 33

IODINE 35

COMPARISON OF WATER PURIFICATION METHODS 35

4. HYGIENE **38**

HANDWASHING 38

HAND SANITIZER 40

QUARANTINE 41

ISOLATION 43

CLEANING 45

DISINFECTING 45

STERILIZING 47
WRAPPING INSTRUMENTS FOR STERILIZATION 48
5. NUTRITION 51
MACRONUTRIENTS 51
VITAMINS 56
MINERALS 70
SECTION 2—MEDICATIONS AND SUPPLIES 82
6. NON-PRESCRIPTION OVER-THE-COUNTER (OTC) MEDICATIONS 82
ANESTHETICS 82
ANTACIDS 86
ANTIDIARRHEALS 87
ANTIFUNGALS 87
ANTIHISTAMINES 87
ANTI-NAUSEA 93
COLD AND COUGH MEDICATIONS 94
EPINEPHRINE 96
PAIN RELIEVERS 97
ALTERNATIVES FOR ADMINISTERING MEDICATIONS 100
SHELF LIFE OF MEDICATIONS 102
STORING SUPPLIES FOR MAXIMUM SHELF LIFE 103
7. PRESCRIPTION MEDICATIONS—ANTIBIOTICS, ANTIFUNGALS, & ANTHELMINTICS 105
ANTIBIOTICS 105
ANTIFUNGALS 131
ANTHELMINTICS 132
PRESCRIPTION BOTTLE SHORTHAND DECODER 135
8. EXPENDABLE SUPPLIES 137
CHEMICAL LIGHT STICKS 137
COLD PACKS 137

COMPRESSED WASHCLOTHS 139
DRESSINGS 139
ENEMA BAGS 140
GLOVES 141
MASKS 142
HEMOSTATIC AGENTS 149
SKIN PREPS AND WASHES 151
SUTURES 159
TAPES 164
WRAPS 165
9. REUSABLE SUPPLIES 166
SAM SPLINTS 167
TOURNIQUETS 168
TRIANGLE BANDAGES 170
10. IMPROVISATIONAL SUPPLIES 172
ACTIVATED CHARCOAL 172
BAKING SODA 173
CAFFEINE 175
COCONUT OIL 177
DUCT TAPE 179
HONEY 182
MAGGOT THERAPY 184
PERMETHRIN 186
PLACEBOS 187
PRESSURE CANNER 196
SUGAR 189
SUGARDYNE 190
11. TOOLS AND EQUIPMENT 192
DIAGNOSTIC 192
LIGHTING 194

TREATMENT 196
12. SUPPLY ACQUISITION 200
PRIORITIZING THE ACQUISITION OF SUPPLIES 200
SOURCES FOR PURCHASING SUPPLIES.... 205
SECTION 3—ILLNESS AND DISEASE 208
13. SUPPLIES FOR DERMATOLOGIC ISSUES.... 208
BLEEDING 208
ABRASIONS 209
LACERATIONS 211
THE BASICS OF SUTURING 213
FIRST-DEGREE BURNS 216
SECOND-DEGREE BURNS 217
THIRD-DEGREE BURNS 221
TETANUS 223
SHINGLES.... 227
14. BITES AND VECTOR-BORNE ILLNESSES 230
INSECTS AND ARTHROPODS....230
VENOMOUS SNAKEBITES 254
DOMESTIC ANIMAL BITES.... 259
RABIES 261
15. COMMUNICABLE DISEASES.... 264
CHOLERA 264
PNEUMONIC PLAGUE.... 266
TUBERCULOSIS....268
TULAREMIA 271
TYPHOID FEVER 273
TYPHUS.... 276
YELLOW FEVER.... 278
OTHER MOSQUITO-BORNE DISEASES....280

16. RESPIRATORY TRACT ISSUES 283
COLDS, INFLUENZA, AND COLD-LIKE ILLNESSES 283
COUGHS 285
CROUP 287
EAR INFECTIONS 290
EUSTACHIAN TUBE DYSFUNCTION 292
FOREIGN BODY IN NOSE 293
INFLUENZA 295
PINK EYE 295
PNEUMONIA 298
RESPIRATORY SYNCYTIAL VIRUS 301
STREP THROAT 302
17. GASTROINTESTINAL AND ABDOMINAL ISSUES 304
FOOD POISONING 304
APPENDICITIS 321
DIVERTICULAR DISEASE 324
BEZOARS 326
CHOLECYSTITIS 328
CHOLANGITIS 329
GALLSTONES 329
ULCERS 330
18. UROGENITAL CONCERNS 334
KIDNEY STONES 334
URINARY TRACT INFECTIONS 337
SEXUALLY TRANSMITTED DISEASES 339
19. ENVIRONMENTAL INJURIES 342
FROSTNIP AND FROSTBITE 342
HYPOTHERMIA 343
HYPERTHERMIA 348
RADIATION 350

20. SELECTED CHRONIC CONDITIONS 354

ASTHMA 354

DIABETES TYPE 1 357

DIABETES TYPE 2 360

HYPOTHYROIDISM 360

LIFE-THREATENING ALLERGIES 363

SECTION 4—MEDICAL RECORDS 365

21. MEDICAL RECORDS 365

PERSONAL MEDICAL RECORDS 365

TAKING AND GIVING A PATIENT HISTORY 367

22. ASSESSING A PATIENT 371

VITAL SIGNS 374

BLOOD TYPES 376

SECTION 5—SAMPLE MEDICAL KITS 378

23. SMALL MEDICAL KITS 379

BOO-BOO KIT 379

IFAK 380

24. LARGE MEDICAL KITS 381

FAMILY MEDICAL KITS 381

ADVANCED MEDICAL KIT 383

SECTION 6—APPENDICES 389

APPENDIX 1. RECOMMENDED READING 389

ALTON'S ANTIBIOTICS AND INFECTIOUS DISEASE 389

ARMAGEDDON MEDICINE 391

SURVIVAL AND AUSTERE MEDICINE, 3RD EDITION 394

THE SURVIVAL MEDICINE HANDBOOK 396

HERBAL ANTIBIOTICS 398

HERBAL ANTIVIRALS 399
THE HERBAL MEDIC 401
NUCLEAR WAR SURVIVAL SKILLS 402
HOW TO OBTAIN THESE REFERENCES 405
APPENDIX 2. .... **406**
THE MASTER MEDICAL SHOPPING LIST 406
APPENDIX 3. .... **410**
TRADE AND GENERIC NAMES FOR MEDICATIONS 410
ENDNOTES 412
INDEX 439

INTRODUCTION

You have picked up this book because you are someone who feels better being prepared. In all likelihood, you've already acquired a substantial supply of food, fuel, clothing, tents, and bedding for your family. You probably have a first-aid kit and maybe even some training from Red Cross or CERT classes. You're well ahead of the crowd.

And yet, you've got some nagging doubts. What if my child gets sick? What if she's got an ear infection? What if my son breaks a leg? My brother had his appendix removed when he was seventeen; what if my child's appendix ruptured and we couldn't get to a hospital? My husband is a type-1 diabetic; how are we going to manage his condition if our society collapses?

Should I do more? *Can* I do more to prepare for challenging times ahead?

The answer is a resounding *Yes!* There is so much we can do to prepare for possible medical needs of our family members, even if we don't currently understand much about medicine or the supplies we should have. Often, well-meaning folks assert that people shouldn't acquire supplies or equipment that they don't know how to use. To them I respond, in all sincerity, "Are you storing up medical supplies for me and my family?"

Naturally, the answer is no. "Who do you think is storing supplies for my family and me?"

"I don't know."

"Are we supposed to suffer or die because we lack officially recognized training to use these supplies?"

In response to that question, there is either some sheepish mumbling or that deer-in-the-headlights look.

Basically, we're on our own for supplies. It doesn't give you warm fuzzies, does it?

The good news is that this book will get you well on your way to being prepared for medical emergencies. It's not medical or nursing school, but what you learn here and store for your family is far beyond a drugstore first-aid kit filled with cheap bandages that doesn't even include some aspirin.

As you go through this guidebook, consider getting some off-grid medicine training. Think carefully about who you are and what you actually want to learn. A tactical combat and casualty course (TCCC or T-triple C) with heavy emphasis on gunshots and chest seals may not be your cup of tea if you're far more interested in how to manage strep throat and dog bites. Wilderness Emergency Medical Training is less likely to benefit Grandpa who isn't hiking in the backcountry anytime soon. Get the training that will let you help the people you will be with, in the situations you are most likely to be in. There are courses out there for lay people who want to be able to give medical care to their family when there is no doctor, and they are offered all over the country.

I'm not a doctor. This isn't a manual for treating any disease, illness, or condition. Any time you have a medical concern, you must seek competent care from licensed medical personnel. This book is a reference to guide you in acquiring necessary medical supplies, to help you understand how they will be used, and when, so that you may acquire those resources your family will most likely need. History has shown us, and COVID-19 is showing us now, that in a long-term crisis, locating a doctor to care for a patient is far easier than obtaining the supplies needed to treat the patient. While it's always a great idea to get more education and know how to use what you have, sometimes we have to make do with acquiring supplies in advance of the education. That's what this book is for. When societies collapse, people have to bring their own bandages to the clinic.

It's a concept many cannot fathom. Doctors' offices are always stocked. So are hospital carts and pharmacies. Drugstores likewise have everything on the shelves, probably because their goods are so overpriced. When society collapses, we'll be in our homes with our families, experiencing the same things people go to the ER and urgent care for right now—coughs, influenza, pneumonia, stitches, abdominal pain. We'll need the same medicines that doctors prescribe or recommend now—antibiotics, OTC pain relievers, antacids, and antihistamines. What will change is easy, rapid access to those medications and supplies. And that's why we need to prepare before disaster strikes.

We don't know what the exact nature of the crisis will be. However, general preparations for the most common and likely things prepare us for what really happens as well. Preparing well for something like typhus, pneumonic plague, or malaria means that we have everything we need when something like COVID-19 occurs—no panic buying of masks, hand sanitizer, or TP.

This guide is incomplete. I know that better than anyone else. There is nothing on dental or mental issues, eyes, orthopedics, obstetrics, or communicable diseases we currently vaccinate for like measles and diphtheria. If I waited until it was perfect, it would never happen. But this first edition is a really good start. It covers the basics of clean water and good nutrition, the common illnesses and injuries, and the medications and supplies needed to have on hand. With the items recommended in this book, you'll have what a doctor needs to address orthopedic and obstetric issues as well.

The endnotes are copious; some would say they are over the top. This is so the reader can do further research on any topic of interest. Secondly, especially with dosing regimens and treatment protocols, it's to provide documentation for what is recommended. Physicians often disagree on treatment, just like experts in other fields. Sometimes there are myths perpetuated by those who really should know better, like tetracycline becoming toxic immediately past the use-by date, people allergic to shellfish being allergic to iodine, or that 10% of people allergic to penicillin have a cross-reactivity to cephalosporins. I have to document all of that.

TEOTWAWKI (The End of the World as We Know It) is not TV. You don't transform from armchair prepper to credentialed physician by turning the page of a script. Storing medical supplies and equipment doesn't make you a doctor any more than having milk and nipples makes you a cow. There are billions of people around the world who wish they'd had the foresight to purchase N95 masks in advance of the COVID-19 pandemic. There are millions of people in Venezuela today who wish they'd acquired some essential medicines and supplies. For them, finding a doctor right now is far easier than finding a little penicillin or Cipro.

A little closer to home, Hurricane Maria wiped out Puerto Rico's plants responsible for producing the bags and critical intravenous fluids used in hospitals all over the United States. Currently, elective surgeries in the US and Europe are currently being postponed to make sure every possible bed is available to treat COVID-19 patients. China, the behemoth with whom we keep playing trade-war chicken, manufactures all of our antibiotics. Every last one.

Not only does developing knowledge and skills to use medical supplies properly take time, whether it's first-aid courses or medical school, but it also requires constant review. In the meantime, the window for acquiring supplies narrows or closes entirely. It is essential to gather supplies while we can. The antibiotic window is gradually narrowing as far as legally obtaining them in US. Of course, letting China take over world production of all antibiotics was foolish in the extreme, and war with China (whether trade war or hot war) or perhaps COVID-19 will effectively cut off those supplies entirely.

Having considered life in Venezuela, the situation with China, and political and economic instability here and throughout the world, let's consider the most common killers in third-world countries, because that's what conditions become like in a societal collapse.

- Diarrhea
- Malaria
- Pneumonia
- Typhoid
- Childbirth

Deaths due to these causes have been almost unheard of in the US due to clean water, sanitation, and advanced medical care. You've got to know how to provide clean water and sanitation. Beyond that, know how to manage your own medical conditions and those that run in your family. Prepare for these eventualities first by gathering the supplies. Keep in mind that it will be easier to find a doctor than to locate critical goods in a collapsed society. Don't let anyone dissuade you from obtaining them. Your family is depending on you.

And finally, work with a like-minded friend or family, if possible. While each family should acquire their own medications, some of the diagnostic tools can easily be shared. Strep test strips are less expensive if they can be shared between a few families. Group buys allow purchasing of gauze and tapes in bulk while reducing shipping costs. Keeping in contact and discussing acquisitions keeps everyone moving forward on the path to preparedness.

SECTION 1—BASIC HEALTH AND NUTRITION

1. THE RATIONING OF MEDICAL CARE AND SUPPLIES

In emergencies today there is little concern about using up resources; medical personnel give no thought to this. The carts and cabinets are always stocked and most of the common medical supplies are relatively inexpensive. There will always be more. When our circumstances change for the worse, most people won't understand that life will never be the same again, or at least for a long time. Doctors will continue to utilize precious medicines at the same pace. Supplies will quickly become depleted. They probably won't be there when you need them.

We must stock and maintain supplies for our own families. We are responsible to provide for our loved ones. While none of us possesses limitless resources or is able to prepare for every problem, we can acquire the supplies to care for most needs. We've got to. No one else is doing it for us.

The purpose of this book is to motivate readers to prevent health problems from occurring in the first place, and to acquire the supplies necessary to manage conditions that will inevitably develop. The aim, if we are prepared, is to prevent needless suffering and death. It is not a pocket guide for medical care nor a substitute for official training.

When society collapses, what you have stored for your family is what you have. There will be no resupply, because manufacturing and transportation will cease. Many of the existing supplies will be wasted; even those that could have been reused will be discarded. While the black market works well in Hollywood, reality dictates a different scenario.

However, like on TV, medical supplies will be a target, as will anyone perceived as being able to provide care. Unfortunately, the supplies run out sooner or later. The importance of learning how to use herbal medicine with herbs local to your area cannot be over-emphasized. But that's a topic for another book. Items that can be improvised will be addressed later. Of great importance now is gathering reusable medical tools and supplies. Glass syringes are hard to locate, but still possible. And they can be autoclaved and sterilized repeatedly. Plastic syringes cannot. Needles can also be reused indefinitely, but you'll want a way to sharpen the tip. Rayon gauze, unlike cotton, can also be sterilized for reuse.

If people are aware that you have medical supplies, they will be requested, demanded, or confiscated from you. Like with a lot of preparedness activities, you may wish to keep a low profile regarding your supplies. As long as possible, anyway.

Bear in mind that your supplies are just that—they're *your* supplies. You decide how, when, and for whom they are used. That is going to be difficult, even heart-wrenching at times. Even if you are only dealing with your own family, you will have to accept that:

- Some are going to die no matter what you do.
- You will have to decline using resources on them, to spare them for others later who can be saved.
- This may include your spouse, children, or grandchildren.
- You can't change reality.

Currently, when someone is wounded and taken to the hospital for treatment, the whole staff and supply stockpile can be devoted to that individual, especially with insurance to cover everything and a functioning manufacturing and delivery system for resupply. When there is a large-scale disaster with more wounded than can be cared for with available staff and supplies, treatment is rationed. In medical terms, it's called *triage*. Different systems include from three to seven colors for categorization of care. We'll just use three:

At its most basic level, there are three categories of triage:

- Patients likely to survive, regardless of what care is given (green)
- Patients likely to die, regardless of what care is given (black)
- Patients for whom immediate care may result in a positive outcome (red)

Advanced triage processes include up to three more classifications, including white (walk away, simple home care at most is required), and yellow and orange (degrees of care between green and red, above).

People need to know who can be helped and whom to help first, based on a layman's assessment and the limited resources available.

With all that being said, people must prepare mentally for death. After the first few days, if people realize that the crisis is going to be a long-term event and recovery will take months or years, the death rate is going to skyrocket. Faced with the reality of a horrible situation, some will opt for suicide. They'll be joined by those afflicted with chronic pain who can no longer get the relief they desire and would rather die. Individuals dependent on life-preserving drugs will also perish as those supplies dwindle. Overcome by stress, others will succumb to heart attacks.

Cardiopulmonary resuscitation today keeps many patients alive until they reach the hospital, but without advanced care available in a functioning hospital, these people will not survive. If an individual suffers a heart attack, that person already has underlying conditions that will only be managed with pharmaceuticals and advanced technology. That equipment will not be available. CPR generally isn't performed in a disaster when there is no hope of further advanced care, but there are three exceptions to this rule. Those are for people who were electrocuted (including by lightning strikes), who choked, or who drowned. These individuals were healthy beforehand and have good chances of making a complete recovery.

Finally, there are those injuries or conditions which aren't automatically terminal right now, but will be without the care that can only be offered in a fully operational hospital. These include pelvic fractures with substantial bleeding, as in car accidents, and those with substantial burns. When advanced care is not accessible, these patients may live for days or even weeks, but they'll exhaust supplies that could be preserved to save so many other people. And these patients will die anyway.

The triage system currently used by emergency responders is for a society where medical care is a right. In a collapsed society, the situation is a whole lot different. Medical care becomes a privilege for those who contribute to society and who chose to prepare.

It's sometimes beyond our ability to comprehend.

How do you tell your child or grandchild to accept the pain of an excruciating ear infection (which can be as painful as kidney stones or labor and delivery) because it will eventually get better? How do you tell your friend that you can't spare your antibiotics to save his elderly father, who, even though he's a nice guy, isn't contributing to the survival of the group? On the other hand, maybe someone comes to you and wants the few antibiotics you have that must be reserved for children or pregnant women.

Your supplies are extremely limited. A soft-hearted individual likely to succumb to a sob story isn't the one to have the medical supplies under his control. They need to be in the hands of someone who can make those hard, rational decisions. Maybe the medications at least need to be very inaccessible. Maybe no one should know what you have. It's yours. It's for your family, not society. It's your call. And it's going to be a hard call.

2. THE GREATEST MEDICAL ADVANCES

It is said that 95% of self-defense is threat avoidance. The same idea can be applied to disease. We need to do everything possible to avoid getting sick.

The top four greatest medical advances, in the opinion of physicians surveyed in 2007, were clean water and sanitation, antibiotics, anesthesia, and vaccines.[1] Notice that three of those four deal with threat avoidance. Now, some may dispute putting antibiotics in that category, but the truth of the matter is that oftentimes antibiotics are given prophylactically, as a preventative measure. Sometimes, however, even when they are given to treat an illness, they are not actually needed. More on that will be discussed in specific cases later. Water, sanitation, and anesthesia will also be addressed in subsequent chapters.

The development of vaccines was ranked fourth in the list of greatest medical advances. What vaccines you choose for your family is your business entirely. However, a tetanus vaccine really should be on everyone's list to stay current on. In a natural disaster or societal collapse, there will be a significant number of dirty wounds. Measles is making a strong comeback now. Keep current on the vaccines you are comfortable receiving. And bear in mind, that if you do not vaccinate, you need to be especially sure you can identify the illnesses you don't vaccinate for, and have all the supplies to deal with them. In all likelihood, the physician you find to help you will *never* have seen a case of measles, diphtheria, tetanus, or rubella.

Hopefully, you're in good physical condition and have addressed your known personal medical issues. If you haven't done it yet, now's the time to plan for the potential medical problems that could face your family. All the advances in modern medicine are of little value to us if we fail in the following.

Most are common sense practices that our mothers pounded into our heads since birth:

- Exercise regularly
- Wear shoes, especially when outside
- Brush your teeth at least twice each day
- Floss
- Lose excess weight
- Eat a balanced diet
- Quit all addictions
- Get adequate sleep
- Watch infants and children carefully
- Wear sunscreen
- Wipe from front to back
- Wash your hands
- Keep hydrated
- Be nice to others

Careful observance of these practices and other preventative measures will keep your family healthy and go a long way towards keeping you out of the "Bring Your Own Bandages Clinic."

But when this fails, and inevitably something will go awry, we want to be sure we're prepared.

3. WATER

The Rule of Threes reminds us that while we can live three weeks without food, we can only go three days without water. And drinking contaminated water can have serious or fatal consequences.

Being able to purify water in a disaster is a critical life skill all people should learn. Everyone should have the supplies necessary to remove contaminants from water using different methods depending on the situation. Boiling and distilling water are the best and most effective methods to render the safest water. Chlorine dioxide tablets are also excellent, but they're pretty expensive. Bleach and calcium hypochlorite are next on the list, followed by SODIS and iodine.

BOILING

When the water supply is compromised, the most common method of purifying contaminated water is boiling. After all, if we're at home, we've got the pans and the stove to accomplish the task quickly, and everyone knows how to boil water.

One of the emergency preparedness classes I taught when we lived in Missouri focused on the entirely unglamorous subject of water. No one gets excited about water sterilization, purification, filtration, distillation, whatever term you want to use (and no, the words are not interchangeable). It's a miracle anyone showed up.

We used the same scummy pond water everyone in our area would have to use in a disaster. I presented the class with four examples of treated water:

- Water that had only gone through a regular paper coffee filter
- Water through the coffee filter and boiled
- Water through the coffee filter and bleach added

- Water through the steam juicer, in effect, distilled

No one wanted to taste test the appropriately treated samples, and yet, what would happen if there were no water coming out of the tap?

The clearest water looked just like it came from the tap. That was the water that only went through the coffee filter. Looks can be very deceiving. The other three treated water samples were all pretty much equally uninviting. They had a kind of dull look to them, like I had started off with dirty pans or something. (My pans were most definitely not dirty.)

The absolute safest method for making drinking (and cooking and washing) water safe is to first run it through a coffee filter, cheesecloth, or some other cloth to remove the larger contaminants. Then boil it at a hard boil for one minute (three minutes for altitudes above 5,000 feet, according to the CDC and FDA).[2] To be extra safe, some recommend boiling for an additional minute for every 1,000 feet above sea level. I am at 5,600 feet altitude, so I would need 6 minutes of a hard boil. Unfortunately, that's going to take a bit of fuel, which we may not necessarily have in excess in a crisis.

BLEACH

If boiling is not an option, common, unscented household bleach may be used. Chlorine, in the right concentration, will kill pathogens in water to make it safe for drinking and cooking. Because liquid chlorine bleach is readily available at stores and often used in the home, it is an ideal prep item that can be easily rotated to have fresh stock at all times. This is important because liquid chlorine bleach does not have a long shelf-life. While bleach does not become toxic with time, it does lose potency such that about six months after purchase it is only 50% effective. After a year, it should be discarded.

The first thing to do when treating contaminated water, regardless of the method you are using, is to filter the water through a coffee filter, dishtowel, or clean cloth of some sort. Removing the solids facilitates purification and improves the appearance. People don't want floaties in their water.

Pour the filtered water into a clean bottle. (Containers may be sanitized by adding one teaspoon of unscented bleach to a quart of water in the container. Shake well, coating the entire interior surface. Let sit for at least thirty seconds and then drain. Rinse well with clean, treated water or let air dry.)

With the chart below as a guide, use a clean dropper to add the amount of bleach to your water. If the water is cloudy, colored, or cold, double the amount of bleach.[3]

Amount of bleach to add to treat water					
	1 quart	1 gallon	2 gallons	4 gallons	8 gallons
5.25-6% bleach	2 drops	8 drops	16 drops or 1/4 teaspoon	1/3 teaspoon	2/3 teaspoon
8.25% bleach	2 drops	6 drops	12 drops or 1/8 teaspoon	1/4 teaspoon	1/2 teaspoon

Stir the bleach in well and let the water stand for 30 minutes. There should still be a faint odor of bleach in the water. If there isn't, repeat the procedure and let the water stand another 15 minutes.

The water is now safe to use. However, if the chlorine smell is too strong, let the water stand longer. The odor should dissipate within a few hours. Removing the chlorine odor can be hastened by pouring the water back and forth between clean containers several times. Flavored drink mixes can help mask the taste as well.

CALCIUM HYPOCHLORITE

Unfortunately, liquid bleach is volatile, resulting in a pretty short shelf life, a serious disadvantage for long-term preparedness. Clorox recommends only using bleach that is less than four months old for water purification purposes; the CDC and EPA both state that bleach up to six months old may be used. Replacing bleach that frequently can become a bit of a challenge. There are so many items we need to rotate and only so much money to go around.

Calcium hypochlorite to the rescue!

The usage of dry calcium hypochlorite powder to purify drinking water isn't some quack doomsday prepper notion of questionable efficacy. Instructions for its usage are included in the Sanitary Control and Surveillance of Field Water Supplies publication issued by the military in 2010.[4] In fact, it is the preferred option for military members away from a secure supply of clean water. Iodine, purification tablets, chlorine, and boiling the water are much further down on their list.

What is calcium hypochlorite? It is very closely related to sodium hypochlorite, common household bleach. Unlike liquid bleach, however, powdered calcium hypochlorite is very stable, with about a ten-year shelf life when stored in a cool, dark place. Because it is powdered, it takes very little space and stock solutions can be made on demand instead of storing liquid bleach that deteriorates rather quickly. This powdered calcium hypochlorite powder is commonly referred to as HTH, high test granular calcium hypochlorite. It can be a bit confusing when you're shopping for it and trying to research the matter.

Use the chart at right to create a 5% stock solution from your HTH calcium hypochlorite. Then use that 5% stock solution to you created to purify drinking water using the chart below.

5% Calcium Hypochlorite Stock Solution	
Amount of water	Amount of HTH
1 ½ cups	1 teaspoon
1 quart	2 ¾ teaspoons
2 quarts	5 ½ teaspoons
1 gallon	10 ¾ teaspoons

Amount of HTH Stock Solution to Purify Water		
Amount of water	Amount of HTH stock solution for clear water	Amount of HTH stock solution for cloudy, cold, or questionable water
1 quart	2 drops	4 drops
2 quarts	4 drops	8 drops
1 gallon	8 drops	16 drops
4 gallons	32 drops-1/2 teaspoon	3/4 teaspoon
5 gallons	1/2 teaspoon	1 teaspoon
6 gallons	2/3 teaspoon	1 1/3 teaspoons

Calcium hypochlorite powder may be used directly to purify larger quantities of water. For example, 1/8 teaspoon of the HTH powder may be stirred into a 55-gallon barrel with 50 gallons of water in it. Cover and let stand for at least 24 hours.

The Environmental Protection Agency suggests a different method on its website, as follows:

Add one heaping teaspoon (approximately ¼ ounce) of high-test granular calcium hypochlorite (HTH) to two gallons of water and stir until the particles have dissolved. The mixture will produce a chlorine solution of approximately 500 mg per liter. To disinfect water, add one part of the chlorine solution to each 100 parts of water you are treating. This is about the same as adding 1 pint (16 ounces) of the chlorine solution to 12.5 gallons of water. If the chlorine taste is too strong, pour the water from one clean container to another and let it stand for a few hours before use.[5]

So where exactly does one purchase this wonder chemical, and what exactly should be purchased? It can be pretty confusing. Lots of times you'll see people saying to get pure calcium hypochlorite. That's where most of the confusion comes from. The strongest you can purchase is about 68-70%. Because this is serious stuff, and because so much misinformation abounds on the internet, here is a direct quote from the Sanitary Control and Surveillance of Field Water Supplies publication:

> "Calcium hypochlorite is a white granular or powdered chemical. When fresh, it typically contains 68 to 70% by weight available chlorine. It is commonly referred to as HTH and is frequently used as a disinfectant in swimming pools."[6]

It can be purchased through Amazon, at Walmart, and at pool supply stores. Due to my experience with bags disintegrating, I opted to buy calcium hypochlorite packaged in a plastic bottle. It is easier to use from a bottle that can be recapped. It cost a few dollars more, but I think the extra expense is worth the convenience. You don't need to buy a lot; a single bag or bottle will treat ten thousand gallons of water.

As a hazardous chemical, calcium hypochlorite can chemically burn the eyes, skin, and mucous membranes. Wear gloves and safety glasses when using this product.

Storage: Calcium hypochlorite has a ten-year shelf life when stored in cool, dark conditions. It should be stored away from food. Off-gassing will make the plastic packaging brittle within a few years, after which time the bags will simply disintegrate with even the most careful handling. Even the plastic bucket we stored ours in shattered after about five years. You may wish to transfer the granules to a glass jar and tape the instructions and label to the outside.

WATER PURIFICATION TABLETS

Katadyn Micropur MP1 Water purification tablets, which are individually packaged for maximum shelf life (five years from date of manufacture, so if ordering online, make sure you're getting current stock), satisfy the US EPA guidelines for safe drinking water. They're really easy to use; just drop one tablet in a liter of water. Micropur tablets kill viruses and bacteria in 15 minutes in all water, and *Giardia* and *Cryptosporidium* in 30 minutes in 60°F clear water. If the water is cloudy and/or cold, eliminating the *Cryptosporidium* requires four hours.

The significant advantages of Micropur chlorine dioxide tablets is that these tablets are effective against *Cryptosporidium*. Unlike some pump filters, Micropur tablets eliminate bacteria and viruses. They are an excellent small and lightweight back-up in case the primary water purification method fails. Because the active ingredient is chlorine dioxide, the same chemical used in municipal water treatment, the taste should be the same for those who drink city water. Most reviewers say it tastes and smells like pool water. If that's a problem, carry some drink flavor packets for your water, especially for children.

Let's address some of the cons:

- Adding chemicals to drinking water. This isn't a "lifestyle choice." This is about preventing dehydration and diarrhea. It's not a long-term solution.
- Floaties. The tablets do not eliminate floaties in your water. If that's an important issue, pre-filter the water through a coffee filter, bandana, or clean t-shirt.
- Long time for eliminating *Cryptosporidium.* The four-hour purification time is only for cold, cloudy water. Run the water through a pre-filter and let it warm up before adding the Micropur tablet to hasten purification.
- The individual foil packets are hard to open. Use nail clippers or small scissors on a multi-tool to open the packets. If you do this in advance, mark the slit with a Sharpie to make the slit easier to find.

Additional thoughts:

- Katadyn Micropur tablets are inexpensive for the short-term or for an emergency or back-up. They're a bit pricey for long-term use.
- For the best protection, use a water filter first to eliminate *Giardia* and *Cryptosporidium,* and then the tablets take only 15 minutes to purify water from bacteria and viruses.
- Don't keep Micropur tablets in the car. They need to be stored below 80°F.
- Store the tablets in their original foil packets in a small plastic or metal mint container to keep them from getting crushed.
- Laminate the instruction card and keep it with the tablets. In a crisis, it can be difficult to remember instructions and think clearly.
- These tablets can be used in a hydration reservoir (water bladder).

SOLAR DISINFECTION

When it comes to prepping supplies and gear, "two is one, and one is none" is good advice to keep in mind. It doesn't matter whether it pertains to having multiples of the exact same item or different skills or methods of achieving a desired goal. It's always having Plans B, C, and D in case Plan A doesn't work out.

SODIS (SOlar water DISinfection) utilizes plastic water bottles and the sun to eliminate pathogens from drinking water. It's about as low-tech and inexpensive as possible. Developed in the 1980s as a means of purifying water in third-world countries, it's a method that can be applied to any disaster situation, keeping in mind the following:

Choose the right bottle material. The best containers are clear, uncolored polyethylene terephthalate (PETE) plastic or glass juice or soda bottles. The distinct advantages to PETE are that it is lightweight and highly resistant to breakage. (PETE bottles in the US are designated by the number *1* in the recycling triangle symbol.) These materials allow ultraviolet radiation to pass through the container to kill bacteria, viruses, protozoa, and other nasties. Contrary to popular belief, it is not the heat, but rather the ultraviolet radiation that does the work here.[7]

Choose the right size bottle. Use one- to two-liter bottles, no more than four inches in diameter. The more water the ultraviolet light has to pass through, the less effective it becomes. For this reason, larger water bottles are not effective.[8]

Clean the bottle. Remove the paper labels and clean the bottles. They must be free from dust and dirt so that the light can penetrate. They must also be relatively free of scratches, as scratches diffuse light and prevent UV radiation from passing into the bottle.

Pre-filter the water if necessary. If the water is cloudy, pass it through a bandana, dishtowel, clean t-shirt, or coffee filter to remove particulates. Adding a pinch of salt is also helpful to bind solids in the water. If you are not sure whether you should have filtered the water first, hold your hand up or put a newspaper on the other side of the bottle. If you can't distinguish your fingers or read a newspaper headline through the bottle, the water needs to be pre-filtered, or disinfection may not occur.

Fill the bottles. Fill the bottles 75% full and shake well for at least 30 seconds. Fill more bottles than you think you will possibly need. In ideal conditions, SODIS takes only six hours. But it can also take up to two days.

Lay the bottles out. The filled bottles need to be laid on their sides to maximize exposure. For best results, lay them on a white or reflective metal (mirrors, corrugated roofing) surface to increase the amount of light passing through the bottles. The bottles must also be outdoors. Laying them in front of a sunny window will not work. Residential housing glass doesn't let enough ultraviolet radiation pass through to pasteurize water.

Wait. The requisite exposure times vary in the literature, but it takes careful research to figure out why. SODIS was developed for lower-income people in third-world countries. The vast majority of these people live within 35° north or south of the equator.[9] They've got the most optimal sun exposure for using SODIS to the fullest extent possible. At these latitudes, SODIS will do its job within six hours on a sunny or partly sunny (more than 50%) day.[10]

However, most of the US is above 35° latitude. You can take a look at a map to see where you fit in, but here's a rough idea:

- Louisiana, Florida, Mississippi, Alabama, South Carolina, Georgia are all good.
- The southern halves of Arizona, New Mexico, and Arkansas are good.
- Most of Texas is good.
- The southern third of Oklahoma and the southern quarter of California are good.

In these areas, solar disinfection can be achieved in six hours on sunny or partly sunny (more than 50%) days. But as you move north, the water needs more time to become pasteurized, up to 48 hours. And remember, it is the ultraviolet radiation doing the job, not the temperature. Just like it is the ultraviolet radiation producing a sunburn. And just like it is possible to get sunburned on a cloudy day. It takes a little longer, but it's still entirely possible.

Keep in mind that the SODIS method is not perfect. It's about 98-99% effective in killing pathogens. Still, it's better than nothing and has been scientifically proven to work. Both the World Health Organization and the Centers for Disease Control recommend it as an option for achieving clean drinking water.[11]

IODINE

In an emergency, an iodine wipe (Betadine) can be dropped into a one-liter bottle of water to purify it for drinking. This generally takes about 15 minutes, but cooler or cloudy water should be permitted to stand 30 minutes. Betadine will not kill protozoa like *Cryptosporidium*. If you have a vitamin C tablet or water flavoring, add it after 15-30 minutes to reduce the iodine taste. This method of treatment is not recommended for long term use (say, more than a few months) due to the risk for developing goiter.

COMPARISON OF WATER PURIFICATION METHODS

This chart covers fourteen different methods of treating water. Some are approved and useful, and others should probably be avoided.

As far as how well water purification and filtering methods work, or to what extent, you need to decide what is important to you, or what you might be able to yield on or compensate for in other ways. The following three contaminants must be dealt with properly to prevent illness.

Bacteria. You've got to eliminate or kill them. If you don't, they might be killing you. If they don't kill you, you might wish they did (*Cholera, Shigella, Campylobacter, Salmonella*, etc.).

Viruses. Same as for bacteria (enterovirus, norovirus, rotavirus, hepatitis A, etc.).

Protozoa. *Giardia* and *Cryptosporidium* are no fun for anyone, but especially for those with weakened immune systems. Make sure your chosen treatment method will eliminate this risk. Most people are satisfied to deal with the first three issues and call it good. The better you can eliminate the following contaminants from your water, the better it will taste.

Chemicals. These are actually the hardest to deal with, but if it makes you any happier, your city water doesn't deal with them well, either. Every time you take a drink from your tap, you're drinking antibiotics and other medications that municipal water treatment plants do not remove.

Cloudiness. Cloudy water in and of itself won't make you sick, but we just feel better drinking clear water.

Taste. Some treatment methods leave an off taste in the water. Activated charcoal excels at improving the taste of treated water. Another option is to consider having some Kool-Aid or similar flavoring to mask off-tastes and cloudiness.

Distillation is the gold standard for any water being given to infants and small children. They are at the highest risk for adverse effects of chemicals in the water.

For the rest of us, making certain bacteria, viruses, and protozoa are eliminated is the minimum standard. To get the cleanest water and best taste, we'll probably have to make sure to have an excellent water treatment system or combine two methods. There are loads of products on the market, and each has its advantages.

Water is pretty critical to life. Make sure you've got a lot stored and the knowledge and equipment to treat it in a few different ways.

Comparison of various water treatment methods						
Method	Bacteria	Viruses	Protozoa	Chemicals	Cloudiness	Taste
Distillation	Yes	Yes	Yes	Yes	Yes	Yes
Boiling	Yes	Yes	Yes	No	No	No
Chlorine	Yes	Yes	No	No	No	No
Iodine	Yes	Yes	No	No	No	No
SODIS (Solar pasteurization)	Yes	Yes	Yes	No	No	No
Stabilized oxygen	Yes	Yes	Yes	No	No	No
UV light	Yes*	Yes*	Yes*	No	No	No
Reverse osmosis	Maybe	Maybe	Maybe	Yes	Yes	Yes
Ceramic filter	Yes	No	Yes	No	Yes	No
Activated charcoal filter	Yes**	Maybe**	Yes	Maybe	Yes	Yes
Sand filter	No	No	No	No	Yes	Maybe
Grapefruit seed extract	Maybe	Maybe	Maybe	No	No	No
Straining through coffee filter	No	No	No	No	Maybe	No
Katadyn Micropur tablets	Yes	Yes	Yes	No	No	Maybe

Yes=eliminates contaminant. No=does not eliminate contaminant. *starting with clear water only **starting with new filters only

4. HYGIENE

The current COVID-19 crisis has brought the hygiene issue front and center to the American public. Hand sanitizer was the first thing Americans rushed to purchase after masks sold out. It makes you wonder what they did before. We're now living the quarantine and isolation life, even as we learn to distinguish between cleaning and disinfecting.

HANDWASHING

We've all seen those people leaving public bathrooms without washing at all, or children who try to get away with a quick rinse. Statistically, only 60% of women and less than 40% of men wash their hands after using a public bathroom. Disturbing, isn't it?

The Centers for Disease Control and Prevention lists when hands should be washed[12]:

- Before and after preparing food
- Before and after eating
- Before and after caring for anyone who is sick
- Before and after treating any injury or changing bandages
- Before touching your face, especially the eyes, nose, or mouth
- After returning home
- After using the toilet or helping a child use the toilet
- After changing a diaper
- After blowing your nose, or coughing or sneezing into your hands
- After touching any animal, including pets, animal waste, or animal feed
- After handling garbage or taking out the trash

- After touching any surfaces in an ill person's room

Washing hands thoroughly and every single time it is called for will dramatically reduce the spread of contagious disease. Even if we are meticulous about washing our hands, we have to do it well and frequently for the best protection. Regular bar soap is all that is required; antibacterial soap is not any more effective and has actually been shown to contribute to antibiotic resistance.

What exactly is involved with effective handwashing? There are five steps:

- Wet hands with clean, warm (it's more comfortable), running water, and then turn off the tap. Leaving the water running makes people rush because they don't want to waste water.
- Lather hands by rubbing them together with the soap. Be sure to cover the hands, wrists, between the fingers and under the nails—especially under the nails. The undersides of fingernails are like miniature Petri dishes perfect for breeding microbes. Keeping nails trimmed and using a nail brush will automatically eliminate a lot of opportunities for infection.

> Artificial nails of any kind can harbor all sorts of microbes. Keeping with the natural look is safest.

- Scrub hands vigorously for 20-30 seconds. Teach children to sing "Happy Birthday" slowly, all the way through, twice, making sure all the while that they wash between their fingers, the knuckles, and under the nails.
- Then rinse well under running water. Rinsing in standing water risks recontamination of your hands. Use a paper towel to turn off the faucet.[13]
- Finally, dry hands using a clean towel or an air dryer. Also, use the paper towel (or the hem of your shirt) to open the bathroom door to avoid the recontamination of your hands.

HAND SANITIZER

You've heard people say that hand sanitizer works just as well as soap, but are they right? Is hand sanitizer as effective as washing hands? Is it better? Or is it worse?

The answer depends on several factors.

First, whether hand sanitizer is effective depends on whether the alcohol content of the hand sanitizer is adequate. The hand sanitizer must contain at least 60% rubbing alcohol. Fifty percent alcohol is not strong enough. The alcohol content should be indicated on the hand sanitizer label. However, if the hand sanitizer is older, some of the alcohol content may have evaporated, and it may not be as strong as when it was manufactured. This is one of the few instances in medicine where the use-by date must be taken seriously. Maintain a careful inventory of your hand sanitizer and rotate it well. If older hand sanitizer is all you have, make sure to apply it two or three times and rub it in well.

Secondly, the hand sanitizer must come into direct contact with the microbes. If there is visible dirt or other waste on your hands, it must be removed first.[14] Use a baby wipe, washcloth, or clothing if necessary to remove all visible dirt and particles. Then apply the hand sanitizer.

Next, hand sanitizer that is applied and rubbed in like lotion is not sufficient. To do its job, hand sanitizer should be applied liberally and rubbed in vigorously for at least twenty seconds, just as for washing hands with soap and water.[15] However, that is just for regular, garden-variety viruses, not the real bad guys (which is what you really want protection from). A study published by Japanese researchers showed that hand sanitizer being rubbed in for two full minutes did not kill the influenza A virus. It took four full minutes of rubbing in hand sanitizer to completely disable that virus. However, handwashing for thirty seconds was effective.[16]

Finally, hand sanitizer really should not be used as a substitute for routine handwashing. Yes, in some cases hand sanitizer works just as well as soap and water. But in others, like with influenza A, it definitely does not. In addition, the alcohol in hand sanitizer is very drying to the skin, and excessive use may result in dry, cracked skin, which is more vulnerable to infection.[17] Hand sanitizer should not be used in place of regular washing in the home. Washing with soap and water is the gold standard and should be used whenever possible.

QUARANTINE

There is a substantial difference between quarantine and isolation; these terms are not synonyms. Isolation is for those known to be ill with a contagious disease, to separate individuals who are sick from those who are not. Quarantine is practiced in relation to people exposed to a contagious disease but who may or may not become ill. In theory, it separates and restricts the movement of people who were exposed to a disease, to see if they become sick. Both actions are taken to protect the group or community.[18]

The diseases listed in the text box on the side are basically the only ones that the government screens for at our borders, ports, and airports. Each of these diseases has the potential to be fatal. Beyond these diseases, however, there are a whole lot more illnesses you might be concerned about and which you should prevent coming into your home, afflicting your family, and using up your medical supplies.

Ideally, anyone with hepatitis, MRSA, pneumonia, fevers, or any other disease or symptoms should have the decency to stay away

> Federal law authorizes quarantine for following diseases:
>
> Cholera
> Diphtheria
> Infectious tuberculosis
> Plague
> Smallpox
> Yellow fever
> Viral hemorrhagic fevers
> SARS
> Pandemic influenza
> COVID-19
>
> Note that Ebola is not on the list. Neither is measles. Previous to the COVID-19 outbreak, the last time a federal quarantine was enforced in the United States occurred during the 1918-1920 influenza epidemic.

from others and practice self-isolation. In our society, that's nothing more than a pipe dream. Parents pressure doctors for antibiotic prescriptions so that they can send their children back to daycare as soon as possible, even though the disease is probably viral and the antibiotic won't work anyway. Public schools have attendance laws. If students aren't completely well but are doing ok, they go back to school, still contagious, and spread disease further. When we're sick, we take cold remedies or other things to feel better, so that we can go to work. Sick people are more susceptible to catching other illnesses and spreading the joy even more.

Of course, there are a whole lot of other communicable diseases to be aware of and screen for than those listed above:

- Everything for which we have immunizations right now, because a lot of people are not immunized
- STDs
- Parasites like lice, scabies, fleas, and bedbugs
- Vector-borne diseases like malaria and dengue fever
- And the list goes on

How do you practice quarantine now? Do you? What will change in a societal collapse or TEOTWAWKI? What if the people at your door are family or close friends? What if they all appear healthy? What if, like with COVID-19, some people are asymptomatic?

Is the runny nose, cough, or itchy eyes really just allergies? Is the rash contact dermatitis, or something a bit more ominous? Does the toddler really have only a cold, which probably won't have serious consequences for anyone who catches it, or is it infectious mononucleosis, which only causes a runny nose in small children for a few days (and has an incubation period lasting up to five to six weeks), but which can be extremely debilitating in an older teen or adult?

It's best to determine in advance how you are going to handle quarantine of any outsiders, and that includes family and close friends. If society has collapsed, and it's been more than a few weeks, even a few days, the potential for all kinds of nasty diseases is out there. The lack of advanced medical care if someone does fall sick is concern enough to practice quarantine.

Are you letting them into your house? Do you have a barn they can use? What about a nice size tent and camping equipment? Maybe an RV? Determine how long you're going to enforce this quarantine. Even five days of quarantine will decrease the transmission risk for most diseases by nearly 90%. Unfortunately, some of those nasties have much longer incubation periods. Are you prepared to keep the quarantine in place for up to ten days, or three weeks, or better yet, five weeks? It's your call, but prepare yourself. These people seeking refuge will probably be angry.[19]

Remind people that if someone breaks quarantine, the quarantine period starts over from the very beginning.

If, however, the people at your door do not look healthy or something nasty is circulating, you definitely don't want to let them in. Maybe the barn or a tent, but not with the rest of your family. Your first responsibility is your family. That means keeping them and you healthy.

Even if people appear healthy and if you decide to admit them, complete physical checks are warranted to be sure. Lice? While they make adults itch, often children do not itch, and it's only when someone spies the bugs crawling around that they realize they've got an issue. Scabies and bedbugs can also be difficult to identify, and a lot of people aren't going to 'fess up about having them.

ISOLATION

In an ideal situation, the ill individual is completely isolated from the rest of the family, with the exception of one caretaker, who is also isolated as much as possible from the household. The patient should have a separate bedroom, preferably with a window that can be cracked for proper ventilation, as well as a separate bathroom, or lacking that, two buckets to substitute for a toilet. Food should be served with paper and plastic ware so that there is no need to wash dishes and less risk for spreading germs.

Further measures to be taken will likely depend on the nature of the illness and how exactly it is transmitted. Is it airborne (tuberculosis, chicken pox), foodborne, or bloodborne? Vector-borne (mosquitoes, ticks), fomite-borne (doorknobs, counters, faucet handles, toys), or droplet-borne?

For airborne diseases, you'll want to be able to seal off duct work and add a rolled towel along the bottom of the sickroom door to prevent air from being sucked into the rest of the house. Any person at risk for the disease, and especially the caregiver, should wear personal protective equipment, most especially a mask, preferably an N95 or better.

In the case of droplet-borne diseases, the patient should also have a simple face mask to prevent spreading the disease to others. While a face mask on the patient does nothing to halt the spread of airborne diseases, it does help prevent the spread of droplet-borne diseases.

With all diseases, the caregiver should have nitrile gloves. Latex gloves don't have a great shelf life, and some people are allergic to it. Both latex and vinyl gloves tend to stick together and melt with time, especially in humid areas. Nitrile gloves, though a little more expensive, are really the only way to go.

The time the patient needs to be in isolation will vary depending on several factors. If electronic devices are no longer working, as the patient recovers, boredom is going to become a huge issue and the temptation to release a patient from isolation will be great. Consider having some really good books available, or perhaps working everything out so a child will be able to watch a movie.

Keep in mind that the most important medicine you can offer may be showing true concern for the patient. That's part of the placebo effect, and while placebos don't work on microbes, a sympathetic caregiver can definitely improve patient morale and thus speed recovery.

CLEANING

In a situation of a prolonged collapse of society, there will possibly come a point when we need to sterilize some medical instruments or equipment. Yeah, this is the kind of stuff we really don't want to think about, the kind of stuff we sure hope won't ever apply to us. We certainly hope no one needs stitches or an appendectomy. While I'm pretty confident we have stored an excess of syringes for my diabetic husband, we also have glass syringes and reusable needles just in case.

And just in case that day comes, we need to know the difference between cleaning, disinfecting, and sterilizing.

Cleaning is what we do when we wash the dishes or the laundry. Using soap or detergent and water, scrub the object clean, and hand dry it or let it air dry. *Clean* means there is no *visible* dirt or debris or food or tissue of any kind. Any gross contamination—visible blood, dirt, or debris—can harbor bacteria and viruses and protect them during disinfection or sterilization. There may still be all kinds of bacteria and viruses on whatever you just cleaned, because the item has not been disinfected or sterilized.

DISINFECTING

Disinfecting comes next. (Actually, in the real world right now, disinfecting is the first step—it helps prevent those handling the medical instruments from picking up any diseases from the blood or debris on the instruments. The order is switched in a more challenging environment to save time and resources.) The disinfection process kills most of the bacteria, viruses, and fungi, but not necessarily all. There are several different ways to disinfect instruments and other items, and each has their pros and cons.

Thermal Disinfection

Boiling water is probably the most popular method for disinfection. Distilled or soft water is preferred to lessen the degree of rusting. Boil instruments and other items in water for 30 minutes. Start timing when the water comes to a full rolling boil. As boiling will rust the edges of scissors and knives, using distilled water is preferred to minimize this issue. Instruments that have been boiled for 30 minutes are disinfected but are not considered sterilized.[20]

Iron textiles, like fenestrated drapes, operating room towels, and clothing with a very hot iron. First, cover the ironing board with a clean cloth that is larger than the object to be disinfected and iron that cloth first. Then carefully lay the object to be ironed over the base cloth. Use several slow passes with the iron and steam well.[21]

Solar power has been used for centuries to disinfect fabrics. Simply hang the textile in full sun for at least six hours for each side. Make sure the item is pinned to the top of the clothesline and that it is not doubled over.[22]

Chemical Disinfection

Rubbing alcohol (70%)

- Does not kill bacterial spores, so sterilization is not achieved[23]
- Wipes are used to disinfect oral and rectal thermometers, scissors, stethoscopes, and small surfaces of the rubber stopper of multi-dose vaccine or medicine vials, like insulin[24]
- Evaporates quickly, so items must be fully immersed for 12 hours to achieve better disinfection[25]

Hibiclens

- Kills some bacteria, but not spores
- Use in conjunction with rubbing alcohol and soak instruments for 24 hours[26]

Betadine

- Soak instruments in a solution of one part of a 10% solution of Betadine to three parts water for 15 minutes[27]

Chlorine (household bleach, 5.25-6.15% sodium hypochlorite)

- 1 tablespoon bleach to 3 cups water OR
- 20 ml bleach to 1 liter of water

- Make this solution just prior to use[28]
- Soak instruments for 15-30 minutes, no more and no less (chlorine corrodes metal instruments)[29]

STERILIZING

Unlike disinfection, which kills *most* organisms on an object, sterilization kills *all* microorganisms. There are several methods that can be employed to sterilize medical instruments. Fortunately, you probably already have the equipment to implement at least one of these options.

First, it's best to cover the conditions where sterilized equipment will be used. Basically, anytime the skin is broken or will be broken. And anytime we are inserting anything into the body, like sutures, tubing, catheters, needles, scalpels, etc. Fortunately, at the time these are purchased they arrive in sterile packages, so we don't have to worry about sterilizing them ourselves. However, we could find ourselves in some interesting situations down the road with the need to reuse instruments.

Electric oven. Two hours at 325°F or one hour at 340°F will sterilize medical instruments. Temperatures in excess of 340°F may damage delicate instruments. Wrap the instruments in aluminum foil or place them on a metal tray.[30]

Sun oven. This will sterilize just as well as an electric oven; however, it must be constantly monitored for temperature drops. If the temperature drops below 325°F, the timing must start over.

Open flame. If there is no other choice, an instrument may be held in the flame until it turns red. And if the handle is also metal, then you'll want a clean cloth to hold it while it's being heated and sterilized. There's no point in creating a burn victim here. This method has the disadvantages of the time it takes for the instrument to cool down prior to use, and there is the potential for damaging delicate instruments.[31]

Pressure canner. This works very similar to the autoclaves that hospitals use. To be considered sterile, the interior temperature of the canner must reach 250-273°F. This is achieved at 15 psi, and that pressure must be maintained for at least 30 minutes.[32]

By way of reminder, instruments must be clean before undergoing sterilization. Any debris, tissue, blood, or whatever on the instrument must be removed; otherwise, it could hinder or completely prevent sterilization. Also, instruments such as clamps and scissors should be in the open position when being cleaned, disinfected, and sterilized.

WRAPPING MEDICAL INSTRUMENTS FOR STERILIZATION

Most YouTubes and written instructions for preparing medical items for sterilization in an autoclave feature the usual instruments—clamps, needle drivers, forceps and the like. But in a crisis there are also some daily use items that may need to be sterilized for diabetics and others whose lives depend on regular injections or the use of catheters and other items. Maybe someone in your family had some kind of traumatic injury and dressings need to be changed frequently—and you don't have an inexhaustible supply of those dressings. Needles, syringes (glass—the plastic won't hold up to the high heat of the pressure canner), rayon gauze dressings, etc., also need to be sterilized. And if you are using a pressure canner, these supplies and instruments need to be properly wrapped. Items sterilized in an oven using dry heat are generally not wrapped because the wrappings may incinerate at oven temperatures.

In an ideal world we would have autoclave paper or sterilization pouches. They're not that expensive through Amazon. But in an ideal world we'd also have hospitals and someone else doing this job. In an austere situation, we'll probably have to make do with clean towels and paper or foil.

Here's what you need:

- Autoclave or sterilization indicator tape (available through Amazon)
- Tightly woven towel, like a flour sack dish towel, or other fabric
- Paper (parchment, kraft, newsprint) or aluminum foil

- Cotton gauze

Before wrapping, it is important to remember to maintain the proper balance in wrapping the items being sterilized. If the wrap is too loose, the package will come undone. If the wrap is too tight, the steam will not penetrate to achieve sterilization.

Gather all the supplies, including the washed and disinfected items to be sterilized, to your work area. Lay a 12-15" square of paper or foil down in front of you in the diamond orientation—so the bottom corner is pointing at your belly and the top corner is pointed away from you. Lay the towel or other fabric on top of the paper in the same diamond orientation.

Take any sharp or pointed instruments, including hinged items, and wrap each point (like for a pair of scissors or forceps—tweezers for us non-medical people) or blade with a piece of sterile gauze to prevent these items from puncturing the package. Set the wrapped item horizontally in the center of the diamond. All hinged instruments are to be completely open. Set those down horizontally next, but not touching any other items. Also set down a small strip of indicator tape. Each package will contain only a few items.[33]

Pick up the bottom corner of the sterile towel, the one pointing at your belly, and fold it over the instruments, almost touching the top corner of the towel, but short by about two inches. Then fold this top corner that is short from meeting the other corner back down halfway towards you again.

Fold the left corner to the right corner, again leaving it short by about two inches. Then fold that left corner back again to the left, leaving it short from meeting the side by about one inch. Do the same for the right side, but when the right corner gets folded back, it overhangs the right side by about an inch.

Now pull the top corner down over the package. It may wrap to the other side. Fasten it securely with indicator tape so that it does not come loose while being processed. Write the date and the contents of the package on the tape.

The sterilization tape is temperature sensitive and shows only that the proper temperature was reached. It does not prove sterilization actually occurred because it doesn't indicate how long that temperature was maintained or whether it was sufficient for actual sterilization. Some instructions may state that the pressure canner only needs to run for 15 minutes to sterilize the instruments. That is true when using autoclave paper or sterilization bags. When using paper or foil and cloth, it takes longer for the steam to penetrate and sterilize and will require at least 30-40 minutes.

5. NUTRITION

While clean water and hygiene are perhaps the most critical elements of avoiding disease, good nutrition isn't far behind. Eating a well-balanced diet will go a long way towards keeping our loved ones out of the Bring Your Own Bandages Clinic.

MACRONUTRIENTS

Good nutrition encompasses more than just making sure people are getting all the essential vitamins and minerals. Believing that a multi-vitamin is going to cover all the bases would be a colossal mistake with possibly grave consequences. In addition to the essential vitamins and minerals, we also need to pay attention to the macronutrients—carbohydrates, protein, and fat—as well as dietary fiber. We need to be aware of what medications can affect the body's ability to assimilate these essential nutrients from our foods.

Carbohydrates

Carbohydrates should comprise 50% of the diet for most people. The best healthy carbohydrate sources are whole grains, fruits, and vegetables. Less healthy sources of carbohydrate are sugars, including honey, molasses, corn syrup, and maple syrup, etc.

Carbohydrates are the high octane fuel that the central nervous system requires for optimal performance. Carbohydrates, like protein, have four calories per gram. However, unlike protein, carbohydrates are needed to digest fat completely. In the absence of carbohydrates, fat breakdown is incomplete, and the waste product is ketones. This may result in a condition called ketosis, which can cause nausea, among other things. Carbohydrates play a valuable role in sparing protein and preventing ketosis. Furthermore, a low carbohydrate diet may make people fatigued, irritable, and lethargic.

One of the functions of carbohydrates is to protect protein so that it is available for building tissue. When carbohydrate intake is insufficient, protein gets broken down and used in its place, and nowhere near as efficiently. Why is this? Because protein can serve as a source of energy if carbohydrate intake is too low.

Fortunately, a lack of carbohydrates in the diet is extremely rare, even among the impoverished, because carbohydrate sources are generally the least expensive foods.

Fat

Fat is an essential macronutrient, just like protein and carbohydrates. We've got to have it. With nine calories per gram, fat is the most energy-dense macronutrient, compared with protein and carbohydrates which have just four calories per gram. Fat's major function in the body is as an energy reserve; it is converted into adipose tissue. In exercise, carbohydrates are utilized for energy for about the first 20 minutes, and then fat starts getting metabolized. However, fat has a few other important jobs. Not only does it help the body absorb fat-soluble vitamins, but it also slows digestion so that the digestive tract can absorb other nutrients. Fat is critical to regulating body temperature, protecting the vital organs, functioning and development of the brain, and producing regulatory hormones. It keeps the hair and skin healthy.

Too much fat in the diet, yeah, makes us fat. Too little fat in the diet, however, doesn't make us skinny. A complete lack of fat in the diet leads to a condition called protein poisoning. It's also known as rabbit starvation, protein starvation, and *mal de caribou*, and it occurs because the body cannot utilize protein in the complete absence of fat and carbohydrates. There's a common misconception that rabbit starvation is a result of eating rabbits. The problem arises from eating *only* rabbits, such as someone surviving in the wild might attempt to do. If the person eating rabbits is also consuming fats and carbohydrates, there is absolutely no risk of developing protein poisoning.

Symptoms of protein poisoning, or a complete absence of fat in the diet, include diarrhea, fatigue, headache, low blood pressure, slow heart rate, and a hunger that is satisfied only by the consumption of fat. Onset of the symptoms of protein poisoning may be accelerated by an extremely cold and dry environment and may occur in as little as one week.

To correct the problem, eat fat. To the body, from the point of view of being able to utilize carbohydrate and protein, fat is fat, regardless of the source. Any fat will do the job.

However, the debate still rages in science and medicine (and society) regarding which fats are healthier. Enter canola and vegetable (soybean) oil, both of which are grown with Roundup, and margarine and oleo. They're polyunsaturated or monounsaturated and have a shorter shelf life. Saturated fats have a longer shelf life, they're more natural, they taste better, and they haven't been grown with Roundup. Regardless, just make sure you have adequate supplies of some kind of fat in your storage.

Protein

Protein is consumed only to build and repair tissue in an ideal diet; it is not used for calories or energy. Yes, protein *can* be a source of energy because, after all, it has calories, the same four calories per gram as carbohydrates. However, it should not be considered a primary source of energy for a few good reasons. First, the body does not need excess protein. In fact, consuming too much protein may contribute to the formation of kidney stones. Also, protein is generally more expensive than carbohydrate sources. In addition, unlike carbohydrates and fat, the body can't actually store surplus protein. What happens to the excess protein that we consume? It goes to the liver and undergoes conversion therapy—into carbohydrates.

On the flip side, insufficient protein consumption forces the body to start breaking down muscle. This even happens when the body is injured, if protein consumption is not increased to meet the elevated demands of the body to repair and build tissue. Anyone recovering from surgery or physical injury requires a lot of protein. Insufficient protein consumption may also interfere with some medications because protein is not available to transport the drugs.

Protein deficiency is detrimental at any age, but particularly to developing fetuses and infants and small children. The effects of insufficient protein are irreversible and include decreased brain size and diminished function and increased stress sensitivity. In older children and adults, a lack of protein contributes to deficiencies in the immune system which may, and often do, become life-threatening.

Kwashiorkor is severe protein deficiency seen in children. The classic symptom of this condition is the swollen belly you see in images of starving children in third world countries. Apathy, stunted growth, fatigue, and flaky skin are other symptoms. This condition very rarely occurs in the developed world and almost always involves small children being fed fad diets or ignorance of the parents regarding nutritional needs of children with milk allergies.

While true protein deficiency is rare in the industrialized world, as we age we sometimes need more protein to maintain muscle mass (because if we don't get enough protein from our food, our body starts to rob our muscles) and prevent bone fractures. The changes that occur in the body as we age and due to insufficient protein consumption are gradual and are often considered part of the normal aging process.

Protein deficiency leads to cataracts, heart problems, and muscle atrophy, conditions most often seen in the elderly. On the way there, people may experience slowed metabolism, difficulty losing weight, muscle and joint pain, slow wound healing, and poor immunity to illnesses. We may not see a whole lot of kwashiorkor, but we do see the consequences of insufficient protein in the diet in our country and even in our families right now.

So how do we insure that we have adequate protein in the future?

We can make sure that we have complete proteins in our diet. By *complete* we mean foods that contain all the essential amino acids for building protein. And this pretty much comes only from meat, fish, dairy products, eggs, and soy. Other complete proteins that are plant-based include quinoa, hemp, and buckwheat. Chickens and rabbits are the most economically feasible way of securing a fresh protein supply when the grid goes down.

Fortunately, it's pretty easy to combine foods that are considered *incomplete* sources of protein to make a complete protein. Examples of these food combinations are beans and rice, wheat and milk, lentils and barley, and peanut butter and whole wheat bread. Even more fortunately, these foods do not need to be combined within the same meal, just within the same day. Getting adequate protein in the diet isn't really rocket science. A well-balanced, varied diet will meet all your protein needs for optimal health under normal circumstances. Just remember, however, as was mentioned above, that when the body is injured, especially with burns and fractures, substantially more protein is required.

Dietary fiber

Dietary fiber is another item that we need to take a look at. It's included on the nutrition facts label of all packaged foods sold in this country.

Dietary fiber occurs in soluble and insoluble forms. Both come from plants, but those well-meaning supplement manufacturers also provide fiber in a bottle. Don't succumb to the temptation of getting your fiber from a bottle. It is far better for the body to obtain the necessary dietary fiber from foods.

It shouldn't be surprising that dietary fiber is sorely lacking in the average American diet; the recommended daily dietary fiber consumption for Americans is about half of what is needed. People know they should be eating more fruits and vegetables, whole grains, and beans, and doing so will provide all the fiber the body needs each day.

All aspects of planning our food storage to meet dietary needs for vitamins and minerals, as well as fats, carbohydrates, and proteins are important. Fiber is no different. For optimal health and well-being, adequate fiber intake needs to be assured as well.

VITAMINS

Vitamin A

Vitamin A is a fat-soluble vitamin essential for proper vision and strong immune system, among other things. It is found in meat, fish, eggs, dairy products, and vegetables.

Vitamin A deficiency, like most vitamin deficiencies, is common in poorer countries, especially Western Africa and Southeast Asia. It is rare in developed countries because we are blessed with food manufacturers adding essential vitamins to their products. What happens when people don't have access to those foods anymore? Any guesses?

Because vitamin A is fat-soluble and thus able to be stored in the body, it usually takes a while, even up to a year if the individual enjoyed a particularly healthy diet, for deficiency to develop.

The classic sign of vitamin A deficiency that most are familiar with is, of course, night blindness. If we or members of our family become so deficient in vitamin A that night blindness develops, we've got a big problem. Severe vitamin A deficiency affects up to a third of the children in the world. That's a lot of kids. It is the leading cause of preventable childhood blindness, and half of children who go blind for this reason die within one year. Vitamin A deficiency is high among pregnant women in poorer countries and is a significant cause of maternal death and problems in pregnancy, gestation, and lactation.[34]

While some symptoms of vitamin A deficiency can be reversed with the addition of vitamin A to the diet, most of the time it's not as simple as eating a carrot. Sub-clinical deficiencies (before night blindness develops) are especially detrimental in children. A deficiency in vitamin A decreases the body's resistance to and ability to fight respiratory and diarrheal infections and increases susceptibility to other diseases, particularly measles. It diminishes the growth rate, slows bone development, and increases the mortality rate and ability to survive illnesses.[35]

Unfortunately, night blindness isn't a sure sign for diagnosing vitamin A deficiency. A person may be severely deficient in vitamin A without experiencing night blindness. Bitot's spots are keratin spots that appear superficially in the eye, usually between pupil and corners of eye, and are oval, triangular, or irregular in shape. They are rather foamy-looking and white to yellowish in color. These spots don't always resolve with treatment and may become permanent. These spots are peculiar to vitamin A deficiency and are not seen in any other disease or condition. They can appear in the absence of night blindness, or before or after. They are evidence of a severe vitamin A deficiency, but because they don't necessarily resolve with treatment, they are not necessarily evidence of a current deficiency.[36]

Other symptoms of vitamin A deficiency include dry skin, dry eyes and inability to produce tears, infertility, poor wound healing, and acne.

In addition to pregnant and lactating women, infants, and children, others at risk for vitamin A deficiency include alcoholics, people with giardiasis, celiac disease, duodenal bypasses, cystic fibrosis, Crohn's disease, ulcerative colitis, and cirrhosis. Iron and zinc deficiencies as well as not eating enough vegetables high in beta carotene also contribute to vitamin A deficiency.[37]

Historically, vitamin A deficiency was treated with animal livers, which, shocker, are very high in vitamin A. From a preparedness standpoint, we need to know which foods are highest in vitamin A content and be sure to consume them regularly and perhaps tank up on the super-vitamin-A-rich foods seasonally. Beef and lamb livers are particularly high in vitamin A, as is cod liver oil (yum). Fish, especially mackerel, tuna, salmon, and trout, are good sources, as are butter, cheese, and eggs. These sources are particularly good because animal sources also have at least a little bit of fat with them, which is necessary for the body to be able to assimilate vitamin A, and because *all* people can assimilate them.[38]

Studies have shown that up to 45% of people are carriers of a gene that significantly reduces their ability to convert pro-vitamin A (which is what vegetables have) into a form that the body can use. If you have this gene, you really need to have your animal-based sources of vitamin A in place. Vegetables such as sweet potatoes, winter squash, and kale provide your daily requirements in a single one-cup serving. Collards, turnip greens, carrots, and sweet peppers are also high in vitamin A. However, keep in mind that in order to make these available to the body, at least a little bit of fat needs to be consumed at the same time.[39]

What if the situation has really deteriorated and for whatever reason your regular sources of vitamin A are not available? Look for dandelions. You can blow on them and make a wish for some vitamin A to appear before your very eyes, and then you can look down and see the dandelion leaves and eat them. One cup of chopped dandelion leaves provides 112% of the recommended daily allowance of vitamin A. Impressive, huh?

One possible option if you are concerned about your plant or animal sources of vitamin A is to supplement with 25000 IU of beta carotene (or mixed carotenoids) every day for a month. You'll then be set for six months.[40] (Not for use by pregnant women—too much at once risks miscarriage and birth defects.)

Vitamin B1

Vitamin B1, also known as thiamine, is routinely added by food manufacturers to enrich breakfast cereals and breads. But what happens when Kraft and Nabisco and Kellogg's aren't working for us anymore? How quickly will thiamine deficiency, also known as beriberi, return?

Ten days. The human body doesn't store thiamine. Symptoms of mild to moderate deficiency may occur in just ten days.

Due to the fortification of foods, cases of nutritional thiamine deficiency in the United States are extremely rare. However, it remains common in parts of Africa and outbreaks occur in refugee camps. While thiamine deficiency has been described in historical records for thousands of years, it only became common in the late nineteenth century with the increased processing of grains, particularly rice in the eastern hemisphere and wheat in the western hemisphere. As researchers observed increasing incidences of disease in populations that consumed more white rice and white flour, governments mandated the addition of essential vitamins back into these foods that processing had stripped away.

Mild to moderate thiamine deficiency is marked by malaise, weight loss, irritability, and confusion. Risk factors for thiamine deficiency in a functioning society include dialysis, bariatric surgery, diabetes, large numbers of diuretics, and alcoholism.

Diagnosis of beriberi in a collapsed society without access to laboratory blood tests is going to be based on symptoms and improvement with good nutrition, specifically whole grain bread, because conventional treatment with thiamine administered intravenously is unlikely.

Unfortunately for caretakers, beriberi is expressed in different forms, which could make diagnosis difficult. Common symptoms include impaired reflexes, droopy eyelids, lack of coordination, and difficulty walking.[41]

Wet beriberi affects the cardiovascular system and is marked by an increased heart rate, shortness of breath, and swelling of the legs due to vasodilation.

Dry beriberi affects the nervous system and is exhibited by confusion, numbness in the limbs, trouble moving the feet, and pain.

Gastrointestinal beriberi causes abdominal pain, nausea, vomiting, and lactic acidosis.

Infantile beriberi occurs primarily in infants two to six months in age whose mothers are deficient in thiamine as well. It may present in either the wet or dry forms, and in addition to an increased heart rate, edema, and vomiting, the infant may also have diarrhea and pale skin. Shortness of breath and convulsions are noted in the terminal stages.

There are also some genetic conditions that make thiamine absorption from food difficult, but they're beyond our ability to diagnose and treat post-collapse.

How do we ensure that we are getting enough thiamine in our diet on a daily basis? Building up a generous supply of supplemental vitamins is one way, but when that supply is exhausted, what next? What foods are high in thiamine?

- Whole grains, especially brown rice (which doesn't have a long shelf-life)
- Beef, pork, fish, liver, eggs, dairy (food from animal sources is only a good source of thiamine if their diet has adequate thiamine)
- Legumes
- Vegetables such as acorn squash, asparagus, spinach, beet greens, and Brussels sprouts

Vitamin B2

Vitamin B2, riboflavin, deficiency doesn't have a common name; probably because it wasn't historically common. However, riboflavin deficiencies are found in more than half the population of third world countries and refugee camps. Deficiency is uncommon in the United States due to government regulations requiring the fortification of milled grains and cereals with essential vitamins. Currently, even with the relatively unhealthy and overly processed diet Americans consume, over 97% of us meet the minimum requirements.

What happens when the government is no longer in place to make sure processed foods are enriched with riboflavin? What happens with riboflavin deficiency?

Even mild to moderate riboflavin deficiency may cause anemia. Severe deficiency, ariboflavinosis, is marked by inflammation of the mouth and lips, sore throat, painful tongue, and chapped and cracked lips. There may also be oily skin rashes on the scrotum or vulva, the little cleft above the lips (anatomically known as the philtrum), and/or the nasolabial folds ("laugh lines" between the nose and the mouth). The eyes may become itchy, watery, bloodshot, and light-sensitive. In pregnancy, riboflavin deficiency may cause congenital heart defects and limb deformities in the fetus.

Riboflavin is water-soluble, which means the body does not store it; it has to be consumed every day. Riboflavin is found in milk, cheese, yogurt, and eggs; legumes; lean meat, liver, and kidneys; leafy green vegetables, beet greens, broccoli, and Brussels sprouts; winter squash, sweet potatoes, mushrooms and almonds.

When basic nutritional needs fail to be met, riboflavin deficiency may become something we see in those around us, but it's likely that they'll have other consequences of nutritional deficiency appear first, especially those related to the other B vitamins.

Vitamin B3

Vitamin B3, also known as niacin, is another vitamin added to foods to boost their nutritional content. That's because not too long ago, a lack of niacin in the diet caused thousands of deaths in the United States.

Pellagra is the common name for the condition known as vitamin B3 deficiency. How many of us even know what this really is? We may have heard of it, but it's not a disease that currently affects our society. We don't pay attention to it.

Pellagra caused over 100,000 deaths in the US alone, almost exclusively in the South, between 1906 and 1940. That's a rather substantial number. Why don't we hear more about it? Well, for one, it's a condition that afflicts the poor. Secondly, it isn't contagious. Third, we don't have any deaths from it now in this country; it really only occurs in third world countries. Fourth, the state governments in the South didn't want to admit that it was their greed that caused a lot of these deaths. When the US descends into third-world status, we'll see it again here. So let's learn about it now to prevent it in the future.

A mild vitamin B3 deficiency slows the metabolism, causing decreased tolerance to cold. That occurs in many conditions, so decreased tolerance to cold will not necessarily indicate niacin deficiency. A more moderate niacin deficiency may result in nausea, skin and mouth lesions, anemia, headaches, and fatigue. A severe niacin deficiency will cause pellagra (Italian; *pelle*=skin, *agra*=sour), the classic signs of which are the four D's: dermatitis, diarrhea, dementia, and death. Where do we get niacin? Foods that have the highest niacin content include meats (specifically tuna, turkey, pork, and venison), plants (ginger, tarragon, sweet peppers, Portobello mushrooms, dehydrated apricots), and whole grains (fortified cereals, rice, whole wheat, barley).

Why did pellagra suddenly start appearing in such large numbers in the US in the early 1900's? And why was it called the *spring sickness*? Pellagra occurred wherever corn (maize) was the predominant food crop because maize is low in digestible niacin. And if you are thinking, "Gee, wasn't maize a staple food for Native American and South American cultures? Didn't earlier Southerners eat a lot of grits (which are from corn)?" you'd be absolutely right. They most certainly did consume a whole lot of it, and it wasn't a problem *then*. Southerners and Native and South American populations knew to use a process called nixtamalization to increase the bioavailability of niacin, meaning the niacin becomes nutritionally available.

> For the curious, lye or wood ash is used to nixtamalize corn. Soaking the corn in water alkalinized with wood ash softens the outer covering, also known as the pericarp, and makes niacin nutritionally available (and the corn easier to grind). Today calcium hydroxide, also known as pickling lime, is used for nixtamalization.

Why did pellagra suddenly start appearing in the US in the early 1900s? After all, Southerners had been consuming maize for years. What changed?

As the farmland in the South became entirely turned over to cotton production, the poor sharecroppers couldn't raise their own food. It was available more cheaply from the Midwest. The problem was that corn from the Midwest was qualitatively inferior to the traditional cornmeal that Southerners had eaten for centuries. The disease appeared in the spring because the niacin-rich pork was only available to the poor during hog slaughtering season—fall and winter. The pellagra victims were always in a state of moderate niacin deficiency, but when the cheap pork was no longer available in the spring, the pellagra symptoms returned.

What does all this mean for us? We better be sure that we are storing some niacin-rich foods for our family. If we don't have a lot of meat, we had better have whole grains. If we're planning on growing corn (field corn or dent corn, not the sweet corn that we eat fresh, frozen or canned), we better be able to nixtamalize it ourselves. We can't just buy a lot of food and put it on the shelves. We have to know that we are supplying all the essential vitamins and minerals and we need to know about additional sources of each of these nutrients.

Vitamins B5, B6, and B7

Vitamins B5, B6, and B7 are up next. (Vitamins B4, B8, B10, and B11 lost their status as vitamins.) Dietary deficiencies of B5 (pantothenic acid) and B6 (pyridoxine) are extremely rare; B5 is found in almost every food. B6 occurs in a wide variety of foods and deficiencies really only occur in the face of other B vitamin deficiencies which are more likely to be identified sooner and hopefully treated and thus resolve B6 deficiency at the same time.

Biotin (B7) deficiency is rare, mostly because intestinal bacteria synthesize B7 for us. However, scientists do not yet know whether these bacteria synthesize adequate amounts of B7 in general. Pregnant women are at particularly high risk for biotin deficiency, so supplements might be a consideration for those of child-bearing age. Biotin is found in a wide variety of foods; beef liver, butter, split peas, lentils, peanuts, walnuts, pecans, sunflower seeds, and brewer's yeast are particularly rich sources of biotin. Symptoms of deficiency include brittle fingernails, hair loss, and conjunctivitis. The patient may also present with dermatitis in the form of a scaly red rash around the eyes, nose, mouth, and genitalia.

Vitamin B9

Vitamin B9, also known as folate, is a naturally occurring essential vitamin found in a wide variety of foods. Folic acid is a synthetic form of folate that is added to supplements and fortified foods. Over twenty years ago, the US Food and Drug Administration mandated that food manufacturers add folic acid to all breads, cereals, flours, cornmeal, pasta and rice. Unfortunately, if we lack a specific enzyme for metabolizing folic acid, the supplement will do little good.

Folate and folic acid are water soluble, meaning that they cannot be stored in the body. In children, symptoms of folate deficiency may develop within a month of inadequate folic acid intake. Deficiencies in folate may cause anemia, fatigue, shortness of breath, heart palpitations, open sores on the tongue, and changes in the color of the skin and hair (gray). With the exception of the change in hair color, most of the symptoms are pretty generic and common to a myriad of diseases and conditions. All are reversible with medication and improvement in diet.

However, there is that one group of people for whom a deficiency in folate can be catastrophic and irreversible—pregnant women and their developing babies. A deficiency in folate has been implicated as the reason for approximately half of all neural tube defects (NTDs) in infants. In this situation, an ounce of prevention—ensuring adequate vitamin B9 intake for all women of child-bearing age—is worth a ton of cure. Treatment of NTDs with the best of modern medicine is limited now. There's just not a whole lot that can be done to reverse the irreversible.

Others at risk for developing folate deficiency include individuals with celiac disease, Crohn's disease, excessive alcohol use, and certain genetic conditions.

Most industrialized nations require the fortification of grain products with folic acid and among those populations there has been a substantial decrease in the number of live births with NTDs. When we no longer have access to fortified foods and our supplies of vitamins are exhausted, where do we obtain the necessary folate?

Brewer's yeast and lentils have the highest amounts of folate. Brussels sprouts, kale, spinach, broccoli and other leafy green vegetables (folate comes from the Latin *folium*, which means *leaf*) are excellent sources of folate. Green beans, beets (not pickled), and organ meats are also good. High heat decreases the amount of folate, so these foods are best eaten raw, if possible. Having a lot of beans in the pantry and the ability to grow leafy green vegetables is critical.

Vitamin B12

Vitamin B12, also known as cyanocobalamin, is water-soluble. However, in contrast to the other B vitamins, B12 has some surprising differences that we better pay attention to. Vitamin B12, unlike the other B vitamins, can be stored in the body for up to two years, which is really nice. But B12 deficiency is also the most common vitamin deficiency seen in the developed world. While most of us get adequate B12 from our diets, as we age our bodies have an increasingly difficult time absorbing B12, so supplementation may become necessary.

Risk factors for vitamin B12 deficiency include heavy alcohol use, gastric bypass surgery, Crohn's disease, pernicious anemia, celiac disease, parasites, Graves' disease, and lupus. Vegans and vegetarians who do not consume eggs and dairy products (plants do not provide B12) are also at high risk.[42]

But those at highest risk are the elderly and anyone taking proton-pump inhibitors or H2-receptor antagonists. B12 deficiency is found in 20% of the population over the age of 60 years in the US, and in 6% of individuals under the age of 60. Those are pretty high numbers. Proton-pump inhibitors such as Prilosec and Prevacid as well as H2-receptor antagonists like Tagamet, Zantac (which the FDA recalled in April 2020), and Pepcid all interfere with the body's ability to assimilate B12 from dietary sources. The same holds true for metformin. Fortunately, these drugs do not affect the body's ability to utilize supplemental B12. Stocking a generous supply of supplemental B12 will be very wise for anyone taking the aforementioned drugs (or who may in the future) and for all those approaching the age of 60 (or past it).[43]

Recent studies show that an early sign of B12 deficiency may be glossitis, a painful swelling of the tongue, with long, straight lesions.[44] [45] Mild deficiency is marked by fatigue, depression, heart palpitations, shortness of breath, pale skin, smooth tongue, numbness, tingling, vision loss, difficulty walking, memory loss, and behavioral changes. More moderate deficiency may manifest as irritability, easy bruising, bleeding gums, and anemia. Nerve damage due to B12 deficiency may be irreversible. In children, B12 deficiency may stunt growth and development, and without treatment this may be permanent.[46]

Where do we get B12? It's all from the animals, or from supplements. Meat, including fish and seafood, eggs, and dairy. B12 is also found in some seaweed, algae, and tempeh, some kind of fermented soybean product originating from Indonesia. It's probably best to turn to the animal sources and supplements, especially if on the aforesaid medications or over the age of 60.[47]

Vitamin C

Vitamin C, also known as ascorbic acid, is most commonly associated with citrus fruits and was the first vitamin to be chemically produced. Because it is water-soluble, vitamin C needs to be consumed on a daily basis for optimal health. Also, cooking lowers the vitamin C content of foods by about one-third, so eating fresh fruits and vegetables whenever possible is best.[48]

Currently, vitamin C deficiency most commonly occurs among the severely malnourished, especially in refugee camps, where up to 45% of the population may be affected. Even in developed countries today it affects 5% of individuals. Severe vitamin C deficiency, scurvy, is rarely seen in the developed world.

Historically, throughout the fifteenth to nineteenth centuries, it was planned that half the sailors on long voyages would die from scurvy. During the eighteenth century, when Britain was engaged in wars the world over, sailors were far more likely to die from disease, especially scurvy, than in battle. Historically, disease and famine always kill more people than military conflicts. Also worth mentioning is that throughout this period, sailors and naval surgeons (the ships' doctors) were convinced that citrus fruits could prevent scurvy. The formally trained physicians, who knew more because they went to school, disregarded the evidence because it didn't conform to their ideas of disease.[49]

Initial signs of vitamin C deficiency, which take from five to twenty weeks to appear, include fatigue, red gums, easy bruising and bleeding, joint pain, and rough, bumpy skin. As time goes on and a diet devoid of vitamin C continues to be consumed, any of the following may be observed: corkscrew-shaped body hair (but these are brittle and may fall out before being observed); bright red hair follicles; spoon shaped fingernails and red spots or lines in the nail bed; wounds very slow to heal; bleeding gums; and teeth falling out. Ultimately, scurvy is fatal if untreated.[50]

Fortunately, the symptoms of scurvy are completely reversible. While meeting the minimum recommended daily allowances of vitamin C (as generally found in five servings of fruits and vegetables per day) is needed for optimal health, very little is needed to prevent scurvy. Just a tablespoon of fresh bell pepper or juice from half a lemon will do the job.

Genetic or other conditions that increase the risk for vitamin C deficiency include anorexia, alcoholism, smoking, dialysis, Crohn's disease, ulcerative colitis, and severe mental illness.[51]

In addition to citrus fruits, other common sources of vitamin C include fruits such as berries, melons, tomatoes, and pineapple; vegetables such as spinach, kale, broccoli, cabbage, potatoes, and bell peppers (which are actually much higher in vitamin C than citrus fruits); fresh milk;[52] and herbs such as rose hips, pine needles, juniper needles, and wheat grass.

Vitamin D

Vitamin D, the sunshine vitamin, is one of those lovely fat soluble vitamins that can be stored in the body. Unfortunately, many of us fail to build up our stores. A 2011 study showed that 42% of American adults are deficient in vitamin D. This number goes up to 69% for Hispanics and 82% for blacks.[53]

We get vitamin D from some foods, but our bodies synthesize most of our vitamin D from exposure to the sun. Ten minutes in the sun can make up to 10000 IU, but this varies widely based on skin color and the amount of skin exposed. While ten minutes will suffice for fair-skinned individuals, those with darker skin may need up to forty minutes per day. How do you determine if you're getting enough any particular day? In general, the best sun exposure occurs between the hours of 10AM and 3PM, but that also varies widely by season of the year and latitude. Go with this rule of thumb that works whenever and wherever: If you are taller than your shadow is long, you're good; if not, you're going to need to be in the sun a lot longer.[54]

This is why it's important to build up the body's store of vitamin D in the spring, summer, and fall; no one wants to sunbathe when it is literally freezing outside. Lying down for a nap in front of a sunny window won't work, either. The UV-B radiation necessary to synthesize vitamin D doesn't actually penetrate through household glass. Also, cloud cover reduces exposure by 50%, and using sunscreen lessens the exposure. Even though vitamin D is synthesized by and stored in the body, it's best to get your sun in small daily doses, rather than trying to do it once a week. Sunburns are no fun. Unfortunately, little research has been done on exactly how much sun is needed and how much of the body should be exposed. Some researchers suggest that 5-30 minutes of sun twice a week to the face, arms, legs, and back will be sufficient.[55]

What happens when we don't have enough vitamin D? Poor immune system function (people are especially susceptible to colds and other upper respiratory infections); bone pain and muscle weakness; chronic lower back pain; fatigue (one study showed that 89% of nurses were deficient in vitamin D—it's not something that just affects lower socioeconomic classes or the uneducated); depression (seasonal affective disorder is quite prevalent in the Pacific Northwest); dementia; irritable bowel disease; cardiovascular disease.[56]

Rickets, a severe vitamin D deficiency, occurs only in children. While it was probably noticed much earlier, cases were recorded in the 1600s in Great Britain. In the early twentieth century, 90% of children in New York and Boston had rickets. It is still found in the US today among the poorer classes particularly, but also in children whose caregivers are overzealous about using sunscreen and preventing exposure to the sun. Symptoms include bowed legs, stunted growth, bone pain, enlarged forehead, and trouble sleeping. Intellectual impairment, bone fractures, and muscle spasms signal more serious complications. Also, younger children will exhibit thickened wrists and ankles; older children will have knock-knees. Rickets usually begins in children between three and eighteen months of age. Those at greatest risk are breast-fed infants whose mothers do not get enough sunlight; breast-fed infants that get little to no sunlight; any child whose diet lacks vitamin D; and adolescents, especially during growth spurts.[57]

Risk factors for developing vitamin D deficiency include vegan diet; dark skin; limited sunlight exposure due to northern latitudes, indoor work, clothing covering most or all of the body, always being inside, always using sunscreen; old age; reduced kidney function; Crohn's disease; cystic fibrosis; celiac disease; obesity.[58]

Sunlight is the best option for getting adequate vitamin D. It's free, doesn't need to be rotated in the food storage, and goes where you go, unless you go too far north (or south, as the case may be) during a certain time of year. In case you want to add some to your diet, what are the best sources? You can choose fortified foods like milk, yogurt, breakfast cereals, and orange juice. With the exception of nonfat dry milk, the rest are going to be pretty hard to come by post-collapse. You also have fish, with wild being loads better than farmed, and fresh being better than canned (though canned is still good). Small amounts are found in beef liver, butter, some mushrooms, and egg yolks. Then there's the vitamin D powerhouse—everyone's favorite—cod liver oil.[59]

The last non-sunlight option is vitamin supplements. The supplement should be vitamin D3, not D2, and should be taken with a meal containing fat for maximum absorption. Vitamin D isn't absorbed as well without fat, and which is also why if drinking nonfat milk fortified with vitamin D, it's important to eat something with fat to aid absorption. Otherwise, most of it is wasted.

MINERALS

Calcium

Calcium is important for strong bones and teeth. Most of us remember that from grade school. Lack of calcium will result in osteoporosis and other things as horrible as the zombie apocalypse. We remember that from watching all those commercials on TV.

Not only does deficiency in calcium cause osteoporosis, but it also results in poor blood clotting, stunted growth, and rickets in children. A severe deficiency, hypocalcemia, manifests with symptoms such as confusion and memory loss, depression, hallucinations, muscle spasms, numbness or tingling in the hands and/or feet, weak and brittle nails, and, of course, brittle, easily fractured bones. Calcium regulates blood pressure, cholesterol levels, heart rhythms, and muscle contractions.[60]

The risk for calcium deficiency increases with age, due to a variety of factors: insufficient dietary intake, medications that prevent the uptake of calcium, hormonal changes (primarily women), and intolerance to calcium-rich foods, mostly dairy products. Consuming too much protein can also cause a calcium deficiency (so that plan to live off what you shoot may not work out so well). If vitamin D intake is inadequate, calcium cannot be absorbed either. They work together.[61]

Risk factors for calcium deficiency include hypoparathyroidism, malnutrition, malabsorption, low levels of vitamin D, pancreatitis, septic shock, celiac disease, chronic kidney disease, gastric bypass surgery, and veganism. Being a post-menopausal woman is the greatest risk factor of all. Women need to increase their calcium intake as they age, especially before menopause begins, because decreasing estrogen levels cause bones to thin faster. Along those lines is having amenorrhea, when body fat levels drop so low that women cease menstruating. This happens with extreme athletes and women who do not get enough to eat.[62]

You need to consume calcium every day. However, you won't see signs of deficiency if you miss a day or two or five. The body maintains proper calcium levels by taking calcium from the bones. But if the bones become depleted, then you've got troubles.[63]

Unfortunately, calcium deficiencies are best diagnosed with lab tests, which are not likely to be available post-collapse. Great care needs to be taken if you suspect a calcium deficiency, because over-treating with supplements may cause kidney problems. Calcium deficiency solutions include taking calcium, vitamin D (increases the calcium absorption rate in the body; getting in the sun, without sunscreen, is also helpful), and/or magnesium supplements.[64]

Calcium supplements work best when they are taken with food, with the maximum dose per meal being 500 milligrams. If more is needed, take it with another meal. Calcium supplements are available in three forms:

- Calcium carbonate, which has the most calcium and is the least expensive
- Calcium citrate, which is the most easily absorbed by the body
- Calcium phosphate, which is easily absorbed *and* does not cause constipation[65]

Foods rich in calcium are dairy products, canned sardines in oil, canned salmon, almonds, pistachios, white beans, black beans, wheat grass, cooked collard greens and broccoli, kale, dandelion leaves, okra, and eggshells. Eggshells can be washed, dried, ground into powder, and then mixed into food or water, if necessary.[66]

There are a number of medications that can have a negative consequence when taken with calcium. Calcium is essential to basically the entire operation of most every cell in the body. It's just not something to be messed with, however minor you think your problem is. You really need to consult with a physician, even if in a grid-down situation. These medications include, but are not limited to, the following:

- Some antibiotics, especially the tetracyclines (anything that ends in -cycline) and the fluoroquinolones (anything that ends in -floxacin), as their absorption may be decreased by calcium
- Diuretics, which may increase or decrease calcium levels in the blood, depending on which particular diuretic is being used
- Antacids containing aluminum
- Digoxin
- Estrogen medications
- Blood pressure beta blockers67

Iodine

Iodine deficiency, like many nutritional deficiencies, is not something we generally give much thought to. We don't see it personally; we don't hear about it. That's because the deficiency has been eliminated in most western countries. However, it does remain a problem in Australia, New Zealand, and several European countries. Iodine deficiency is most common in areas where the soil is deficient in iodine, especially islands and mountainous regions. Statistics vary; somewhere between 33% and 70% of the world's population is deficient in iodine to some extent.[68]

Here in the US, iodine deficiency hasn't been an issue since the introduction of iodized salt in 1924. However, change is in the air. For the past several decades, Americans got sufficient iodine in their diets from bread, dairy, and meat. But as commercial bakeries have more recently transitioned to bromine-based conditioners for their bread, iodine levels started dropping. In addition, as a whole, Americans are also consuming about 33% less salt that we used to. Most food processors—the manufacturers of frozen, canned, and boxed foods—do not use iodized salt. Many individuals are limiting their salt intake to prevent cardiovascular disease.[69]

So iodine deficiency is a common worldwide problem, on the verge of becoming a possible problem in this country, and people in general don't know much about it. Why should we care? What does iodine deficiency cause?

First, it gives rise to hypothyroidism, symptoms of which include extreme fatigue, goiter, mental slowing, depression, and weight gain.[70] In pregnant and nursing women it can cause intellectual disability, stunted growth, and deafness in their children. Iodine deficiency has been correlated to a 12 point loss on the IQ scale, while iodine supplementation in the diet in the US has been found to increase the IQ of children 15 points.[71] Note that this is in the diet of pregnant and nursing women; there is nothing you can do to reverse the intellectual disability that occurs in children who lack sufficient iodine for proper brain development.[72]

Risk factors for iodine deficiency include low dietary iodine (especially due to vegan/vegetarian diets and paleo diets), pregnancy, exposure to radiation, gender (women), smoking, alcohol consumption, and oral contraceptives.

Adults need to consume 150 micrograms of iodine per day. Women of childbearing age should have 200-300 micrograms per day. Iodine is found in iodized salt, seafood, milk, eggs, baked potatoes, navy beans, and cranberries.[73]

What's this mean for the average person who prepares for interesting times? Clearly, the best prevention of iodine deficiency is to use iodized salt. Keep in mind this little tidbit of info: According to Morton Salt, the shelf life of iodized salt is about five years. After that, the iodine breaks down and you have plain salt. So even the salt that we thought we didn't have to worry about rotating has to be rotated.

Of course, achieving a definitive laboratory diagnosis of iodine deficiency is going to be difficult post-collapse. Laboratory facilities will likely be limited; however, there is simple, if crude, test you can do on your own if you suspect iodine deficiency. Paint a 3x3 inch square of iodine solution on the inner arm, inner thigh, or abdomen. Let dry completely before replacing clothing. Check the iodine patch 24 hours later. Is it still the same color? Lighter? Gone? If it's gone, that suggests a serious deficiency. If it's lighter, there is a mild to moderate deficiency. And if it's the same color, keep doing what you're doing. Unfortunately, this test will be difficult to perform on people with darker skin.

Note. Some suggest that iodized salt impedes yeast fermentation in bread, but I have not been able to find any definitive references for this. In an effort to reduce iodine deficiency in their countries, some governments mandate the use of iodized salt in their bread. Iodized salt is not to be used in fermenting vegetables, as in making sauerkraut.

Iron

Iron deficiency is the most common nutritional deficiency worldwide. While most cases of iron deficiency anemia are mild, the consequences are far-reaching because mild to moderate deficiency results in poor school performance and lower IQ. In the US, the most common cause of iron deficiency anemia is bleeding, especially from the gastrointestinal tract. Worldwide, the most common causes are parasitic in nature—whipworms, hookworms, schistosomiasis, and amebiasis.[74]

A severe iron deficiency results in anemia, and if left untreated, can stunt growth in infants and children and can cause heartbeat irregularities and complications in pregnancy for others. Iron deficiency can also lead to fatigue, dizziness, hair loss, muscle twitches, and irritability.[75] In severe anemia, there may be increased cardiac output, as well as palpitations, angina, and symptoms of heart failure.

Unfortunately, symptoms of anemia are common to many conditions. Fatigue, weakness, diminished ability to exercise, and shortness of breath characterize anemia that develops slowly. Anemia that comes on quickly is marked by confusion, lightheadedness, thirst, and loss of consciousness.[76] In iron deficiency anemia, the sclera (white) of the eye may take on a bluish tinge;

spoon nails (normally convex nails become flat or concave) may also develop. Interestingly, anemia must be rather significant before a person actually looks pale. In general, the causes for anemia can be broken down into three classes:

- Blood loss—major trauma, menstruation, pregnancy, and gastrointestinal bleeding
- Increased breakdown of red blood cells (diseases like malaria and sickle cell anemia and autoimmune diseases—these have symptoms of bone deformities and leg ulcers)
- Decreased blood cell production (iron deficiency, vitamin deficiency; thalassemia—a genetic disease; and tumors of the blood, lymph, or bone—symptoms include jaundice)

The focus here is on mild, moderate, and severe iron deficiency, the latter of which results in anemia due to inadequate dietary intake or absorption. The other causes of anemia are not related to iron deficiency and will not be discussed here.

Anemia is a common blood disorder affecting about one-third of the population worldwide. Anemia stemming from iron deficiency afflicts about one billion people worldwide and accounts for approximately 200,000 deaths each year. In the developing world about two-thirds of women and children are iron-deficient; one-third of these are severely deficient or anemic. In the United States, 12% of *all* women of child-bearing age are iron-deficient, while this is true for only 2% of men in the same age group. Up to 20% of African-Americans and Hispanics are deficient in iron as well.[77]

Anemia is a condition marked by a decrease in the number of red blood cells circulating in the body. Hemoglobin, which is what makes red blood cells red, is composed of iron. Without enough iron or hemoglobin in the blood, the red blood cells can't bind oxygen. Without adequate oxygen, we fatigue easily and the body is unable to carry out many essential functions.[78]

Iron deficiency anemia is due to insufficient dietary intake which is essential to compensate for gastrointestinal bleeding, heavy menstrual bleeding, or frequent blood donations. Iron deficiency anemia may also be due to inadequate folate (vitamin B9) and/or cyanocobalamin (vitamin B12) intake or absorption which can be attributed to a wide variety of causes—age, autoimmune diseases, gastric bypass, hypothyroidism, or alcoholism. Inadequate folate intake/absorption does not normally produce neurological symptoms, while insufficient intake/absorption of B12 normally does.[79]

Chronic iron-deficiency anemia may cause behavioral problems in children who as infants lacked adequate iron. It results in reduced academic success in school-age children, and it causes restless leg syndrome in adults.

Risk factors for developing anemia due to iron deficiency include inflammatory bowel disease, untreated celiac disease, gluten sensitivity, *Helicobacter pylori* infections and stomach ulcers, Crohn's disease, vegetarianism, pregnancy, and being over the age of 65.[80]

Foods high in iron include red meat, lentils, beans, poultry, fish, and leafy green vegetables. The bioavailability of iron (the ability of the body to absorb iron) is increased when iron is consumed at the same time as vitamin C.[81]

Foods to avoid to increase iron absorption include excess sugar, coffee, black tea (herbal is fine), soda, and dark chocolate.[82]

Supplement use is generally acceptable in pregnant women, women with heavy menstrual bleeding, and those who frequently donate blood. Otherwise, supplemental iron should not be used unless the specific cause of anemia has been ascertained and supplementation is warranted and recommended by a physician.

Magnesium

Magnesium is used by every cell in the body. Hundreds of enzymatic processes in the body depend on it. Without it, you die. Magnesium doesn't work alone. It's like one of the three musketeers of essential minerals—the body also has to have adequate levels of potassium and calcium for magnesium to do its job properly.[83]

Surprisingly, even in the United States, about 68% of the population fails to get the minimum recommended daily allowance of magnesium. This is primarily attributed to insufficient dietary intake as well as taking proton-pump inhibitors. And magnesium deficiency is increasing for a number of reasons:

Soil depletion. Leafy green vegetables and whole grains are the primary dietary sources of magnesium. If our veggies don't get enough magnesium from the soil they grow in, they don't have it to give to us. Most farmers do what it takes to get a good product to market, but they do it at the minimum level.[84] They aren't adding any more magnesium (in the form of fertilizer) to their soil than they have to. Even the organic, non-GMO stuff, isn't as nutritious because of the soil.

Digestive problems, due to disease or aging. Several digestive diseases make it difficult for the body to absorb vitamins and minerals, including magnesium. We also become at greater risk of nutrient malabsorption as we age.[85]

Chronic disease and medicine use. It's a vicious cycle. Many chronic diseases can be traced to magnesium deficiency, but instead of correcting the magnesium deficiency, drugs are prescribed. These drugs have their side effects, one of which is inhibiting nutrient absorption in the digestive tract.

Lab work probably isn't going to be an option post-collapse; you're going to be on your own to figure out if you need more magnesium in your diet or need to take supplements. Some of the most common symptoms of magnesium deficiency include:

- Leg cramps and restless leg syndrome[86]
- Insomnia (take 400 mg magnesium with dinner or before bedtime to sleep better)[87]
- Anxiety[88]
- High blood pressure
- Heart arrhythmias and palpitations[89]

- Type-2 diabetes (magnesium deficiency is a cause of it, but also a symptom)
- Migraines
- Osteoporosis
- Severe asthma[90]

Individuals most at risk for magnesium deficiency include type-2 diabetics; those who drink a lot of soda, caffeinated drinks, or alcohol; the elderly; and those with gastrointestinal issues such as celiac or Crohn's disease or those who have had gastric bypass surgery.[91]

That's just people who are *most* at risk. The rest, unfortunately, are not off the hook. There are some people that are genetically disposed to absorb magnesium poorly, and then there is the afore-mentioned problem of soil depletion. There are also the people on acid blockers (including Tagamet, Pepcid, and Prilosec), antacids (like Tums, Maalox, Milk of Magnesia, and Alka-Seltzer)[92], corticosteroids, antibiotics (all the ones commonly stored, except penicillin and Keflex), blood pressure drugs, hormone and birth control medications, and ADHD drugs.[93]

So where do we get magnesium? What are the best sources, especially post-collapse?

Magnesium is found in leafy green vegetables, whole grains (especially popcorn and oats), cocoa (in the form of dark chocolate), and nuts (particularly almonds, peanuts, and cashews). We need to be able to grow these vegetables and store a whole lot of the rest. If eating a balanced diet high in leafy greens and whole grains still doesn't provide enough magnesium as is often the case, we need to store supplements. Magnesium chelate and magnesium citrate are the most common forms. Physicians all seem to have their preferences; you will too. The supplements aren't that expensive. Try a few to see which works best for you. If you don't need it now, acquire it for the future, just in case. Remember, every cell in the body uses it, and many chronic diseases are associated with inadequate magnesium levels.

For those who truly have difficulty with digestive malabsorption of magnesium, magnesium chloride flakes can be used in a bath or made into magnesium oil that is applied externally.

Potassium

Potassium deficiency is common amongst Americans, but severe potassium deficiency, known as hypokalemia, is not. Fortunately, all forms of potassium deficiency and hypokalemia are rarely due to insufficient dietary consumption of potassium.

The most common causes of potassium depletion in the body are due to fluid loss as a result of excessive bleeding, vomiting, diarrhea, diuresis (urine production), or sweating. Unfortunately, any one of these can be fatal, and that's why excessive vomiting and diarrhea, particularly in the very young and very old, is taken very seriously by medical personnel and hospitalization is often recommended.

Potassium levels are entirely regulated by the kidneys, and anyone with kidney disease or taking diuretics is at risk for potassium problems. Potassium levels in the body affect numerous biological processes, including those involving nerves and muscles, hormones, blood pressure, kidneys, glucose and insulin metabolism, and the fluid and electrolyte balance.[94]

Low potassium levels are most common in the following:

- Those on a very low calorie diet
- Alcoholics, smokers, and drug abusers
- Extreme athletes who exercise a lot in hot weather or people with physically demanding jobs
- People with uncontrolled diabetes or Crohn's disease
- Those taking diuretics or laxatives
- Anyone with kidney or adrenal gland conditions

Low potassium levels are also sometimes the result of a magnesium deficiency, bronchodilators, NSAIDs, and some antibiotics.[95]

Moderately low potassium levels are common among Americans and Europeans. Symptoms include trouble concentrating, difficulty sleeping, hypertension, muscle weakness, and joint pain. Individuals with moderately low levels of potassium are at greater risk for developing type-2 diabetes and kidney stones and have reduced levels of bone formation.

Like many conditions, potassium deficiency can cause weakness and fatigue due to weakened ability of the muscles to contract and move. It can also diminish insulin production and cause elevated blood sugar levels. It can cause muscle cramps and spasms, heart palpitations, and persistent tingling or numbness in the arms and legs. Severe potassium deficiency, hypokalemia, can be fatal if not corrected immediately.[96]

All fruits, vegetables, most meat and fish contain potassium. Foods with high amounts of potassium include yams, beet greens, spinach, parsley, milk, dry beans (especially white), chocolate, nuts, bananas, potatoes (with the skin), and dried apricots.

Potassium supplements are not recommended due to the potential for overdosing and damaging the intestines or causing abnormal heart contractions, either of which could be fatal.

If an individual is suspected of having a severe potassium deficiency, and especially if that person has experienced excessive vomiting, diarrhea, bleeding, sweating, or urination, he needs potassium as quickly as possible. Oral rehydration salts may be the only way to go at that point.

Zinc

Zinc is one of those essential trace minerals we need to be healthy and happy. It's second only to iron in its concentration in the body.[97] Without adequate zinc in the diet, you're susceptible to a whole host of problems, especially anything involving the immune system and the healing of wounds. Zinc is essential for proper growth and development during pregnancy, infancy, and childhood, and the consequences of deficiency during this period are irreversible.[98]

Fortunately, zinc deficiency is rare in the United States. It is most commonly found in people with poor diets, as in third world countries. Zinc deficiency is a major factor in diseases worldwide with high mortality rates attributed in part to the role zinc deficiency plays in pneumonia and childhood diarrhea.[99]

In addition to frequent infections and slow-healing wounds, symptoms of zinc deficiency also include poor appetite, problems with the senses of taste and smell, depression, irritability, lethargy, skin sores, trouble seeing in the dark, migraines, and loss of hair. In men and boys, impotence and hypogonadism may develop.[100] Zinc deficiency is also found in individuals with psychological disorders like anxiety, panic attacks, and obsessive-compulsiveness.

Risk factors for developing a zinc deficiency include vegetarianism, alcoholism, celiac disease, Crohn's, ulcerative colitis, chronic kidney or liver disease, pancreatic disease, diabetes, chronic diarrhea, old age, bariatric surgery, and limited diet.[101]

The body does not store zinc so you need to get enough from your diet every day. Where do you find it?[102]

The best sources of zinc are animal proteins like beef, pork, and lamb. Fish, not so much, but oysters are great (one oyster—100% of the USRDA). The dark meat of chicken has more zinc than the light meat. Yogurt, milk, beans, nuts, and oatmeal are also good choices.[103] Pumpkin seeds are actually one of the richest sources of zinc (assuming the soil they grow in is not depleted of zinc), but they aren't high on the list of items for most people to store.[104] However, it's a good thing to keep in mind when it's time to plant those gardens.

A couple little tips: Soaking beans in water before cooking them makes the zinc more available to the body. Leavened grain products have more bioavailable zinc than unleavened.[105]

SECTION 2—MEDICATIONS AND SUPPLIES

6. NON-PRESCRIPTION OVER-THE-COUNTER (OTC) MEDICATIONS

We are fortunate to live in a time when there are so many medications to relieve pain, calm coughs, kill bacteria, and eliminate parasites. Many of these wonder drugs have multiple actions and don't fit neatly into a single category. Benadryl is a fantastic antihistamine, but it's also an anesthetic and a sedative. Aspirin is a pain reliever and an anticoagulant. Because these medications have multiple actions, you may not find them listed in the category you would expect. The vast majority of these common OTC medications are known by their trade names. Appendix 2 provides the trade names and generic names of OTC medications listed in this book. For simplicity, only the trade names will be used in the text.

ANESTHETICS

Just because we find ourselves in challenging times, we aren't necessarily going to want to "suck it up" when it comes to pain. We'll want relief every bit as much then as we want it now. So will our children.

Here are the legal options, ranging from the simplest and cheapest to the most difficult and expensive.

Ice. This is what mothers used to numb their daughters' ears before piercing them with a needle in days gone past. Let's just say I didn't find it very effective and I didn't want her to pierce the other ear. I lost that battle. Ice works better post-injury.

Benzocaine. This is most commonly used in a cream or gel, especially in an oral gel for dealing with toothaches (Anbesol, Orajel). It's also an active ingredient in lozenges for soothing sore throats; Cepacol is one brand. Finally, benzocaine is the active ingredient in topical creams like Lanacane for use on irritated skin and in creams like Vagisil for vaginal itching.

Benadryl. In addition to being an antihistamine, Benadryl cream and spray also provide some anesthetic relief for bug bites and stings.

Alcohol. I took off-grid medicine classes from two different doctors, one who was Jewish and one who was a member of the Church of Jesus Christ of Latter-day Saints, also referred to as Mormons or LDS, people who abstain from alcohol. And they had very different opinions on the use of alcohol as an anesthetic. The Jewish doctor said all you get is an angry drunk who doesn't want to be hurt; the LDS physician didn't have a problem with it. Use your own judgment.

I'm guessing that, so far, you are less than impressed with the options. The following are more effective.

Lidocaine cream. This is most commonly available in strengths of about 2-2.5%. It will provide very minor numbing of the skin. However, there is also tattoo numbing cream with 5% lidocaine. This is the maximum strength of lidocaine cream that can be purchased without a prescription. And it works pretty well for some of the more substantial, yet still minor issues. There are several brands available in stores and online.

Cold Spray. Isobutane, N-butane, and propane are the active ingredients. This topical freezing spray anesthetic instantly numbs the skin, but it wears off rapidly, like 30-90 seconds. It is often used for dealing with ingrown toenails. It's probably better for placing staples than sutures, unless your doctor is *really* fast putting those stitches in. It's not so commonly used, so it will probably be easier to find on Amazon than at the drugstore.

Injectable Benadryl. This is especially useful for those who are allergic to lidocaine.[106] The physicians I visited with said they would have no objection to opening a Benadryl capsule and mixing the powder with sterile saline for injection.

Lidocaine + epinephrine. This option is probably the best you can hope for without a prescription. It is extremely effective and often used in emergency rooms for placing stitches. Again, getting the epinephrine is a bit of a challenge, but you might persuade your doctor or veterinarian. The good news is one little vial should suffice for the entire family for all of TEOTWAWKI. It is normally added to 2% lidocaine in a 1:1000 ratio. The combination amplifies the anesthetic effect as well as significantly reducing the bleeding. Because it constricts blood vessels so well, it is never used on the fingers, toes, ears, nose, or penis.

> I wasn't sure how much to purchase for our family. Medical Numbing Agents only sells three drugs—caffeine, benzocaine, and lidocaine. Their primary clients are hospitals and medical offices.
>
> So I went with the smallest amount, 25 grams, for $22.00 at the time. But I wasn't sure this was sufficient. So at our class a few months later, I asked Dr. Steve what he would recommend for my family of seven.
>
> "Five-hundred grams." I was sure he hadn't understood me. I about choked. So I asked again, emphasizing it was just for my family of seven. Yep, the answer was still the same.
>
> Fortunately, it is much less expensive to purchase in bulk. If you have a few families you can get together with on this purchase, so much the better.

Injectable lidocaine. This is great stuff to add to your medical kit. It's not a controlled substance and doesn't require a prescription but you might have a hard time persuading your doctor to supply you with some vials. However, making your own under a doctor or pharmacist's supervision is an option. Read on:

Lidocaine

Lidocaine is an anesthetic used for topical numbing of the skin prior to suturing and for minor surgeries. It's in topical creams for relieving itching and available in pain patches.

In addition to use as a local anesthetic, lidocaine finds application as a nerve block. It also works synergistically with epinephrine so that the numbing effect lasts longer with less lidocaine and decreases bleeding.

The topical creams often used in tattooing contain up to 5% lidocaine, the strongest available without a prescription. It usually takes 10-15 minutes before the area is fully numb.

Unfortunately, injectable lidocaine is available only through a physician. It's not a controlled substance, and it's not by any means illegal to possess it, but it's definitely not easy to obtain. If you have a good relationship with your physician, he may be willing to get some for you. For the rest of us, fortunately, lidocaine powder to make injectable

To make a 1% lidocaine HCL solution:

1. Weigh 150 mg of lidocaine HCL on the scale.
2. Cut off the top of a 15 ml sterile saline vial about halfway down the neck.
3. Insert the funnel securely into the neck of the vial.
4. Pour the lidocaine into the funnel. (If the powder sticks to the funnel, squeeze the vial gently to move some saline into the funnel. Then release so that the saline drains back into the vial, taking the lidocaine with it. This procedure may need to be repeated a few times to get all the lidocaine into the vial.)
5. Remove the funnel.
6. Close the neck of the vial using the surgical clamp.

To make a 2% lidocaine HCL solution:

1. Weigh 300 mg of lidocaine HCL on the scale.
2. Follow steps 2-6 above.

For both 1% and 2% lidocaine solutions:

1. Create a double boiler with a small canning jar almost filled with water placed in a pan of water over the stove. Clean tap water is fine; it doesn't need to be sterile or distilled.
2. Place the vial in the canning jar, but be especially careful not to submerge it near the openings. Do not let any tap water enter the vial, which would contaminate the solution.
3. Heat the water past 176°F. (Lidocaine dissolves in water, but it doesn't melt until it reaches 176°F. Melting ensures even distribution.)
4. Remove the vial from the jar. Do not remove the clamp.
5. Let cool.
6. You now have a 1 or 2% solution of lidocaine HCL.
7. This solution should be used within 24 hours and discarded thereafter.

solutions can still be purchased without a prescription. (One supplier is Medical Numbing Agents.com.)

How is this lidocaine going to be used? This is only for physicians and pharmacists to use. Trained personnel will make and administer the lidocaine. They have the training to do it safely. They just need the equipment and supplies.

Making injectable lidocaine is not at all complicated, but it is essential to be careful and very precise. In addition to scissors, a surgical clamp, a candy thermometer, and the lidocaine HCL, the following will also be required:

- Sterile saline, preferably labeled as being for injection. But that can be hard to come by. A grid-down, out in the wilderness hours or days away from a hospital solution is the single-use vials of sterile saline.[107]
- A scale that can accurately measure milligrams. Digital scales start at about $20. Non-electronic scales start around $30. I have no experience with either yet. A lot of reviewers on Amazon indicate that they use both scales for reloading ammunition.
- A tiny funnel to add the lidocaine HCL into the bottle of sterile saline.

Before beginning, make sure all the instruments are sterilized—clamp, scissors, funnel. Disinfect the scale thoroughly, especially the pan that will hold the lidocaine. Wash and scrub your hands thoroughly and put on gloves to assist the doctor. [108]

To use this solution, with the clamp still in place, clean the top of the vial with an alcohol pad. Invert the vial, insert the needle through the top of the vial, and draw out the desired amount of lidocaine into the syringe.[109]

ANTACIDS

Calcium carbonate (Tums) has been used to treat heartburn since the 1930s. It provides immediate relief from heartburn and is entirely safe for use during pregnancy. And it comes in lots of flavors. For best shelf life, get the regular chewables. Calcium carbonate may decrease the absorption of some drugs, including tetracycline antibiotics like minocycline and doxycycline and fluoroquinolone antibiotics such as Cipro and Levaquin.

Effervescent antacids (Alka-Seltzer) contain aspirin, sodium bicarbonate, and anhydrous (dry) citric acid to treat inflammation, fever, headache, and minor aches and pains, in addition to heartburn, indigestion, and acid reflux.

Contraindications: Not for use in individuals with heart failure or kidney failure.

ANTIDIARRHEALS

Imodium treats loose stools due to gastroenteritis, irritable bowel syndrome, and mild traveler's diarrhea. It is NOT used for treating cholera, salmonella, typhoid, or *Clostridium difficile*; you want to get the bacteria causing these conditions *out* of the body ASAP. Imodium slows intestinal motility and keeps fluids *in* the body. Imodium should not be used by pregnant or nursing women or in children under the age of five years.

ANTIFUNGALS

Lamisil, **Lotrimin**, and **Tinactin** are all OTC topical creams that work well to treat common fungal infections like athlete's foot and ringworm (which isn't actually caused by a worm). The trick is to use them until the rash is completely resolved, plus one additional week.

Gyne-Lotrimin is effective for vaginal yeast infections.

Unfortunately, as these items are creams, they don't have a great shelf life. Stock needs to be checked and replenished with fresh supplies.

ANTIHISTAMINES

Antihistamines are a class of drugs that block the release of histamine from cells. Their primary usage is in treating cold and allergy symptoms, and as such they do not cure colds or allergies. They just help people feel better. If people in the family suffer from seasonal allergies, stock plenty of what works for them. As far as what works best for drying up runny noses, physicians generally agree that Benadryl and Zyrtec work well.

However, the following three over-the-counter antihistamines have other uses, many of which are quite valuable for long-term preparedness.

Zantac is an antihistamine that, prior to April 2020, was commonly used for treating heartburn, GERD, and peptic ulcers to reduce acid production in the stomach. It was used in conjunction with other medications in treating *Helicobacter pylori* ulcers. It was also used together with Benadryl as a second-line treatment for mild anaphylaxis. (First-line is always epinephrine, and Zantac and Benadryl aren't going to save someone with a life-threatening anaphylactic reaction, but in a disaster, you work with what you've got.) With Zantac, there was an increased risk of developing pneumonia or a *Clostridium difficile* infection. Zantac was generally regarded as safe to use in pregnancy but not for nursing women. Zantac was available in the United States over-the-counter in 75-mg and 150-mg tablets; 300-mg tablets were by prescription only.[110] (Zantac was recalled due to contamination with N-nitrosodimethylamine (NDMA), a probable human carcinogen. Subsequent testing revealed that when Zantac is stored at room temperature, the amount of NDMA increases with time. Furthermore, it increases at a greater rate when stored at high temperatures. I opted to retain the information on Zantac due to the possibility that some people may not have gotten the message about the recall, and because some may wonder about the safety of occasional use. It is also still in use countries outside the US.)

Zyrtec is very similar in action to Benadryl but has the advantage of not usually causing drowsiness. It is especially suited for runny noses, hay fever, hives, and dermatitis. It is usually only taken once a day. The off-label, or alternative uses, include treating mild anxiety. It is considered safe in pregnancy, but not for nursing a baby. In the US, Zyrtec is available over the counter in 5-mg and 10-mg tablets; 20-mg tablets are available by prescription only.[111]

Benadryl is the most valuable of all the antihistamines from a preparedness standpoint. It is used as a mild sleep aid and in treating anxiety and mood swings. In addition, it is used as an anesthetic, especially for people allergic to lidocaine. Benadryl is also an active ingredient in creams and sprays for treating allergic reactions and bug bites and stings.[112]

For this reason alone, some physicians believe the most critical drug a layperson can carry in an emergency kit is Benadryl. Pain relievers may be used more frequently, but Benadryl can save a life. It is not a substitute for epinephrine, but it can work in mild to moderate anaphylaxis, and it can buy you some time. It is the most commonly used antihistamine for addressing acute allergic reactions in emergency rooms.

> My husband and I were camp cooks a few years back, and one of the girls, who had no known allergies, fell ill after eating some candy-coated sunflower seeds the campers were given before heading out on a hike. She returned to camp and was attended by our camp nurse and EMT. Of course, the medics had epinephrine, but most choose to avoid using it if possible. In this case, the girl was given several doses of Benadryl to stop the anaphylactic reaction. She has since tested positive for numerous food allergies and must carry an Epi-pen at all times.

The above is reason enough to stock and carry Benadryl; however, there are many other uses as well.

Alternative Uses of Benadryl

Sleep aid. The most frequent use of Benadryl is for treating allergies and runny noses, but it is also widely sold as a sleep aid.[113]

- Tylenol PM contains Tylenol and 25 mg (one regular pink pill) of Benadryl
- Advil PM is Advil and 25-38 mg of Benadryl
- Vicks' ZzzQuil is merely 50 mg of Benadryl

Of course, all of these cost a whole lot more. To save money and space, store straight Tylenol and Advil. When in pain and having trouble sleeping, add in some Benadryl.

Nausea, anxiety, Parkinson's. Physicians also use Benadryl in treating nausea due to motion sickness, vertigo, and other illnesses. It can be used in the treatment of mild anxiety and mood swings in addition to some symptoms associated with Parkinson's.[114]

Anesthetic. Benadryl is marketed in lotions and sprays for topical pain relief from:

- **Rashes**, **insect bites** and **stings**
- **Contact dermatitis** due to **poison oak**, **poison ivy**, and **poison sumac**
- **Hives** and **eczema**[115]

It is critical to control itching, because scratching may compromise the integrity of the skin, our most important defense against infection. Scratching increases the possibility of introducing *Staphylococcus* bacteria that are typically present on the skin into the body. And this may cause cellulitis, a potentially fatal infection if left untreated.

Injectable. Benadryl is also used as an injectable or topical local anesthetic, especially for individuals allergic to lidocaine.

Dogs. Veterinarians also sometimes suggest Benadryl tablets to help dogs with allergies or anxiety.

Forms of Benadryl

Tablets and **capsules** are the most common and least expensive. Tablets have the longest shelf life and can be split in half if necessary. Capsules are a little faster-acting than tablets. They can be opened and sprinkled over food or mixed in liquid for individuals who have difficulty swallowing pills. The powder inside the capsules can also be combined with saline or dextrose for an injectable anesthetic, with cream for a topical anesthetic, or with water for a topical spray or paste. Unless the capsules are well-protected from moisture and stored properly, they can melt together and become an unusable mess.

Syrups have a much shorter shelf life, not much beyond the use-by date on the packaging. But they get into the bloodstream faster and are easier for children to swallow.

Chewables and **rapid melts** are a compromise between the solid and liquid forms. Their significant advantages are that they get into the bloodstream faster and store better than liquids. They are the best choice for first aid kits when getting into the bloodstream quickly is critical. While they are relatively expensive, only a few are needed for emergency purposes in medical kits.

Spray, **lotion**, and **gel** forms of Benadryl for topical use don't cause as much drowsiness as the oral forms do. Creams and sprays have a shorter shelf life because they are liquids. These topical forms grant almost immediate relief, quite the blessing in taming the urge to scratch. The topical forms not only treat insect stings and bites, rashes, and poison oak, poison ivy, and poison sumac, but they also help with the itching that occurs during the healing of minor burns (including sunburns), cuts, and scrapes. Benadryl powder from capsules can also be used to make lotion or spray by merely mixing with cream or water. Combine the powder and a small amount of water to make a paste that can be applied in and around the edges of a wound to numb it prior to cleaning and closure.

Injectable Benadryl acts faster than any of the other forms. This is absolutely critical when it is used as an adjunct in treating anaphylaxis. It is also used as a local anesthetic, especially in individuals allergic to lidocaine. Unfortunately, the injectable is only available for purchase by licensed health care providers. In a true emergency, it can be mixed under a physician's guidance. Having the supplies on hand will be critical, and in addition to having Benadryl powder from capsules, sterile saline or dextrose solutions and syringes will also be needed.[116]

Dosage

An adult dosage of Benadryl is one or two pills for a total of 25-50 mg every four to six hours. Children six to twelve years are prescribed one 25-mg tablet. Prescription-strength Benadryl is 75 mg. A physician should be consulted before using oral Benadryl products in children under the age of six years. Topical lotions and sprays may be used in children two years or older.[117]

Cautions. Drug screens may produce false-positive results for methadone use in people who have recently taken Benadryl. A typical 50-mg dose can create impairment equivalent to a 0.10 blood alcohol level, which is why each bottle contains a warning about driving and operating heavy machinery. In some children, Benadryl can have a paradoxical effect, where instead of having a sedating side effect, the side effect is stimulating. This is particularly true for children who have ADHD.

Interactions. Benadryl may interact with other medications, so a drug reference should be consulted before medication is administered.[118]

Contraindications. Benadryl is not recommended for use in people over the age of 60 without a physician's care. It is especially contraindicated for those with enlarged prostate and hypertension. It should not be used by nursing mothers because it is excreted in breast milk (it can also dry up the milk supply).

H2 (Histamine) Blockers

Pepcid is an antihistamine that inhibits acid production in the stomach and is thus used in treating gastric and duodenal ulcers and gastroesophageal reflux disease (GERD). This H2 blocker may also be used to treat *Helicobacter pylori* infections, though Prilosec seems to be more effective. It is even used to prevent the development of NSAID-induced ulcers. It was discovered in 1979 and has a significant advantage over other similar medications in that it does not seem to interact with other drugs. It is available over-the-counter in 10-mg and 20-mg tablets. Prescription strengths are sold in 20-mg and 40-mg tablets.

Zantac is also an antihistamine that was developed for treating heartburn; gastric, duodenal, and *H. pylori* ulcers; and GERD. It may be administered to help prevent NSAID-induced ulcers,[119] but proton-pump inhibitors are generally more effective in this role.[120] It is used for preventing stress-induced ulcers in critically ill patients. According to Dr. Cynthia Koelker, author of *Armageddon Medicine*, Zantac may be taken one hour before taking over-the-counter pain medications if the latter cause stomach discomfort.

Zantac may be used by physicians in conjunction with Benadryl as a secondary treatment for anaphylaxis, after epinephrine.

The use of Zantac may increase the risk of developing infectious diarrhea, may lead to an elevated risk of developing food allergies, and may lead to a risk of developing pneumonia. The FDA issued warnings in January 2020 that Zantac was contaminated with the NMDA carcinogen. As previously stated, the FDA recalled Zantac in April 2020. It is still in use in other countries outside the US.[121]

Prilosec may be used to treat frequent heartburn (two or more days per week). However, it takes 1-4 days to start working, so heartburn is not relieved right away. As a proton-pump inhibitor, it decreases the amount of acid produced by the stomach to let the stomach and esophagus heal from damage done by acids. It is used to treat GERD and gastric and duodenal ulcers, especially those caused by aspirin, NSAIDs, and *H. pylori*.[122]

Contraindications for all PPIs and to a lesser extent, the H2 blockers: These drugs may interfere with the bioavailability of vitamin B12, so a supplement should be taken to prevent adverse effects on the nervous system. In addition, these drugs also increase the risk of osteoporosis. Do not use any of these drugs for more than 14 days unless directed by a doctor. Also, consult with a doctor before using more than once every four months.

ANTI-NAUSEA

While anti-nausea medications are desirable just for treating nausea alone, they're critical in helping a patient to keep from vomiting the precious medicine that itself makes a person nauseous. Anti-nausea medications are cheap. Antibiotics and prescription pain relievers aren't necessarily expensive now, but the time may come when they will be very precious, and the supply will need to be wisely used.

Pepto-Bismol, the pink stuff, was initially sold over 100 years ago in the US as a remedy for diarrhea in infants. It's probably not the best choice for stockpiling, at least in the liquid form. All "use-by" dates on liquid medications should be taken seriously. And it can cause constipation, never fun in any situation, but particularly not fun in a bad situation. Some pediatricians advise against using it in children.

Zofran (prescription only) is administered for nausea, especially when needed to help a patient keep other medicines from causing nausea or being vomited.

Bonine (**Antivert**—prescription strength) comes in 12.5-, 25-, and 50-mg tablets and is used to prevent nausea, vomiting, and motion sickness. If OTC pain medications cause nausea, a dose of Bonine may be taken one hour prior to taking the pain medications. It may also help with dizziness and is a mild sedative as well. For these reasons, it is also used as a sleep aid and an anti-anxiety remedy. Doctors generally advise adults to take one 25-mg tablet an hour before traveling, or up to 50-100 mg per day in divided doses for anxiety, dizziness, or sleeping. While a licensed physician should be consulted before anyone takes any medication, Bonine really should not be taken by anyone under the age of 12 or over the age of 65 without a doctor's recommendation.

Dramamine comes in 12.5-, 25-, and 50-mg tablets and is used to prevent nausea, vomiting, and dizziness in children over the age of two and adults. It is also a mild sedative.

COLD AND COUGH MEDICATIONS

These are the medications medical professionals most often suggest for alleviating the symptoms of colds and coughs.

Sudafed ("real" Sudafed--pseudoephedrine). Due to its illicit use in manufacturing methamphetamine, real Sudafed is over-the-counter but behind-the-counter in most US states. One must show identification, sign for it, and get entered into a database. There are limits to how much can be purchased each month. Sudafed works really well. It is only available in blister packs.

Sudafed PE (phenylephrine). It definitely does not work as well as the real Sudafed. It's a bit cheaper, and can be stored more easily. It is also only available in blister packs.

Benadryl, **Zyrtec**, and **ChlorTrimeton** are antihistamines that dry up secretions.

Mucinex expectorant thins the mucus, so the throat is less irritated. If an antihistamine isn't working to alleviate a cough caused by drainage, Mucinex may help.

Afrin nasal spray clears stuffy noses and makes it easier to sleep at night.

Vicks VapoRub (or generic equivalent) is rubbed on the chest to calm coughing. Some also note that it can be rubbed on the soles of the feet (and then covered with socks) for additional relief.

Codeine, a controlled substance, is difficult to acquire. If nothing else is working, and you have some available and a doctor to prescribe it for you, a small dose of codeine may help. Usually, one-fourth of a pill of Tylenol-3 or Vicodin will do the job.

Tylenol. If a cough is accompanied by fever, reducing the fever may help. This is because a fever increases the metabolism, which increases the respiration rate. Lowering the body temperature should lower the respiration rate, and may thus decrease the irritation that causes some coughing.

Caffeine, however one takes it, through coffee, tea, soda, or pills, is a bronchodilator that helps open the airway and diminish coughing.

As with all medications, tablets or capsules are the best for the longest shelf-life. Obviously, that's not an option with a nasal spray, but everything else is available in a dry form.

EPINEPHRINE

Epinephrine, a hormone produced in the adrenal glands, is also a medication. It's the fight or flight response people experience when startled or scared. It makes the heart beat faster, widens air passages to facilitate breathing, raises the blood pressure, and dilates pupils. (Epinephrine and adrenalin are the same thing; the former is derived from Greek and the latter from Latin. Americans favor the term *epinephrine*, and the rest of the world uses *adrenalin*.)

The use of epinephrine in treating anaphylaxis is addressed in chapter 20.

Epinephrine is a vasoconstrictor that helps stop bleeding. In this case, epinephrine is usually combined with lidocaine in a 1-2% solution. It is not used on fingers, toes, noses, or ears because it may cut off circulation entirely. It also should probably not be used in the feet of diabetics or others with compromised circulation. It is excellent when used with lidocaine on superficial wounds with significant bleeding, especially scalp wounds.

Another reason to consider having epinephrine in your medical kit is for treating croup. Detail on this use are covered in chapter 16.

The US FDA took Primatene Mist, a mainstay for treating mild asthma for many years, off the market in 2011 because it didn't like the propellant used in it. It is finally available again, as of November 2018. It would be a really good idea to have this in the kit for treating mild asthma, severe wheezing, coughing, and croup.

Epinephrine is not a controlled substance. It is not illegal to possess it, but it is not so easy to find. If you have a good relationship with your doctor or veterinarian, you may be able to get a vial that way, and one bottle is all you should need to get you through TEOTWAWKI.

The other possibility for obtaining epinephrine is online at Dr Natural Healing.com. It's labeled as being straight epinephrine, with 0.22 mg per capsule. It also comes with the inhaler and instructions on how to use it. It probably won't work for someone who is having an anaphylactic reaction, as that person won't be able to inhale it. It is designed for asthma sufferers. Could it be combined with sterile saline for use as an injectable? That's a question for your doctor or pharmacist. Mine believes it would work.

PAIN RELIEVERS

Sometimes we get the idea that over-the-counter (OTC) pain relievers are all basically the same. While occasionally any one of two or three choices will work for what ails us at times, it really behooves us to gain a better understanding of which pain medications work best in any given situation. Let's review the most common OTC pain relievers.

Advil (Motrin) is taken for reducing pain, inflammation, fever, painful periods, rheumatoid arthritis, osteoarthritis, kidney stones, dental pain, migraines, and even treating patent ductus arteriosus in a premature baby. Side effects include heartburn and rash, and it may worsen asthma. Advil may increase the risk of heart, kidney, and liver failure and should not be used during pregnancy. It can interfere with the antiplatelet effect of low-dose aspirin and is a weak photo-sensitizing agent. Chronic use is associated with an increased risk of heart attack, stroke, and high blood pressure. If poisoning is suspected, treat with activated charcoal. Inducing vomiting is not recommended. One study showed that people who regularly used Advil reported a 38% less risk of developing Parkinson's. However, the effect of long-term use on the urinary and gastrointestinal tract should be noted. **Prescription-strength** Advil is 800 mg per dose taken at 6-hour intervals for a maximum of 3 doses in a 24-hour period. The maximum total daily dosage is 2400 mg.[123]

Aspirin is one of those drugs that would not be approved by the FDA today because it does too many things. Because it is an anticoagulant and can be used to stop a heart attack, chewable baby aspirin should be part of every medical kit. Aspirin can cause stomach upset and may worsen asthma. It should not be used in the last trimester of pregnancy and should not be used for children with infections due to the risk of Reyes syndrome. It is generally not as effective against pain as Advil, nor is it very useful for pain due to muscle cramps, bloating, gastric distention, or acute skin irritation. Aspirin works synergistically with caffeine. Effervescent formulations work faster than tablets and are more effective for migraines. Topical aspirin works for some types of neuropathic pain. Aspirin is more effective for tension headaches and less effective on other types of headaches. It is most effective at stopping migraines when they are first beginning. An overdose is treated with activated charcoal and IV saline.[124]

Aleve is similar to Advil and is taken for relieving pain, fever, swelling, and stiffness. It is generally safe for use by nursing mothers. It may cause side effects of rash, heartburn, and stomach ulcers. Aleve is used to treat migraines, osteoarthritis, rheumatoid arthritis, psoriatic arthritis, kidney stones, gout, tendinitis, bursitis, and menstrual cramps. It is not indicated for diabetic neuropathy. Aleve may have antiviral activity against influenza. Aleve may be used to differentiate between infectious fevers and neoplastic (connective tissue) fevers, as in cancer. Heavy use may cause end-stage renal disease and kidney failure. Aleve should be taken with food. It may interact with blood thinners and prednisone. Aleve has been an over-the-counter drug in the US since 1994 in 220 mg tablets but remains prescription only in much of the rest of the world. Regular OTC usage is one 220 mg tablet every 8-12 hours.[125] **Prescription dosage** should not exceed 1250 mg in the first 24 hours; subsequent daily doses should not exceed 1000 mg.[126]

Excedrin and **Vanquish** are combinations of Tylenol, aspirin, and caffeine used primarily for headaches, but also used for arthritis, backache, colds, menstrual cramps, and muscle aches. The Tylenol/aspirin/caffeine combination is as effective in treating migraines as lower doses of sumatriptan. Excedrin has more Tylenol, aspirin, and caffeine per dose than Vanquish. Excedrin is sold in "extra strength" and "migraine" formulas.[127] There is no regular strength. And the "extra strength" and "migraine" dosages and formulas are exactly the same, but if the bottle says "migraine" on it, it costs substantially more.

Mobic is a pain reliever similar to Tylenol but is available by prescription only in the US. However, it is included here because it has an essential advantage over the other OTC pain relievers. US combat troops are issued this pain reliever for their IFAKs (individual first aid kits) because it does not interfere with platelet function, i.e., blood-clotting, it is more effective at relieving pain than Tylenol, and it is taken only once per day. Mobic is an NSAID most often prescribed for treating arthritis and tendinitis. It should be taken with food and is better than Advil for moderate to severe pain. Mobic should not be used by individuals with asthma or by pregnant women. Long-term use may cause liver damage and increase the risk of heart attack and stroke. It may reduce kidney function and should be used with caution in individuals with heart failure. Mobic may contribute to insomnia, bladder infections, and upper respiratory infections. The beginning dose is 7.5 mg/day. The maximum daily dose is 15 mg, taken once per day.[128]

Tylenol is most often indicated for treating pain, fever, allergies, cold, cough, flu, and headache. It reduces the *perception* of pain, but does little to treat the cause of pain. Tylenol is quite safe, as long as it is used as directed. Complications arise from overdoses, usually unintentional. These overdoses most often occur because Tylenol is found in so many OTC medications. Before July 2011, the maximum daily dose listed on the packaging was 4000 mg, but that year manufacturers reduced that maximum to 3000 mg per day. This was a liability defense protection move; the FDA still lists the maximum dose as 4000 mg per day.[129] Tylenol tablets come in several strengths: 325 mg regular strength, 500 mg extra strength, and 650 mg arthritis pain (but this last caplet is extended or sustained release over the day and needs to only be taken every twelve hours). With 300 mg Tylenol and 30 mg codeine, Tylenol-3 is a controlled substance available by prescription only.[130]

Most of the above pain relievers become noticeably effective within 30 to 60 minutes. Children's chewable tablets enter the bloodstream much more quickly and thus begin acting faster. This can be especially important when attempting to stop a migraine, so stocking some children's chewable tablets may be worthwhile.

Furthermore, most of these pain relievers are anticoagulants and should not be administered when bleeding is or could become an issue. For this reason, combat troops are not allowed to use anything but Tylenol or Mobic.

One study showed that any use of NSAIDs, even Tylenol, by pregnant women increased the risk of miscarriage 2.4-fold.

Combining Tylenol and Advil: Yes, it is safe. They have different mechanisms of action. Tylenol is cleared by the liver; Advil is cleared by the kidneys. The combination of these two medications is more effective than Vicodin or Norco for treating dental pain. This is most effective when the doses are alternated, and dosing recommendations depend on the strength of the pill.[131] The same idea goes for combining Tylenol and Aleve. Do not combine Advil and Aleve as they are both cleared by the kidneys.

ALTERNATIVE METHODS FOR ADMINISTERING MEDICATIONS

We normally store tablets and capsules because they have a much longer shelf life than liquids. However, sometimes a patient can't take a medication for any number of reasons. It's most frequently because the individual is an infant or young child that can't swallow pills yet. Sometimes the person is unconscious. The elderly can also have difficulties due to advanced age. Sometimes medications are better administered in a different manner due to the illness being treated.

We've got a few options here. The first step for all of these options is to grind tablets into powder with a small mortar and pestle. In the case of capsules, they just need to be opened up.

- Sprinkle the powder on food. Make sure this is a food the patient will happily eat so that the medication isn't wasted.

- Make a syrup. Use honey (not for infants under one year of age), corn syrup, pancake syrup, or sugar. Just mix enough for one dose at a time.
- Mix the powder into juice or milk. Don't use more than the patient will drink quickly. Do not mix tetracycline family antibiotics with milk.
- Up the bum. Mix the powder into some water—tap water is fine—and put it in an enema bag. Get a little lubricant, send the tubing up the bum, and squeeze the solution in.
- Mix the powder into a tablespoon or so of water, maybe with a little juice or flavoring, and gargle it in the throat as long as possible. This is an especially effective way of administering pain relievers to soothe a sore throat. The pain reliever comes into the fastest possible contact with the inflamed tissue in the throat. After a minute or two of gargling, the medication is then swallowed and enters the bloodstream to facilitate further relief.

Do not grind up time-release tablets. Those formulations are specifically designed for gradual release. Powdering them will defeat the time-release purpose of those medications.

SHELF LIFE OF MEDICATIONS

Have you ever wondered about those "use by" dates printed on the bottles of your prescriptions and over-the-counter medications? Have you ever suspected that if, say, aspirin in a bottle labeled "use by November 2018" was safe to take on November 30, 2018, that it might also be safe to take on December 1, 2018?

Wonder no more. About thirty years ago, the US government began to wonder the same thing and financed some studies. Basically, the government recognized it was wasting money if it threw away perfectly good medicines. Drug manufacturers felt about the same. Results of the "Shelf-Life Extension Program" studies were published in medical journals, but little effort has been made to disseminate this information to the general public.[132]

The gist of the articles is that it's better to use new stuff, but if there is a bioterrorist attack, or a public health emergency like a massive earthquake, or an epidemic, then it's ok to use older stock. If it's going to save the government money or there's a crisis that the government can't handle with what supplies it currently has, then it's safe to use older stock.

Per the articles, there is no hazard *per se* to using expired medications, only that they gradually decrease in efficacy. (But if you have a serious infection and your antibiotic is less effective, that could be hazardous.) This is true even for tetracycline family antibiotics (including minocycline and doxycycline, the latter being a drug of choice in treating anthrax). (The supposed toxicity of expired tetracycline is discussed in the next chapter.)

There is a significant exception, and that is for liquid medications. Those simply do not have the shelf-life of tablets and capsules, but they don't generally become toxic; they just become less effective.

STORING SUPPLIES FOR MAXIMUM SHELF LIFE AND EFFICIENCY

After gathering medical supplies for a while, you recognize the need to store them properly and keep them organized so they can be located when needed, and kept out of the way when they aren't.

Like foods, all these medicines and supplies should be stored in a cool, dry, dark place. But it doesn't mean they should be refrigerated or frozen unless otherwise indicated for individual substances.

Liquid medicines don't have a long shelf life. That's why they are mixed from powders in the pharmacy just before sale to consumers. Hydrogen peroxide has a fairly short shelf life. Rubbing alcohol and Betadine, on the other hand, last indefinitely.

Tablets and capsules store well; however, capsules must absolutely be protected from humidity, or they'll melt together into an unusable mess.

Any medications with the potential for abuse must be well-hidden. All medications should be kept out of the reach of children.

Plastic and latex products should be kept cool, dry, and dark to avoid melting and deteriorating. The same goes for vinyl and nitrile gloves.

Fragile items, such as glass thermometers and syringes, should be carefully wrapped to protect from breakage, and likewise for wind-up watches.

The foregoing doesn't present much of a challenge. It's the actual storage that becomes an issue for many. After a while, there are a lot of different items to store! As we prepare for a years-long grid-down situation for our large family, we have accumulated a lot of supplies. It would be nice to be able to store everything in just a few totes. However, in my experience using totes for camping gear, they just don't keep out dirt and bugs. And there's no way I want to risk spoiling precious medical supplies.

Six-gallon buckets work well for this purpose, especially when outfitted with gamma lids for easy access to the contents. And while the six-gallon buckets are no longer favored in this family for food (because six gallons of wheat, beans, or rice is just too much for me to wrangle), they are perfect for medical supplies, most of which are pretty light-weight. The buckets protect everything from dirt, bugs, mice, and moisture.

Before going into the buckets, most items get re-packaged in Ziploc bags to keep them extra clean and get rid of the boxes. It also helps to keep like items together for finding them more easily and rotating better. Some buckets hold the truly TEOTWAWKI-type items like sterile gloves, gowns, and towels, lidocaine powder, ether, and the glass thermometers and syringes. This keeps these items out of the way until they're needed, which is hopefully never. Other buckets are dedicated to just gloves, masks, or gauze. Some hold vitamins, supplements, or OTC pain relievers.

7. PRESCRIPTION MEDICATIONS—ANTIBIOTICS, ANTIFUNGALS, & ANTHELMINTICS

These life-saving medications have drastically extended and improved millions of lives over the past century. Without them, much of the care we provide our families would be limited to nineteenth century offerings. Some of these industrial pharmaceuticals have herbal counterparts that will serve us well (and that's a topic for another book); others do not yet have any known herbal options.

ANTIBIOTICS

How antibiotics work and how bacteria respond is a complex topic. Countless researchers devote their careers to studying just one aspect of bacteria or plants or compounds. That's far beyond the scope of this book, and yet acquiring a very basic understanding of how they work, what they can and cannot do, may help us use our limited supply of industrially manufactured antibiotics and natural herbal antibiotics as best as possible for our families. What follows is a gross simplification of how bacteria and antibiotics work.

Imagine a bacterium as a house. There are different ways to get into the house and destroy the inhabitants. Direct access (doors—front, back, garage, balcony, doggie), ventilation (windows, heating, air conditioning, dryer vent, chimney, cracks), water (plumbing, leaking, flooding). The agents of death can be bullets, falling trees, hurricanes and tornadoes, air-, insect-, or human-borne disease, carbon monoxide, radiation, fire. There are all kinds of options here.

Just as there are different ways to enter a house and kill the residents, there are also different ways that substances enter bacteria and kill them. Bacteria differ in what they are susceptible to. That's why antibiotics, natural or synthetic, have to be selected for the specific condition they are treating.

When bacteria encounter an antibiotic, they begin to respond. Most die pretty quickly, but due to genetic diversity, some hang on a bit longer. They learn what the threat is. They generate possible responses. Those bacteria in the meantime make more bacteria, with their specific genetic advantages, and some of their descendants are even better adapted to the antibiotic, and the cycle continues. Bacteria reproduce quickly, as fast as twenty minutes per generation, and they adapt. While most bacteria may die, if the chosen antibiotic doesn't wipe out all the bacteria quickly, the species as a whole survives. They become resistant. Those resistant bacteria rebound with a vengeance and seek to share knowledge they acquired in the recent battle with other bacteria far and wide.

Some of the earliest antibiotics worked by **disrupting the cell wall**, either by breaking down the wall or by preventing the bacteria from repairing the wall. They specifically work on the peptidoglycan layer of the cell wall and are thus effective on Gram-positive bacteria. Penicillin family antibiotics (penicillin, ampicillin, amoxicillin) and cephalosporins (Keflex) act in this manner.

Another way antibiotics operate is by **disrupting the cytoplasmic membrane** (which is distinct from the cell wall mentioned above). Polypeptides like polymyxin B and bacitracin work this way. These antibiotics work like a harsh detergent roughing up the cytoplasmic membrane of Gram-negative bacteria. The membrane isn't destroyed, but is so shaken by the experience that it lets the antibiotics through to do their work. Eventually, the bacteria respond by altering the amount of antibiotic that penetrates through the membrane, so that little to nothing gets through. The bacteria do this by changing the locks, so to say. They modify the size of the door or increase security.

Other antibiotics **interfere with the bacterial DNA replication** process or inhibit DNA enzymes. Bacteria don't actually live all that long. If they can't make babies, the little community they have sought to colonize in or on you dies out. Fluoroquinolone family antibiotics (-ofloxacins like Cipro, Levaquin, and moxifloxacin) work this way.

Some antibiotics impede or **prevent bacterial RNA protein synthesis**. This includes several classes of antibiotics—lincosamides (clindamycin), macrolides (Zithromax, Biaxin, erythromycin), and tetracyclines (doxycycline, minocycline, tetracycline). The antibiotics bind to the RNA. No protein can be made. No growth. No offspring. To combat this threat, the bacteria make internal adjustments such that the targets of the antibiotics, the RNA, aren't affected. They drank the poison, but it didn't matter because Poison Control was already on the scene.

Carbapenem antibiotics (end in *-penem)* greatly **inhibit some bacterial enzymes** to prevent cell wall synthesis. They're often used when all else fails. Kind of like Indiana Jones in the *Raiders of the Lost Ark* using his whip to escape his foes in the marketplace. He fights on and the bad guys keep coming. He finally whips out his pistol and dispatches the last assassin without a second thought. The bacteria are learning to make their own compounds to disable these broad-spectrum antibiotics of last resort. Which means the antibiotics of last resort are losing this battle.

Inhibiting folate synthesis, a process essential to nucleic acid synthesis, is another way antibiotics work. These antibiotics don't kill the bacteria; they just don't let the bacteria reproduce. This includes the sulfonamides like Silvadene and trimethoprim-sulfamethoxazole (TMP-SMZ).

By producing **toxic free radicals**, nitroimidazoles like metronidazole work against anaerobic bacteria.

Over the millennia, bacteria have evolved different mechanisms to protect themselves. One of these mechanisms involves **efflux pumps**. They're basically sump pumps, varying in sophistication from the entry-level ones that act on only a single substance to the highly complex that remove all kinds of foreign matter.

Sometimes bacteria take a "if you can't beat them, join them" approach, like when they decide to live in cleaning solutions. They can even adapt themselves to digest antibiotics as if they were food. This **extreme adaptability** and all the other adaptations bacteria make don't bode well for us. Unfortunately for us, the bacteria don't stop there.

Once they learn how to adapt, they have **massive bacteria networking parties** and share all they know with each other so that they can kill us more efficiently.[133]

It's a wonder any of us are still alive.

The following chart suggests common antibiotics to have on hand for a variety of conditions, and the quantities required for a standard course of treatment. It provides a general idea for what a family might wish to store. People living in tick country might wish to store a lot more doxycycline. Individuals lacking a spleen should consider stocking more amoxicillin and Keflex. Moxifloxacin could be added to the list for those who may be in particularly hazardous situations far from home. Someone frequently plagued by urinary tract infections may desire to store more TMP-SMZ. The medical shopping list at the back of the book suggests acquiring approximately 100 tablets of several different antibiotics.

No, we should not need all these within a year, especially if we have stored good quality food and have proper sanitation and hygiene practices in place. A specific antibiotic may be prescribed due to a contagious illness. A few family members may require treatment. Also, while some antibiotics can be substituted for others, many cannot. Don't just get one and plan on using it for everything. It won't work. Remember, these are antibiotics to have on hand for a licensed physician to administer appropriately.

Antibiotic Acquisition Charts

These charts outline the typical illnesses treated with antibiotics and the usual adult dosages (unless otherwise indicated) per course of treatment as a means of calculating the quantities to acquire for your family. THIS IS NOT

TO BE INTERPRETED AS A PRESCRIPTION FOR ANY GIVEN MEDICAL CONDITION. A physician will calculate children's dosages based on age and weight.

As you make your decisions about what to acquire, consider the following:

Which of these infections are you and your family members actually susceptible to? We don't have problems with sinus infections, so I don't even look at what's required for treating those. Strep throat and ear infections are pretty common in young children. I'd store a lot more penicillin if I had a young family.

Look at the cost per pill. Doxycycline is cheap. If I've got a choice between using that or just about anything else, I'll go with doxy, after discussing it with my doctor, of course. If I were worried about sun exposure, however, another choice might be better.

Consider the side effects. Not only is Cipro on the more expensive side, it can have some really undesirable side effects. I stock it because it may be the best choice for some conditions.

Remember, you aren't making decisions about what to use and when. You are merely stockpiling these antibiotics for a time of need when a physician can prescribe what is best. You just want to give the doctor the right tools for the job.

Antibiotic Acquisition Guidelines for Bioweapon and Skin Infections			
Condition	**First Line**	**Second Line**	**Notes**
Biological weapons			
Anthrax	Cipro 500 mg/2x per day/60 days	Doxycycline 100 mg/2x per day/60 days	
Plague	Doxycycline 100 mg/2x per day/10 days	Cipro 500 mg/2x per day/10-14 days	OR Moxifloxacin 400 mg/1x per day/10 days
Cholera	Doxycycline 100 mg/2x per day/10 days	Cipro 500 mg/2x per day/10-14 days	
Tularemia	Doxycycline 100 mg/2x per day/10 days	Cipro 500 mg/2x per day/10-14 days	
Skin infections			
Staphylo-coccus	TMP-SMZ DS 2x per day	Clindamycin 500 mg/3x per day Doxycycline 100 mg/2x per day TMP-SMZ DS	(Duration based on how quickly condition resolves)
Strepto-coccus	Penicillin	Ampicillin Augmentin Keflex Clindamycin	(Duration based on how quickly condition resolves, at least 10 days.)
Cat and dog bites	Augmentin 250-500 mg/3x per day/3-5 days Penicillin 500 mg/4x per day/3-5 days	Amoxicillin 500 mg/3x per day/3-5 days Erythromycin 250-500 mg/3-4x per day/3-5 days	Prophylactic treatment begins immediately after cat bite.
Cellulitis	TMP-SMZ DS 2x per day Augmentin 875 mg/2x per day	Clindamycin 500 mg/3x per day Keflex 1000 mg/2x per day	(Duration based on how quickly condition resolves, at least 10 days.)
Tick bites	Prophylactic use: doxycycline 200 mg once; disease treatment: 100 mg/2x per day/10-14 days		
Typhus	Doxycycline 100 mg/2x per day/7-10 days		

Antibiotic Acquisition Guidelines for Upper Respiratory Infections			
Condition	**First line**	**Second line**	**Notes**
Pneumonia	IV/IM antibiotics best	Levaquin 750 mg/1x per day OR Augmentin 1000 mg/2x per day OR Amoxicillin 1000 mg/3x per day PLUS Zithromax OR Moxifloxacin 400 mg/4x per day	
Aspiration pneumonia	IV/IM antibiotics best	Moxifloxacin 400 mg/4x per day	
"Walking" pneumonia	Cipro 500 mg/2x per day Levaquin 750 mg/2x per day	Doxycycline 100 mg/2x per day Erythromycin 400 mg/3x per day	
Bronchitis	Zithromax 500 mg first day, 250 mg per day/7 days	Biaxin 500 mg/2x per day TMP-SMZ DS 2x per day	
Strep throat	Penicillin Amoxicillin	Clindamycin Zithromax Biaxin	
Dental infections	Amoxicillin	Clindamycin	
Sinusitis	Augmentin 1000 mg/2x per day/7-10 days	Levaquin 750 mg/1x per day/7-10 days	
Otitis media (ear infection)	Amoxicillin Augmentin		Dosage and duration depend on age of patient

Antibiotic Acquisition Guidelines for Gastrointestinal and Urinary Tract Infections			
Condition	**First line**	**Second line**	**Notes**
Gastrointestinal			
Giardia	Metronidazole 250 mg/3x per day/5-7 days		
Post-antibiotic colitis (*Clostridium difficile*)	Metronidazole 500 mg/3x per day/14 days		
Cholera	Zithromax 1000 mg 1x Doxycycline 300 mg 1x	Erythromycin 500 mg/1x per day/3 days	
Traveler's diarrhea	Levaquin 500 mg/1x per day/1-3 days	Zithromax 500 mg/1x per day/3 days	
Salmonella	Levaquin 500 mg/1x per day/7-10 days	Zithromax 500 mg/1x per day/7-10 days	
Shigella	Cipro 750 mg/2x per day/3 days	Zithromax 500 mg/1x per day/3 days	
Diverticulitis	TMP-SMZ DS OR Levaquin 750 mg/1x per day/7-10 days PLUS Metronidazole 500 mg/1x per day/7-10 days		
Appendicitis	Augmentin 500 mg/3x per day OR TMP-SMZ DS OR Cipro 500 mg/2x per day PLUS Metronidazole 500 mg/3-4x per day		Continue taking until 3-4 days after symptoms have resolved.
Urinary tract infections			
Lower UTI	TMP-SMZ DS 2x per day/7 days	Cipro 500 mg/2x per day Levaquin 400 mg/1x per day	
Upper UTI	IV/IM antibiotics best	IV/IM antibiotics best	

Amoxicillin

(Fish-Mox—250 mg and Fish-Mox Forte—500 mg)

This is a newer version of ampicillin that is effective against Gram-positive and Gram-negative bacteria. It is very well absorbed, much better than penicillin, and well-tolerated with fewer side effects.[134]

When treating various bacterial infections with amoxicillin, physicians will prescribe along the lines of the following:

- **Upper respiratory**
  - Bacterial bronchitis, 500 mg, 3x per day, at least 5 days, or until no fever for 2-3 days
  - Bacterial pneumonia, 500 mg-1000 mg, 3x per day, at least 5 days, or until no fever for 2-3 days
  - Sinusitis, 250-500 mg, 3x per day, 5-7 days
  - Strep throat, 1000 mg, once per day, or 500 mg 2x per day, 10 days
  - Ear infection
  - Adults, 500 mg, 3x per day, 5-7 days
  - Children 25-90 mg/kg/day, in two divided doses, 7-10 days (there's a pretty wide range in what doctors recommend for children)
- **Skin**
  - Cutaneous anthrax, 1000 mg, 3x per day, 60 days
  - Mastitis, 500 mg, 3x per day, 10-14 days
  - Dog and cat bites, 500 mg, 3x day (2nd line), 3-5 days prophylaxis or 7-10 days treatment[135]
- **Gastrointestinal**
  - *Helicobacter pylori*, 1000 mg, 2x per day, 7-10 days (combined with metronidazole and Biaxin or tetracycline)[136]
- **Urogenital**
  - Gonorrhea, 3 grams, in a single dose[137]
  - Chlamydia, 500 mg, 3x per day, 7 days

- Bladder or kidney infections, including cystitis, 500 mg, 2-3x per day, 7 days
- with cystitis, it's safe to stop taking the antibiotics 2 days after symptoms are resolved.[138]

- **Other**
  - Lyme disease, 500 mg, 3x per day, 14-28 days[139]
  - Other bacterial tick-borne diseases, 500 mg, 3x per day, 14 days
  - Typhoid fever, for patients 12 years of age and older, 75-100 mg/kg per day for 14 days (second line choice; Cipro is preferred)[140]
  - Dental abscess

Amoxicillin may be taken with or without food.

Side effects. Common side effects include upset stomach, diarrhea, headache, and dizziness.

Contraindications. As amoxicillin is in the penicillin family, do not give amoxicillin to individuals allergic to penicillin. Amoxicillin is safe for use during pregnancy and breastfeeding but is excreted into breast milk. Infants of nursing mothers may develop thrush as a result.

Augmentin

This popular broad spectrum antibiotic combines amoxicillin and clavulanic acid, and is effective against Gram-positive, Gram-negative, and anaerobic bacteria. It's not mentioned as much in preparedness circles because there is no equivalent counterpart amongst the fish antibiotics that are a common work-around for Americans who can't get antibiotics without a prescription. However, it can be obtained through overseas pharmacies. Because it is considered safe for children and pregnant women, it's one to keep in the medicine supply.

Augmentin is available in a variety of strengths to suit pediatric and adult needs. The two sets of numbers associated with the prescription indicate the strength of the tablets. The first number is always the amoxicillin component; the second is the clavulanic acid component. The ratio varies from one tablet to the next, and this is why Augmentin tablets of one strength cannot be combined or divided to substitute for another strength. Doctors often prescribe Augmentin to treat the following conditions:

- **Upper respiratory**
  - Ear infections, dose dependent on weight of child; in adults, 875 mg, 2x per day, 10 days, or 250-500 mg, 3x per day, 5-10 days
  - Sinus infections, 875 mg, 2x per day, or 500 mg 3x per day, 5-7 days
  - Pneumonia, 875 mg, 2x per day, or 500 mg 3x per day, 7-10 days.
  - Tonsillitis
- **Skin**
  - Impetigo, 500-875 mg, 2x per day, or 250-500 mg 3x per day, 7 days
  - Insect bites and stings
  - Dog and cat bites and scratches, 875 mg, 2x per day, or 500 mg 3x per day, 3-5 days
  - Cellulitis, 250-500 mg, 3x per day, at least 5 days, and at least 2-3 days after redness disappears
  - Burns, same as for cellulitis[141]
- **Gastrointestinal**
  - Diverticulitis, 500 mg, 3x per day, until 3-4 days after symptoms resolve[142]
  - Gallbladder, 500 mg, 3x per day[143]
- **Urogenital**

    - Chronic prostatitis, 500 mg, 3x per day, 10 days[144]
    - Pyelonephritis, 875 mg, 2x per day, or 500 mg, 3x per day, 10-14 days
    - Cystitis, 500 mg, 3x per day, until 2 days after symptoms have passed
- Augmentin is also effective against the following bacteria:
    - *Haemophilus influenzae,* 500/125 mg, 2x per day, or 250/125 mg, 3x per day, 10 days for less severe infections; 875/125 mg, 2x per day, or 500/125 mg, 3x per day, 7-10 days
    - Enterobacteria (*Shigella*, *Salmonella*, *E. coli*)

Augmentin is a second line choice in treating chronic prostatitis.

The usual dose of Augmentin in adults is one 500-mg tablet, 2x per day, or one 250-mg tablet 3x per day. With more serious infections, including respiratory tract infections, the dosage is 875 mg, 2x per day, or 500 mg, 3x per day.

The pediatric dosage of Augmentin in infants under three months of age is 30 mg/kg/day in divided doses, based on the amoxicillin component. For infants and children over three months of age, the dosage is 45 mg/kg/day in divided doses for ear, sinus, and lower respiratory infections. For less serious infections, the dosage is 25 mg/kg/day in divided doses.

Cautions. Augmentin should be taken with food. Do not use alcohol while taking Augmentin. It may increase the risk of side effects or make the side effects worse. Two 250-mg Augmentin tablets should not be substituted for one 500-mg tablet, and vice-versa, because the amount of clavulanic acid is the same in both tablets. Augmentin may increase the risk of yeast infections, headache, and blood clotting problems. Side effects of using Augmentin include diarrhea, vomiting, and allergic reactions.[145]

Interactions. Augmentin may increase bleeding in individuals using anticoagulants. It may increase the likelihood of a skin rash in persons taking allopurinol. It may also decrease the efficacy of oral contraceptives.

Contraindications. Augmentin is not for use in those allergic to penicillin.

Cipro

(Fish-Flox—250 and Fish-Flox Forte—500 mg)

Cipro often gets a bad rap; indeed, valid concerns regarding its use do exist. However, just as it would be foolish to hunt squirrels with a shotgun, you don't hunt bears with a BB gun. It just doesn't work. Likewise, amoxicillin works for garden variety upper respiratory infections, but for some TEOTWAWKI-type diseases, you really want the best, most effective weapon. The best often comes at a cost, so to speak. The use of Cipro may have side effects, some quite serious. With Cipro and other quinolones, there is a risk of tendinitis and/or tendon rupture during treatment and for several months afterward. This risk is greatest in men over the age of sixty. Cipro is only used in children under the age of twelve years in the case of anthrax or when there are no other alternatives in a life-threatening situation. The risk is greater for those who take Cipro for longer periods. Shorter courses of treatment have far less risk.

Cipro is a broad-spectrum antibiotic, in the same family as the other fluoroquinolone antibiotics like moxifloxacin, norfloxacin, and Levaquin. It is very effective against most Gram-negative bacteria, and only moderately effective against Gram-positive bacteria.

The following are typical dosages and treatment courses for some TEOTWAWKI-type illnesses. These are not prescriptions. They are only a means of helping you calculate how much Cipro you may wish to have on hand for your family, and so that a physician can treat your loved ones as best as possible. All are adult dosages. Children should not be given Cipro except in extreme situations.

- **Upper Respiratory**

    - Pneumonia, 500-750 mg, 2x per day, 7-14 days
    - Pneumonic plague, prophylactic treatment post-exposure is 500 mg, 2x per day, 7 days; disease treatment is 500 mg, 2x per day, 14 days[146]
- **Gastrointestinal**
    - Appendicitis, 500 mg, 3x per day, plus metronidazole, 500 mg, 3-4x per day, at least 7 days, or until 3-4 days after symptoms resolve[147]
    - Cholera, 1 gram, taken once
    - Diverticulitis, 250-500 mg, 2x per day, 1-3 days, in patients with a prior history of infection or considerable bleeding[148]
    - Typhoid, 500 mg, 2x per day, 5 days
- **Other**
    - Tularemia, 500 mg, 2x per day, 10-14 days.[149] (Doxycycline would be preferred if it's an option.)
    - Anthrax, inhalational and cutaneous, 500 mg, 2x per day, 2 months[150]

Cipro is also used to treat the following infections, but due to the adverse side effects, its use for these conditions is best avoided if at all possible.[151]

- Cellulitis, 500-750 mg, 2x per day, 7-14 days
- Mastitis, 500 mg, 2x per day, 10-14 days
- Dysentery and diarrhea due to *Campylobacter, Escherichia coli,* and *Shigella*, 500 mg, 2x per day, 7-10 days[152]
- Urinary tract infections, 250-500 mg, 2x per day, 7-10 days, or until 1-2 days after symptoms resolve

In addition, Cipro is used to treat gallbladder infections, epididymitis, and ear infections in adults.

Cautions. Cipro should be taken with a full glass of water, with or without food.[153]

Interactions. Common substances that inhibit Cipro include dandelion (in teas or salads),[154] calcium (i.e., milk, calcium supplements, Tums),[155] grapefruit, and Diflucan (for three days after taking it).

Contraindications. Cipro is not indicated for use in pregnancy, but as little is excreted into breast milk, it is safe for nursing mothers, though infants should be monitored for thrush. It is not for use in children except in the case of post-exposure anthrax, or when there are no other alternatives available in a life-threatening situation.

Doxycycline

(Fish-Doxy and Bird-Biotic, both 100 mg)

Doxycycline is a broad-spectrum member of the tetracycline family that also goes by the trade names of Vibramycin or Vibra-tabs. The following are typical treatment regimens for some illnesses. These are not prescriptions. They are only a means of helping you calculate how much doxycycline may wish to have on hand for your family, and so that a physician can treat your loved ones as best as possible. All are adult dosages.

- **Upper respiratory**
  - Inhalational anthrax, 100 mg 2x per day, 60 days[156]
  - Pneumonic plague
    - Prophylactic treatment post-exposure (for those who have been exposed to pneumonic plague, but are not sick), 100 mg, 2x per day for the first day, then 100 mg per day for 7 days
    - Disease treatment, 100 mg, 2x per day for the first day, then 100 mg per day for 10 days[157]
- **Skin**

- Dog and cat bites, 50-100 mg, 2x per day, 3-5 days[158]
- Tick bites, bacterial tick-borne diseases, 100 mg, 2x per day, 10-14 days[159]
- Typhus, 100 mg, 2x per day, usually 7-10 days (until at least three days after the fever subsides).[160] For children under 100 pounds, the dosage is 2.2 mg/kg, 2x per day. Without doxycycline, most patients die. In wartime outbreaks, many of the typhus fatalities were actually among those nursing the ill and wounded.

> If you have the resources, every patient presenting with a tick bite in a high-risk area may be given a single 200-mg dose.
>
> If I had an immediate family member with a tick that had possibly been attached for more than twelve hours, I wouldn't hesitate to use doxycycline in this manner, assuming I had an adequate supply.

- **Gastrointestinal**
  - Cholera, a single 300-mg dose for illness contracted under normal conditions; 100 mg, 2x per day, 10 days when it's a biological weapon.[161]
- **Other**
  - Tularemia, 100 mg, 2x per day, 10-14 days. Unfortunately, there's a good chance for relapse.[162]

Doxycycline is a second line antibiotic for treating pneumonia and infected burns. It is also indicated for some sexually-transmitted diseases—chlamydia, gonorrhea, syphilis, and pelvic inflammatory disease; some urinary tract infections, chronic prostatitis, and epididymitis; upper respiratory infections caused by strep, MRSA infections, and some parasitic worm infections (it kills bacteria in worms that the worms need to survive).

Cautions. Avoid sun exposure between the hours of 10AM and 3PM and wear hats, sunglasses, long sleeves, and pants when outdoors. Finally, doxycycline inhibits the efficacy of oral birth control and other methods must be used when taking this antibiotic.

Interactions. Common substances that inhibit doxycycline include calcium (i.e., milk, calcium supplements, Tums), some supplements (magnesium, iron, zinc), and warfarin.

Contraindications. Not for use by pregnant or nursing women, unless there are no other options in a life-threatening situation. Brief use, i.e., prophylaxis for a tick bite, is "probably safe."[163] It is not for use in children except in the case of typhus, post-exposure anthrax, and Rocky Mountain spotted fever, or when there are no other alternatives available in a life-threatening situation.

Keflex

(Fish-Flex—250 mg and Fish-Flex Fort—500 mg)

Keflex is the most familiar member of the cephalosporin family of antibiotics. This antibiotic is effective against most Gram-positive and Gram-negative bacteria. It disrupts cell wall formation, eventually rupturing the wall, causing all the innards to leak out and the bacteria to die. It's a weapon you want in your war against bad bacteria.

The most common dosing regimen is taking the capsules every 6 hours for 7-14 days, less for bladder infections, and much longer for bone infections. Pediatric dosages range from 12.5 to 25 milligrams per kilogram of body weight.[164]

When treating various bacterial infections with Keflex, physicians will prescribe along the following lines:

- **Upper respiratory**, all for 7-14 days, unless otherwise indicated:[165]
  - Pneumonia, bronchitis, 250 mg, 4x per day OR 500 mg, 2x per day

- Strep throat, 250 mg, 4x per day OR 500 mg, 2x per day, 5-10 days[166]
- Ear infection
- Adults, 250 mg, 4x per day OR 500 mg, 2x per day[167]
- Children 12.5-25 mg/kg/day, in 2 divided doses

- **Skin**:
  - Impetigo, 250 mg, 4x per day, 7-14 days
  - Cellulitis, 500 mg, 4x per day, 7-14 days, continuing until 2-3 days beyond resolution of the redness[168]
  - Mastitis, 500 mg, 4x per day, 10-14 days[169]
- **Urogenital**, all for 7 days
  - Cystitis, 250 mg, 4x per day OR 500 mg, 2x per day, (but may discontinue two days after symptoms pass)
  - Pyelonephritis, 250 mg, 4x per day OR 500 mg, 2x per day
  - Prostatitis, 250 mg, 4x per day OR 500 mg, 2x per day
- **Bone**
  - Osteomyelitis, 500 mg, 2 to 4x per day, 4-6 weeks[170]

Keflex may be taken with or without food. However, individuals with sensitive stomachs should take it with food and a full glass of water.

Metronidazole

(Fish-Zole, 250 mg)

Metronidazole is another one of those antibiotic wonders. As the only member of the nitroimidazole family that is commonly available to non-medical personnel, it's in a class by itself, often doing a job no other antibiotic can. Sold under the brand name Flagyl, metronidazole kills anaerobic bacteria and protozoa by interfering with DNA replication. It is used for a wide variety of diseases in just as wide a variety of dosages and protocols.

BACTERIAL INFECTIONS:

- **Upper respiratory.** Aspiration pneumonia, 500 mg, 3-4x per day, until 3-4 days after symptoms resolve. It is always used in conjunction with TMP-SMZ DS. [171]
- **Skin.** Animal or human bites. Metronidazole is an alternative if the preferred antibiotics are not available, and is used in dosages of 250-500 mg, 3x per day, 7-10 days. Tetracycline or Biaxin may also be prescribed.
- **Gastrointestinal**
    - **Diverticulitis** and **peritonitis**, 500 mg, 3-4x per day, until 3-4 days after symptoms resolve. It is always used in conjunction with TMP-SMZ DS.[172]
    - **Gallbladder infections**. As with diverticulitis and peritonitis, metronidazole is combined with TMP-SMZ DS. However, because the risk of nausea and vomiting is very high, physicians often also administer a single dose of Bonine to reduce the possibility of vomiting.[173]
    - **Colitis** due to *Clostridium difficile* (which may occur from taking other antibiotics), 500 mg 3-4x per day, 5-10 days.[174]
    - ***Helicobacter pylori*** ulcers, 500 mg, 2x per day for several days, in conjunction with Prilosec and amoxicillin, tetracycline, or Biaxin
- **Urogenital**
    - **STDs**, **postpartum infections**, or **miscarriage**, metronidazole, 500 mg, 2x per day, 2 weeks, in conjunction with doxycycline, Levaquin, ofloxacin, or Zithromax[175]
    - **Bacterial vaginosis**, 500 mg, 2x per day, 7 days[176]
- **Other**
    - **Meningitis, cellulitis**, **bone** and **joint infections** are treated with intravenously administered metronidazole

- **Dental infections**, where deep roots and poor oxygenation are an issue, 400 mg, 3x per day, 5 days[177]

PROTOZOAL INFECTIONS:

- **Giardiasis**, 250 mg, 3x per day, 5-10 days[178]
- **Trichomoniasis**, 250 mg, 3x per day, 7 days[179] or 2 grams (four 500 mg tablets) taken at once[180]
- **Amoebic dysentery**, 750 mg, 3x per day, 5-10 days[181]
- **Side effects**. Nausea, loss of appetite, and a metallic taste in the mouth

Contraindications. Not for use in pregnant or nursing women. Do not consume alcohol during treatment or for two days after treatment is completed or there is risk of having an almost instant hangover and vomiting.

Penicillin

(Fish-Pen, 250 mg; Fish-Pen Forte, 500 mg)
Discovered in the 1920s by Alexander Fleming and first used clinically in the early 1940s, penicillin was heralded as the first "miracle" drug. While hundreds and thousands of others have followed, penicillin is the one that started it all. Penicillin works by preventing bacteria from building and repairing cell walls. Water flows into the bacterial cells, and the cells swell up and die. Penicillin-resistant bacteria survived by learning how to defeat that mechanism of action.

Penicillin comes in several forms. They cannot necessarily be used interchangeably.

- Benzylpenicillin (penicillin G) is the original penicillin found in 1928. It is administered by intramuscular or intravenous injection. This is the best for severe streptococcal pneumonia and *Neisseria* infections in the chest, meningitis, and cellulitis.[182]

- Benzathine penicillin acts for a longer time than benzylpenicillin. It is administered by intramuscular injection. The benzathine is a stabilizer that slows the release of penicillin so that it remains in the body for two to four weeks.
- Procaine penicillin also acts for a longer time than benzylpenicillin. This is another slow-release penicillin administered by intramuscular injection.
- Phenoxymethylpenicillin (penicillin V or VK) is the only form that can be taken orally. It is less effective against Gram-negative bacteria. It comes in two different strengths, 250 mg and 500 mg. This preparation works well for strep throat due to *Streptococcus pyogenes* or Group A strep.[183]

Penicillin is a narrow-spectrum antibiotic to which many bacteria have developed resistance. However, it does have a couple of significant advantages. The first is that penicillin penetrates very well into the central nervous system. It's a good choice for bacterial meningitis infections, but it has to be started very quickly.[184] The second is that it is considered safe for pregnant and breastfeeding women. [185]

Penicillin is useful for upper respiratory tract infections due to *Streptococcus pneumoniae*, but it is not the first choice of doctors because there are so many other bacteria that cause URIs, and the antibiotics that treat those will also cover *Streptococcus pneumoniae*. Penicillin is a good choice for dental infections.

When treating various bacterial infections with penicillin, physicians will prescribe along the lines of the following:

- **Upper respiratory**
    - Sore throat due to bacterial infection, 250-500 mg, 4x per day, until there has been no fever for at least 2 days[186]
    - Scarlet fever, 250 mg, 3-4x per day, 10 days[187]

- Ear infection, 250-500 mg, 4x per day, until there has been no fever for at least 2 days[188]
- Diphtheria, 250-500 mg, 4x per day, 14 days[189]
- Cutaneous or inhalation anthrax, 500 mg, 4x per day, 10 days in "normal" situations, or up to 60 days in the case of bioterrorism[190]

- **Skin**
  - Dog and cat bites, 500 mg, 4x per day, 3-5 days[191] (second line choice)
- **Bone**
  - Joint infections, 500 mg, 2-4x per day, 14-42 days[192]

Penicillin is not generally effective for cellulitis, nor does it work well on other skin infections, or insect bites or stings.

A true allergic reaction to penicillin occurs in less than 0.1% of the population.

Side effects. Adverse reactions to penicillin are not uncommon. These include diarrhea, nausea, rash, hives, and secondary fungal infections. An adverse reaction may or may not be a precursor to a future allergic reaction and should be noted in medical records.

Allergic to Penicillin?

Say you are allergic to penicillin. You've been told this, you believe it, the end. Is there any reason to go on?

Well, maybe. Here are some interesting facts:

Ten percent of Americans report having an allergy to penicillin (and ampicillin and amoxicillin are also members of the penicillin family).[193] However, more than 80% of those reporting a penicillin allergy are not *truly* allergic to penicillin.[194]

Often the report of an "allergy" is from parents who indicated that the child had a *reaction*. Often, like with other allergies, the patient outgrows the allergy. Even those who displayed a genuine allergic reaction to penicillin in the past, when tested ten years later exhibited no allergic response.[195]

Signs and symptoms of a penicillin allergy usually begin within one minute to one hour after taking penicillin. These may include:

- Itching or hives
- Numbness or tingling of lips or tongue
- Swelling of lips, eyes, mouth, or tongue
- Wheezing
- Shortness of breath
- Difficulty swallowing
- Low blood pressure
- Fast heart rate
- Dizziness
- Nausea and vomiting

Alternatives for those allergic to penicillin include:

Cipro
Clindamycin
Doxycycline
Erythromycin
Metronidazole
Minocycline
Sulfa drugs
Tetracycline
Zithromax

A localized rash and mild nausea are considered a sensitivity and not an allergic response.

The only way to really know whether a person is allergic to penicillin is to perform a skin allergy test followed by an oral challenge. We can DIY the skin test if we have to, but the oral challenge has to be done with medical supervision. If you believe that you or your child is allergic to penicillin, it would be best to determine this now, if possible. Schedule an appointment with your doctor to find out for sure.

So what if you think there is a penicillin allergy. Can't you just take something else? Does it really matter?

Actually, it might. What if you or your child has an illness that needs an antibiotic, and penicillin is the best choice? What if, due to whatever circumstances arise, penicillin is the *only* choice? Are you going to skip the penicillin because of a supposed allergy? Now, this isn't to mock those who are genuinely allergic. It's just to bring to mind that quite often, as has been stated, more than 80% of people who report having a penicillin allergy are not truly allergic. If a person is truly allergic, penicillin must absolutely be avoided. Anaphylaxis is deadly.

Penicillin is a narrow-spectrum antibiotic that is usually very well tolerated and is safe for pregnant and nursing women and children. The alternatives are often broad-spectrum antibiotics which have more side effects and contribute to antibiotic resistance. *Clostridium difficile* infections actually occur more frequently in patients who report a penicillin allergy. With the ever-increasing number of antibiotic-resistant bacteria, penicillin is still a useful and inexpensive option. Those who believe they are allergic should really be tested now to find out for sure.

If a person is truly allergic to penicillin, what are the alternatives? It is all going to depend on the bacteria that need killing. There is no one antibiotic that will substitute for penicillin in all cases. [196] The substitute antibiotic will have to be chosen based on the disease being treated. In all conditions listed below (and elsewhere), antibiotics will only work on bacterial infections. They never have and never will work on viral infections.

Tetracycline

Whenever two or more preparedness-minded individuals gather, and the topic turns to antibiotics, inevitably the following cautions are offered: "Don't store tetracycline. It becomes toxic." A lot of what's posted online is copied from someone else online, who copied it from another source, and so on. The myth gets perpetuated.

The idea of tetracycline becoming toxic is a myth. Sometimes even doctors, who should know better, are the ones perpetuating the myth.

According to *The Medical Letter*, a professional newsletter,

> "The only report of human toxicity that may have been caused by chemical or physical degradation of a pharmaceutical product is renal tubular damage that was associated with the use of degraded tetracycline... Current tetracycline preparations have been reformulated with different fillers to minimize degradation

and are unlikely to have this effect" (*The Medical Letter*, Vol. 44, Issue 1142, 28 October 2002).[197]

Tetracycline is a broad-spectrum antibiotic used to treat the following infections:

- **Upper respiratory**
  - Ear infections in adults
  - Sinusitis
  - Bronchitis
- **Gastrointestinal**
  - Cholera, 500 mg, 4x per day, 3 days (but doxycycline, Zithromax, or Cipro may be better choices)[198]
  - Enterotoxigenic *E. coli*
  - Gallbladder
  - *Helicobacter pylori*, 500 mg, 2x per day, 10 days, taken in conjunction with metronidazole and an acid blocker[199]
- **Urogenital**
  - Urinary tract infections
  - Trachoma
  - Chlamydia, 7-10 days[200]
  - Gonorrhea, 7-10 days[201]
  - Pelvic inflammatory disease, 10-14 days[202]
- **Vector-borne**
  - Tick-borne relapsing fever, 500 mg, 4x per day, 10 days[203]
  - Typhus, 6-10 days[204]
  - Brucellosis, 2-3 weeks[205]
  - Malaria

Unless otherwise indicated, the adult dosage is 250 mg, 4x per day, 7 days. For children ages 8 to 12 years, the dosage is 125 mg, half the adult dosage. Tetracycline is not used in children under the age of eight years unless there is no other option. Tetracycline can cause problems in developing bones and stain teeth.

Alternatives. Colloidal silver has been shown to be as effective as tetracycline in laboratory studies.[206]

The following herbs have been demonstrated in clinical studies to work synergistically with tetracycline, even against tetracycline-resistant bacteria:

- Berberines like Oregon grape and Japanese barberry combined with tetracycline are extremely effective in treating cholera and *E. coli* infections
- Thyme, in the form of one to two drops of essential oil under the tongue, combined with tetracycline worked well against *Salmonella typhimurium, Streptococcus pyogenes, Escherichia coli,* and *Staphylococcus aureus*[207]
- Bidens;[208]
- Licorice (the herb—*Glycyrrhiza*—not the candy)[209]
- Ginger[210]
- Pomegranate rind and peel[211]

Most cholera strains are resistant to tetracycline alone. It should be combined with an herb to be effective in treating cholera. Furthermore, combining tetracycline with an herb may significantly shorten the treatment period, allowing you to make the tetracycline supply last longer.

Cautions. Tetracycline may cause sun sensitivity and the development of a rash. Avoid sun exposure while taking tetracycline.

Interactions. Tetracycline absorption is significantly (50-90%) impaired by milk and milk products. The issue arises not from the milk itself, but rather the antibiotic binding with calcium. Tetracyclines also bind with iron, zinc, and magnesium. Antacids like Tums and supplements of these minerals also inhibit tetracyclines, as do any other foods rich in these minerals, like oysters, dried figs, and raisins. For this reason, do not use milk products or antacids for two hours before or after taking tetracycline.

Contraindications. Tetracycline should not be taken by pregnant women and children under the age of eight years as it can damage bones and stain teeth.

ANTIFUNGALS

Diflucan

(Fish-Flucon, 100 mg)

Diflucan is a very handy anti-fungal, particularly for women prone to yeast infections and for individuals who develop fungal infections following a course of antibiotic therapy. It is available by prescription only in the US, but is OTC in Canada.

For a yeast infection, a physician will usually prescribe two or three 150-mg pills. The first pill is taken any time, with or without food, and starts working immediately. If symptoms still aren't resolved three days later, then the second pill is taken. If the infection is particularly resistant, a third pill may be taken. They are a little pricey, at about two dollars each, if you are buying them yourself without insurance from an overseas pharmacy. But remember, you're only taking one or two at most. They're way more compact and convenient than over-the-counter creams and have a longer shelf life.

Diflucan is also used to treat thrush, 100-200 mg per day for 7 days. Other illnesses for which Diflucan is used include valley fever, ringworm, athlete's foot, and fungal infections of the toe- and fingernails. However, these all require months of treatment. OTC topical creams will probably be a better way to go.

Caution. Diflucan remains in the body for up to three days. All medications that may interact with Diflucan need to be avoided until 72 hours have passed from when the last dose was taken.

Interactions. There are over 600 medications that interact with Diflucan. If you are taking any medication, do not use Diflucan unless under a physician's direction. The most commonly used drugs that interact with Diflucan include

Cipro, erythromycin, Biaxin, cyclosporins, Zofran, Percocet, Norco, Miralax, Prilosec, and metronidazole.

Contraindications. Absolutely do not use if nursing, pregnant, or trying to become pregnant.

ANTHELMINTICS

With all the medications we acquire for an uncertain future—OTC drugs, antibiotics, antifungals, other prescription medications, etc., no one really gives any thought to treating worms. None of the afore-mentioned work to kill worms. You can have the best medical kit on the planet—all the antibiotics, all the pain meds, lots of antifungals, and they will do nothing against worms.

Now, consider the following. Various statistics from all over the 'net state that pinworms afflict about 40 million Americans. Another put the figure at 20% of the population, which I think would get us closer to 75 million people. They're three times more common than head lice. If those numbers weren't bad enough, consider the fact that one-third of people are totally asymptomatic. They could be spreading it without even knowing.

We get worms from contact with an infected person or from contaminated food or water. TEOTWAWKI will provide us the perfect storm of conditions for getting worms—people with inadequate sanitation and contaminated food and water.

Pinworms cause rectal itching, especially at night, when the female pinworms migrate to the outside of the body to lay eggs around the anal orifice. The pinworms and clumps of eggs are irritating and make the patient itch. To find and definitively diagnose pinworms, wrap a piece of tape around a gloved finger. Stick the finger up the rear end of the patient at night. The pinworms will stick to the tape. Pinworms are easily spread from person to person, especially among young children who don't wash hands after using the toilet or who scratch their bottoms and then go play with other children. ALL close contacts with an infected person should be treated, especially because asymptomatic infection and re-infection often occur.

Roundworms are much larger, like earthworms, and can grow to over 12 inches. We get them from contaminated food. Diagnosis usually occurs when adult roundworms work their way out the mouth, nose, or anus. Other symptoms of roundworms are abdominal pain, intestinal blockage, and malnutrition. Like pinworm infestations, many roundworm infections are asymptomatic, so everyone in close contact with the afflicted individual should be treated.

The treatments listed below also work for tapeworms, whipworms, and flukes.

Albendazole

Albendazole is a sheep and cattle dewormer that is not FDA-approved for human use, but it appears that many physicians would have no problem using it in a crisis. Because it is for livestock, albendazole can be purchased without a prescription in this country. As best I can tell, it is given in a single dose, 400 mg all at once. Check with your physician to be sure.

Natural treatments that claim to be effective against worms include black walnut, garlic, pumpkin seeds, turmeric, cucumber seeds, wormwood, clove, plumeria, and tobacco.

Contraindications: Do not use if you are taking metronidazole. Do not use if nursing, pregnant, or planning to become pregnant.

Ivermectin

Ivermectin for use in people is by prescription only and is sold under the brand name Stromectol. It is an FDA-approved treatment for worm infestations, and as such is taken internally. Stromectol is not FDA-approved for internal use for treating other parasitic conditions. If their blessing is important to you, then you don't need to read any further.

Scabies. The Centers for Disease Control recommends the use of ivermectin to treat scabies in patients for whom other treatments have failed, or who cannot tolerate FDA-approved topical medications for eliminating scabies. Two doses of oral ivermectin are taken seven days apart, in a dosage of

200μg/kg/dose.[212] Usually, it is recommended that ivermectin be taken on an empty stomach; however, scabies researchers indicate that the bioavailability of ivermectin is improved when it is taken with food.[213]

Norwegian (crusted) scabies. With this severe form of scabies, both oral ivermectin and a topical agent should be used. Oral ivermectin in a dosage of 200μg/kg/dose should be taken with food. The number of doses depends on the severity of the infection:

- Three doses taken on days 1, 2, and 8
- Five doses taken on days 1, 2, 8, 9, and 15
- Seven doses taken on days 1, 2, 8, 9, 15, 22, and 29[214]

Scabies patients treated with ivermectin overwhelmingly approved this treatment as being easier, faster, and much more effective. The itching resolved much more quickly and patients were able to sleep better.[215]

Lice. As with scabies, the US FDA does not approve the internal use of ivermectin to treat lice. However, oral ivermectin has been used to successfully eliminate lice. Like the regimen for scabies, it is given in a single dose of 200 μg/kg and repeated 9-10 days later.[216]

Contraindications: Ivermectin is not indicated for use in children weighing less than 15 kg or in pregnant women. The World Health Organization indicates that ivermectin has been used to safely treat younger children in reduced dosages.[217]

Mebendazole

Mebendazole is a dewormer available by prescription only in the US. However, it can be obtained through overseas pharmacies.

None of the physician-authors of *Armageddon Medicine*, *The Survival Medicine Handbook*, or *Survival and Austere Medicine* provided dosages for mebendazole. A few online sites indicated that a single 100-mg tablet is prescribed for children two years and up through adults, and the treatment is repeated two to three weeks later. Of course, you should not use any medication without consulting a physician. Information herein is provided merely to familiarize the reader with what a physician may do for treatment and what medications to have on hand.

PRESCRIPTION BOTTLE SHORTHAND DECODER

This handy reference for interpreting what those abbreviations on prescription bottles mean is for those instances where you saved a bottle of whatever in case you needed it again in the future, instead of turning it in to the authorities for proper disposal—and in case your instructions were written in code which was interpreted for you at the time, but you have since forgotten.

I have to admit, I have never seen or even heard of many of these abbreviations, but I figure there are some areas of the country where their use might be more common, or maybe among some doctors they're more generally used. Most all of these abbreviations come from Latin, and they are used around the world. Theoretically, you could pick up a prescription bottle from Brazil, Bahrain, or Boston and be able to understand the written instructions.

Prescription Bottle Abbreviations			
Gtt	Drop	t	teaspoon or 5 ml
T	Tablespoon or 15 ml	Oz	Ounce or 30 ml
Route of administration			
PO	Per oral—mouth	IM	Intramuscular
SQ	Subcutaneous	PR	Rectal
SL	Sublingual	IV	Intravenous
ID	Intradermal	TAA	To affected area
OD	Right eye	OS	Left eye
OU	Both eyes		
Schedule			
QOD, QD	Once per day	Q4	Every 4 hours
BID	2x per day	Q6	Every 6 hours
TID	3x per day	Q8	Every 8 hours
QID	4x per day	Q4-6	Every 4-6 hours
QH	Every hour	NPO	Nothing by mouth
AC	Before meals	PC	After meals
HS	Before bed	CC	With food
Ad. Lib.	As desired or needed	Dieb. Alt.	Every other day
PRN	As needed		

8. EXPENDABLE SUPPLIES

Expendable supplies are the single-use items involved in caring for patients. They must be stocked in abundance because there will be no replacing them.

CHEMICAL LIGHT STICKS

Just like children only get sick at night and on weekends, most emergencies where we really need a lot of good light are going to happen at night. The power will probably be out as well. A single headlamp probably won't provide enough illumination, so it's chemical light sticks to the rescue. They're lightweight and easy to move around, without the risk of flame or fumes from a lantern. White light is best. Chemical light sticks usually have a shelf life of a few years, which significantly depends on the storage conditions. They don't last as long at high temperatures. On the other hand, freezing them will extend their life substantially. Of course, if they're in the freezer, then they aren't in the medical kit when you need them.

COLD PACKS

Cold packs and ice packs are most often used to reduce swelling following an injury like a sprain or muscle strain. These packs also work well for treating bug bites, arthritis, and tendinitis. In an ideal situation, the cold/ice pack is applied for 10 minutes every hour in the first 72 hours following an injury. After that, it should be applied 3 times per day for 15-20 minutes, and especially after working, exercising, etc.

The cold/ice pack really only works if it actually comes into close contact with the afflicted tissue. The pack should definitely not be applied directly to the skin; there should be a cloth of some sort between the pack and the skin to prevent damage to the skin. That being said, the pack should conform to the afflicted body part as closely as possible for maximum benefit.

Because cold/ice packs are so easily improvised at home, many people don't actually store chemical cold packs. And why would you, when it is so easy to use a:

- Bag of frozen vegetables
- Damp towel, wrung out, and frozen for 15 minutes
- Bag of ice
- Quart-size freezer bag filled with 1 cup of rubbing alcohol and 3 cups of water, and frozen until slushy
- Cloth bag filled with rice and frozen

However, none of these may be an option if there is no electricity, and that's where the chemical cold packs come in. These are NOT ice packs, nor are they designed to be. They should probably be thought of more as "cool" packs. They don't get incredibly cold, one reason for which is to prevent damaging skin tissue. And they don't last forever, just about the amount of time a cold pack is to be applied before taking a break, 10-20 minutes. These chemical cold packs should not be used around the eye to avoid inflicting any damage to the eye in case the chemical cold pack springs a leak.

Chemical cold packs are available in a variety of sizes, configurations (like for neck or back or knee), and disposable or reusable. Lower-end options are sold at dollar stores, but even large ones through medical supply stores are pretty inexpensive, especially if purchased in bulk.

A roll of gauze or vet wrap can be used to hold a cold pack in place.

Every once in a while, you come across the suggestion that these chemical cold packs can be used for treating hyperthermia—heat cramps, heat exhaustion, or heatstroke. Researchers at Stanford simulated a test to determine the validity of the claim. Their results showed that these chemical cold packs are just not effective in such a situation; regular ice packs are five to six times better at rapidly cooling a hyperthermic body. Save the chemical cold packs for physical injuries.

COMPRESSED WASHCLOTHS

Compressed washcloths are tiny, about the size of a Life Saver. They're not too expensive, so it's easy to get a lot so that they can be put anywhere and everywhere, like all the boo-boo kits and medical bags. They take about ten seconds to re-hydrate and then it takes about a minute to unfold, maybe less. They expand to about the size of a regular baby wipe and are about as durable.

Some companies market it as compressed toilet paper. Some are individually wrapped, and others come in tubes. The individually packaged ones stay clean until needed.

DRESSINGS

So what do we want as far as dressing supplies?

Gauze. When purchasing gauze, if it's just at Walmart or CVS, there won't be a lot of decisions to make. But if going with Amazon (not necessarily the best idea) or ShopMedVet (great idea if buying a lot), there will be numerous options. One is going to be the number of plies in the gauze. The thicker, the better, and the generally more expensive. Sterile, of course, will be more expensive, but that's what you want.

Rayon gauze is a bit more expensive than cotton gauze. However, it can be washed and reused. It is *the* gauze to use if you are soaking up blood to re-infuse into a patient. Rayon gauze is sturdier so it can be wrung out and washed out and autoclaved (sterilized) a few times, whereas the usual cotton gauze will not withstand that kind of abuse.

Bandages. Don't buy cheap adhesive bandages unless you have small children who need them for invisible boo-boos. Real Band-Aids adhere better.

Telfa non-stick pads are non-adhering gauze bandages especially useful for wounds that are lightly oozing. They come in two sizes—2x3" and 3x4". They are really nice for wounds like burns or anything where you have delicate tissues re-growing and which you do not want to disturb during dressing changes.

Petrolatum-gauze dressings are used for wounds that need to be kept moist. They are ideal for a number of reasons:

- Faster wound healing
- Less scarring
- Lower risk of infection
- Less painful dressing changes
- Less trauma to the healing wound
- Prevent air and contaminants from reaching wound
- Retain heat, moisture, and medication
- Petrolatum-gauze dressings, sold commercially as Xeroform, find application for a number of conditions:
- First- and second-degree burns
- Slightly weeping wounds
- Donor sites and skin grafts
- New circumcision wounds
- Lacerations and abrasions

DIY Petrolatum Gauze Dressings

Using a small pan and a canning jar as a double boiler, bring Vaseline to a boil in a canning jar to sterilize it. With a sterile instrument, spread the Vaseline on a sterile piece of gauze or food-grade plastic wrap. (Colored plastic wrap, such as is commonly available in grocery stores around Christmas and Easter, is thicker and easier to manage.)

Petrolatum-gauze dressings should not be used on infected wounds.

ENEMA BAGS

Enema bags should be part of each family's medical storage. Here are some of the conditions, beyond constipation, that enema bags are used to treat:

Severe hypothermia. When a person has severe hypothermia, she is close to dying. The patient needs to be warmed up through the usual methods of warming people with mild to moderate hypothermia, but additional measures should be taken. One of those is administering warm fluid through the rectum. This is most easily accomplished with an enema bag.

Dehydration. Like hypothermia, most mild to moderate cases of dehydration (that are not due to diarrhea), can be treated easily using the usual methods of drinking fluids like water or oral rehydration solution.[218] However, severe dehydration necessitates a more comprehensive approach. One way of getting fluids into the body faster is through the other end with an enema bag.

> **Oral Rehydration Solution**
>
> 2 tablespoons sugar
> 1/2 teaspoon salt, regular or lite
> 1 quart of water
>
> Dissolve the sugar and salt in the water. It may take up to two minutes to dissolve completely. Do not alter the recipe, except to add a little more water if absolutely necessary to get the patient to drink.

Medication administration. Sometimes a patient is so nauseous that he can't take medication orally. Reducing tablets to a powder or opening up a capsule and then mixing the medication with saline or tap water and then using an enema bag is one means of getting medication into a patient who cannot otherwise take it.

As enemas appear to be a popular thing to do at home now, there are all kinds of purchase options online and in stores.

GLOVES

Personal protective equipment is designed to minimize the hazards a care provider is exposed to while aiding a patient. It is not to protect the patient, though that also occurs at the same time to some extent. It is not just for use in health care situations. These same masks and gloves can also be used in cleaning up after a disaster or for filtering out airborne contaminants. While heavier gloves are good for cleaning, the ones used in medicine provide an additional layer of protection. The three most commonly used are:

Latex gloves, which were used for years, are not recommended for at least two reasons. The most important is the increasing number of people with allergies to latex. The second is that latex gloves start to deteriorate pretty quickly and become a sticky mess and tear easily within a relatively short period, especially in hot, humid areas.

Vinyl gloves also tear quite easily and become a bit porous and sticky as well.

Nitrile gloves stand the test of time—several years—even when exposed to extremes in temperature. Nitrile gloves are the only way to go.

Naturally, gloves are wanted anytime any level of care is being offered to prevent contact with bodily fluids or contaminated materials. Do not take a one-size-fits-all approach to buying gloves. Buy them by the box in sizes to fit teen and adult family members. If they are not comfortable to wear, because they are too big or too small, people won't wear them. And if you don't have a whole lot on hand, your family may become too cautious about using them up too quickly. As a result, they're less likely to wear them when they should.

MASKS

Procedure or surgical masks do absolutely nothing to protect the wearer from airborne pathogens. They filter nothing, though they are useful for preventing blood or vomit from spraying the nose and mouth. They are for protecting the patient receiving care from any bacteria or viruses the caregiver or visitors may shed. They also remind the wearer not to touch his face—something that is especially important for laypeople to remember when giving care. And importantly, a surgical mask helps hide facial expressions and other involuntary responses to unpleasant sights and smells. Finally, rightly or wrongly, people tend to assume someone wearing a mask has some level of competence.

N95 masks are the next step up. The filters in these masks trap particulates before they can enter the lungs. According to the National Institute for Occupational Safety and Health (NIOSH), the N95 mask traps **95%** of **N**on-oil particles larger than 0.3 microns. They are used for preventing laborers from inhaling dust and protecting people from air pollution in large cities.

N95 masks are not all created equal. Some are better than others. The *filter* portion of the N95 mask does a phenomenal job removing particulates from the air you breathe before it enters your lungs. Where the difference occurs among the various N95 filters is in how well they fit the face. When dirt accumulates *inside* an N95 mask, it is due to a poor conformity around the *outside* of the mask, not dirt penetrating through the filter. Most respectable N95 masks feature elastic straps to hold the mask on and a nose clip that adjusts to create the best possible seal. The best masks, like the 8511V produced by 3M, have a rim that conforms well to the contours of the face, so that there are no gaps in the seal.

What they filter:

- Bacteria
- Viruses
- Allergens
- Pollution
- Dust
- What they do not filter:
- Oil-based substances
- Gases

Other considerations for the N95 masks:

Beards reduce the efficacy of any mask.

Vented or **non-vented**? Vented masks are only a little more expensive than non-vented, so cost isn't an issue. The vent does not improve or diminish the filtering capacity of the filter. The vent itself is a one-way valve that makes wearing the mask more comfortable because it lets the breath exit without condensing inside the mask. On a patient, a non-vented mask will help confine the pathogens to the patient and reduce the risk to others. It's not actually designed to catch stuff coming out of the nose and mouth, but the air still gets filtered (as opposed to the exhaled air from a vented mask, which does not get filtered).

Reusable? While they are lightweight and can be purchased in large quantities, there aren't actually any instructions on how frequently they need to be changed, if at all. People who wear these to filter out allergens use them up to a month before replacing them. In a situation where preventing the spread of disease is the goal, the mask should probably be changed at least every eight hours.

N99 masks filter **99**% or more of particles 0.3 microns or larger that are **N**on-oil based. So they are a *little* more effective than N95 masks. The masks are denser, so your lungs have to work harder. In moderate levels of activity, like tending to a sick patient, this shouldn't be an issue. If doing a lot of physical activity, it will be noticeable. Like with the N95, odors due to gas and diesel still pass through. Amston makes an N99 mask that gets high reviews on Amazon.

- What they filter: same as N95, just at a higher efficiency
- What they do not filter: same as N95

P100 masks filter 99.9% (or almost **100%**) of particles 0.3 microns or larger that are oil-based (oil-**P**roof) or not. Most of what we want to filter out are bacteria and viruses, and the N95 and N99 masks cover that. P100 masks protect you from diesel and gas fumes. These are permanent masks, not disposable, and are rather expensive. Most have filter replacements. They are not vented and can become stuffy, especially in strenuous activities.

What they filter:

- Bacteria
- Viruses
- Allergens
- Pollution

- Dust
- Oil-based substances
- Gases

RZ masks are a step above the N95 and N99 masks, and comparable to the P100. The masks are washable and reusable. However, the replacement filters are not washable; they last about 60 hours each before needing to be replaced. These filters have two layers. The outer layer filters particles down to 0.1 micron in size, so it is more effective than the other masks listed above that only filter to 0.3 microns. The inner layer is active carbon, so it filters out the fumes, like the P100 mask, as well as organic chemicals. The RZ masks come in three sizes and a few colors. Like the others, they do not fit a small child. They run around $30 each.

What they filter:

- Bacteria
- Viruses
- Allergens
- Pollution
- Dust
- Oil-based substances
- Gases

Masks and COVID-19

> **Reusing Disposable Masks**
>
> When possible, use alternatives.
>
> Limit who has access to the patient (which is what they're doing now--relatives are not allowed to visit the patient)
>
> Extended use and reuse of masks do not degrade respiratory protection.
>
> Masks may be used past the date on the package.
>
> Masks may be reused as long as functionality is not compromised, like by a patient coughing on the mask.
>
> Mask functionality can be preserved and extended by using face shields over the masks, like plastic jugs.

If you are lacking masks, they can be made by hand from fabric you have on hand or clean t-shirts. In the wake of the COVID-19 pandemic, dozens of patterns have popped up on the internet.

Numerous questions surround the use and reuse of commercially manufactured masks.

One of the first things we all heard as the coronavirus started being detected in the US was that re-using masks was a horrible idea. That is definitely true in normal times.

The COVID-19 pandemic is not a normal situation. Even the folks at the Centers for Disease Control have finally acknowledged this. And they provide information on their website regarding the reuse of medical masks in a pandemic situation. * [219]

Researchers at Stanford University recently tested five methods for disinfecting masks for reuse. Keep in mind that there are two important factors to consider here. The functionality of the mask has to be preserved in addition to disinfecting it from pathogens.

- Spraying with alcohol was not effective, as the efficacy of the mask dropped below 95%.
- Steam and wet heat also reduced mask efficacy below 95%.

---

* Also, the info on that webpage echoes what the CDC said in with the influenza outbreak in 2009, so it's not necessarily new to this event. They recognized then that they could have problems. They just did absolutely nothing to prepare for them.

- Autoclaving with high pressure and high temperature deformed the masks.
- UV light disinfection results were inconclusive.
- Dry heat at 160°F for 30 minutes was effective. Use a dehydrator or oven set to 160°F.[220]

Another option discussed by Dr. Joseph Alton on his YouTube broadcast about re-using masks is putting used masks in a paper bag to let the virus naturally die. Simply remove the mask and drop it in a paper bag, close the bag, and date both the day you dropped it in and the day to reuse it. Because some sources say the virus can live up to nine days, they're dating their bags for ten days out. You may wish to wait longer. If you are limited on the masks, you might wish to combine with dry heat.[221]

Nothing, not even a P100 mask, is fool-proof. We see medical personnel who know better and suit up and take all precautions falling victim to this virus.

But everything we do, every precaution we take, improves our odds. Nothing improves the odds like not going out in public at all. But if you have to go out, take measures to protect yourself. What the government, CDC, and WHO have totally failed to communicate, and even sought to hide, distort, lie about, is that masks are protective FOR ALL OF US. Not just medical personnel. People do understand about wanting to preserve masks for medical personnel, but that was the responsibility of the hospitals and government. Stock rotation isn't rocket science.

Simply put, the masks are a barrier. How effective a barrier depends on the type of mask and the fit. Surgical masks don't do a whole lot to prevent pathogens from circulating, but they do some good. N95s are good, N99s are better. Then you get into gas masks, PAPR, and other really expensive stuff that's just beyond the finances of most people.

The government agencies and hospitals are telling us that medical personnel need them more. Medical personnel are definitely at greater risk. Everyone should be able to understand that--they're surrounded by sick people coughing and shedding virus particles everywhere. They have to get up close and personal and come into contact with bodily fluids. It's the nature of their work.

Data right now are showing that there is a difference in the course and outcome of the disease between those who have a small inoculum and those with a large inoculum.[222] What are these inocula?

Small inoculum sounds small, right? Like maybe you touch a handle that an asymptomatic carrier who didn't wash well touched previously. You then touch your nose or rub your eyes. You have picked up a little dose of the virus. A small inoculum of just a few virus particles. And so they go to work in your body. But there are so few of them and you are so big. If there is a really small number of virus particles, then they might even die off or be killed before they can do any harm. But even if there are just a few more, the current theory is that the body has time to adjust--the T-cells and the white cells have time to mount their defense before the virus can replicate in sufficient numbers to kill the host.

A large inoculum, on the other hand, would come from a symptomatic patient coughing or sneezing on a healthcare provider. That medical worker just got a boatload of virus particles. So many virus particles that don't need to build up their numbers because they already have a massive invading army sufficient to overwhelm the body's defenses within just a couple of hours.

So what exactly does this have to do with masks, poor masks, mistakes, gloves, and social distancing?

In reality, we will all probably pick up this virus at some point. But if we can slow the transmission, flatten the curve, as they say now, we can avoid overwhelming the hospitals. We can prevent unnecessary deaths due to a shortage of medical care and a lack of beds or equipment available. That's huge. Everything we do to slow the transmission--masks, gloves, and social distancing--also works to reduce the inoculum--the amount of virus we pick up.

Our goal is to make any inoculum we pick up is as small as possible. Masks reduce the inoculum. If you have to go out, wear a mask. If you have the option, first put on an N95 mask, and then cover it with a surgical mask. Another tidbit to keep in mind if you are reluctant to wear a mask when you go out: my husband observed that those wearing a mask were given much wider berth at the store than individuals who were not wearing masks. Social distancing increases. (While the CDC says the safe distance is 6 feet, researchers in China indicate that a better distance is 12-14 feet.)[223]

The mask(s) you wear not only reduce the number of virus particles you inhale, but they also remind you not to touch your face. Big win. Gloves reduce the number of viruses you touch, and again, remind you not to touch your face. If you are willing to ramp it up a notch, add glasses or safety goggles. When you arrive home, leave the shoes in the garage, strip in the garage or laundry room and dump everything into a laundry basket or the washer. Head straight for the shower and wash and shampoo really well.

HEMOSTATIC AGENTS

When faced with treating life-threatening bleeding, military medics have turned to hemostatic agents for years. In conjunction with direct pressure, they stop bleeding in places where tourniquets cannot be used, especially the head, neck, and abdomen and pelvic area. Celox and QuikClot have been around for years; X-Gauze is the new kid on the block. First, let's take a look at the similarities among these three products.

While initially designed for military use, all three products are available to civilians without restriction. Celox and QuikClot can be found in stores and online, but for X-Gauze, you've got to go to their website.

These clotting agents are sold as granules, z-pack gauze, and sponges. The granules are poured onto or into a wound, but if that wound is still spurting blood, the granules are going to be washed away. The clotting agent must be exactly where the blood is coming from to be of any use.

Z-pack gauze (this is just how it's packaged—it's not a brand name) is favored for most applications. The gauze is impregnated with the clotting agent and can be packed very tightly against an internal wound. The clotting agent cannot be washed away. The medic using this product does not have to balance packing the wound while simultaneously sprinkling in the clotting agent. There have not been any reports of allergic reactions to these products.

Now let's see how the three products differ in their mechanisms of action.

QuikClot uses kaolin, a natural clotting agent that accelerates the body's natural clotting abilities. When used in conjunction with direct pressure, it stops life-threatening bleeding within five minutes. It has a five-year shelf-life from the date of manufacture. QuikClot and the kaolin and gauze must be completely removed from the body before the wound is closed.

Celox uses chitosan, a clotting agent derived from shrimp. Throughout extensive clinical trials and field use, there have been no reports of any allergic reactions, even among individuals allergic to shellfish or iodine. Like QuikClot, Celox stops severe bleeding within five minutes when used together with direct pressure. Unlike the kaolin in QuikClot, the chitosan in Celox can be broken down by the body. While it should be thoroughly washed away before the wound is closed, chitosan is less likely to cause a problem if small amounts are not removed. Celox granules have a four-year shelf-life. Like QuikClot, Celox gauze has a five-year shelf-life from the date of manufacture.

Both of these products work to clot blood even in patients taking blood thinners, as well as in cases where hypothermia is an issue.

X-Gauze, in contrast, does not use a hemostatic clotting agent. Instead, it is gauze impregnated with miniature sponges that expand to ten times their size on contact with fluids to stop bleeding by direct pressure. It is ideal in that it conforms to the wound perfectly and exerts pressure everywhere. It is not available on Amazon; you have to go to their website. Because it is new, it does not have extensive field testing, but clinical trials have shown that it is a very promising technology. Unfortunately, at $50 each, they're a little expensive right now.

It must be emphasized that none of these clotting agents substitute for direct pressure. Direct pressure will stop the vast majority of bleeding within 30 minutes. If direct pressure fails to stop bleeding after 30 minutes (without peeking every 5 minutes to check, which may interrupt any clotting that started), then a clotting agent and/or tourniquet may be required.

SKIN PREPS AND WASHES

Because we have been taught that only physicians and nurses should be providing care for anything more serious than simple scrapes and common colds, many don't have a clear understanding of various supplies and their uses. Here are the different solutions used for cleaning skin and wounds.

Benzalkonium Chloride (BZK, BAK, BAC)

BZK is active against bacteria, some viruses, fungi, and, unlike all the other solutions, protozoa. It is the preferred solution when dealing with animal bites, as it has been shown effective against rabies. (In an emergency, if you are dealing with an animal bite, drop a BZK wipe into a bottle of water to make a disinfecting solution. Irrigate with this for ten minutes, and then irrigate with plain clean water.) It is more effective than alcohol, doesn't dry out the skin like alcohol, and isn't messy like Betadine. It's one of the active ingredients of Bactine.

Like all the other disinfecting solutions above, it is used for cleaning around a wound, never in, except for the previously mentioned animal bites. It is ideal for prepping before inserting a catheter and the safest for use around the eyes, but should not be allowed to get into the eyes. It is available in wipes and is the skin prep of choice for wounds received in water because it will kill protozoa. Larger groups may include a box of BZK wipes in their supplies. In our family, we all carry two BZK wipes in our boo-boo kits, more in the larger kits.

Betadine

Betadine lasts forever. While companies are required by law to label their products with "best by" or "use by" dates, Betadine doesn't go bad. It can be twenty years old and still good to use in so many ways.

Wound cleaning. There's a bit of debate about whether Betadine should be used for cleaning in a wound. Physicians seem to split about 50-50 on the issue, so let's consider that for a moment. For one, it's a 50-50 split. Does one risk killing healthy tissue to prevent possible infection? On the other hand, why not just use straight water, which won't destroy tissue? Now consider that in a post-collapse society, Betadine may become a very limited resource. Why use up a valuable resource when plain water will do the job?

Disinfecting solution. For cleaning *around* a wound or in preparing for surgery, or washing hands prior to procedures, and in cleaning umbilical cords, Betadine is a great choice. Fortunately for us, it is available over the counter. Some evidence suggests that alcohol and Hibiclens are better than Betadine for pre-operative skin cleaning.

Sugardyne. See Sugardyne in chapter 10.

Disinfecting medical instruments. When diluted to 2.5% (one part of the 10% solution to three parts water), Betadine can be used to disinfect medical instruments. Instruments should soak for 15 minutes.

Water purification. In an emergency, an iodine wipe can be dropped into a one-liter bottle of water to purify it for drinking. This generally takes about 15 minutes, but cooler or cloudy water should stand 30 minutes. Betadine will not kill protozoa. If you have a vitamin C tablet, add it after 15-30 minutes to reduce the iodine taste. This method of treatment is not recommended for long term use (say, more than a few months) due to the risk for developing goiter.

Radiation exposure. One option that may work if you don't have potassium iodide tablets, and there is the threat of radioactive iodine exposure, is to apply Betadine in place of taking the tablets. See chapter 19 for specific instructions.

Health. The body needs iodine to function properly. That's why we have and why we store iodized salt. Unfortunately, iodized salt doesn't stay iodized and *becomes plain salt over time. To test a person for iodine deficiency, paint a* 3x3" square of iodine on the inner arm, inner thigh, or abdomen. Let it dry completely and then dress as usual. Check the square in exactly 24 hours. Is the patch the same color, lighter, or gone? If it is lighter or gone, then the body is deficient in iodine, and Betadine can be painted regularly on the body to remedy that deficiency. Unfortunately, this test does not work well on those with darker skin.

Cautions. Do not drink Betadine. Do not use Betadine on burns or in puncture wounds. Adverse reactions may occur in those individuals taking diuretics and/or lithium. Do not use iodine for water purification for those with any thyroid condition or for pregnant women.

Contraindications: Do not use Betadine in individuals allergic to iodine.

Clean water

Clean water (just tap water, or even water from a clear stream) is actually one of the best things for irrigating a wound and removing debris. However, irrigating does not mean pouring water over or swishing in a basin. Decent water pressure, which is achieved using a needle-less syringe, a water bladder, or a perineal bottle (like those the hospital sends home with new mothers), is best for irrigating a wound.

Dakin's solution

This simple solution of baking soda and bleach was developed during WWI as a wound antiseptic. It is used to kill germs and prevent the growth of microbes in wounds. It is an excellent solution for irrigating wounds without destroying healthy tissue. It is very inexpensive and easy to make, and thus ideally suited for the difficult circumstances a collapsed society will present.

The full-strength solution is used only on stainless steel medical instruments. Dakin's solution will corrode nickel, chromium steel, iron,

Dakin's Solution

You will need:
Sterile equipment—pan and lid, glass jar(s) and tight-fitting lid(s), measuring cups and spoons

32 oz clean water
1/2 teaspoon baking soda
Regular, unscented, not concentrated or ultra, just regular bleach in one of the following concentrations:

full-strength—3 ounces (95 ml) bleach—for disinfecting instruments
1/2 strength—3 tablespoons plus 1 teaspoon (48 ml) bleach—for debridement of necrotized wounds
1/4 strength—1 tablespoon plus 2 teaspoons (24 ml) bleach—for irrigating wounds
1/8 strength—2 1/2 teaspoons (12 ml) bleach—for mouthwash

Boil water for 15 minutes with the lid on the pan. Remove from heat. Add the baking soda to the boiled water. Measure bleach according to desired strength and add to water. Cover tightly in a glass jar and wrap the jar in aluminum foil to shield it from light. (Do not store Dakin's solution in metal containers.) Once opened for use, it is good only for 48 hours. Discard unused portion. Unopened and protected from light, the solution can be stored for one month at room temperature.

Label the jar with the date and time you made the solution, as well as the date to discard it.

and other metals. Because of its corrosive nature, tools should not be in the bath solution for longer than 30 minutes.

Use only a 1/4 strength solution for acute wound irrigation. Always irrigate very generously with plain water following irrigation with Dakin's solution. If the solution is used for mouth wash, do not swallow it. Do not use in individuals allergic to any of the ingredients.

Hibiclens

This antiseptic is used to disinfect surgical tools and the skin before surgery. More effective than Betadine, it is, however, not effective against poliovirus or adenovirus. It has recently started being used in poor countries for cleaning umbilical cords in newborns and has been shown to reduce the neonatal death rate by 12%. Do not allow Hibiclens to get into the ears as it can damage hearing.

Hydrogen peroxide

Hydrogen peroxide is most commonly available in a 3% solution and is always sold in a brown bottle because it is degraded by light. Even with being in a brown bottle, it still only has a six-month shelf life once it's opened. Hydrogen peroxide can be used to disinfect surgical tools and is effective against viruses, bacteria, and fungi. It is environmentally safe as it degrades to form oxygen and water. It has historically been used for disinfecting wounds; it's been a staple of home first aid cabinets for years and is still used in developing countries because it is cheap and readily available. As it kills newly formed tissue and induces scarring, it should never be used *in* a wound, only *around* a wound for cleaning.

Rubbing alcohol

With a multitude of uses, rubbing alcohol is commonly available in 50%, 70%, and 90-91% solutions. There is also 99% isopropyl alcohol, which is generally for industrial and technical uses, and which doesn't really pertain to us. (Despite extensive research, I haven't quite figured out the purpose of the 50%

rubbing alcohol, which has been stocked in stores the past few years. It's just more diluted than 70%. Most people can add water at home, if necessary.) Rubbing alcohol and isopropyl alcohol are different substances; the former is a mixture of compounds, while the latter is a single compound. Rubbing alcohol is what we use for cleaning the skin. Alcohol does not inactivate some viruses (hydrophilic viruses like polio and Coxsackie).

Rubbing alcohol should never be used *in* a wound, only *around* a wound for cleaning. Using alcohol in a wound kills healthy cells and can delay or prevent healing.

There is a disturbing amount of misinformation about the use of rubbing alcohol, and it's all the more alarming because some of that misinformation can have life-threatening consequences.

The first bit of misinformation is that 70% and 91% can be used interchangeably. While that is fine for fire-starting purposes, it is most definitely not the case with medicine. A 70% rubbing alcohol solution is more effective at disinfecting than a 91% solution. This is because water is needed to carry the alcohol *into* the bacteria to kill the bacteria. A 91% solution of alcohol evaporates faster and has less water to take the alcohol into the bacteria and kill them. [224]

The second, potentially deadly, bit of misinformation perpetuated online is that rubbing alcohol is useful in reducing a fever. Well, actually, it does work pretty well in lowering body temperature. However, one of the basics tenets of medicine is to first, "Do no harm." Using rubbing alcohol to reduce a fever can most definitely be harmful. Remember, alcohol can poison the body by drinking, by absorption through the skin, or by inhaling the vapors. When alcohol is rubbed on the

Treat an Ear Infection with Rubbing Alcohol

Combine 1/4 teaspoon rubbing alcohol and 1/4 teaspoon vinegar or hydrogen peroxide.

With the afflicted individual lying on his side, put 3-4 drops of the mixture in the affected ear.

Have the patient remain in this position for 5 minutes, and then tilt the head and drain out the solution.

Next, place a few drops of plain warm olive oil in the ear. This does not need to be drained.

body to reduce a fever, that alcohol is absorbed into the body at a toxic level. The vapors are also inhaled by the patient. Using rubbing alcohol to lower a temperature was common practice through much of the last century. Unfortunately, the practice persists with some physicians, even with increasing numbers of cases of alcohol poisoning causing coma and death, especially in infants and small children. Having addressed those issues of poor information, let's move on to other ways rubbing alcohol is used.

Making a liniment. As the name suggests, rubbing alcohol is for rubbing, though it is rarely used for this purpose today. It is perfectly safe to apply small amounts of a 70% solution of rubbing alcohol to sore muscles and joints. It can be used alone, or rubbing alcohol can be used to tincture various medicinal herbs to make a liniment for greater relief of aches and pains. In no case should rubbing alcohol be used as a liniment for infants and children. The risk of toxic overload is too high.

Disinfecting instruments. A 70% solution of rubbing alcohol can be used to disinfect instruments. Instruments must soak for at least 12 hours. Note that rubbing alcohol does not kill all bacteria and viruses, so sterilization is not achieved. If, however, you cannot wait 12 hours or you need sterilized instruments quickly, the alcohol containing the instruments may be ignited to produce rapid sterilization. But keep in mind that the intense heat may damage delicate instruments.

Making a reusable ice pack. Combine three parts water to one part rubbing alcohol in a zippered bag or vacuum seal bag and seal. Freeze for three hours. These ice packs are quite flexible and can be shaped around the afflicted body part to reduce pain and swelling. Do not place these ice packs directly next to the skin. Make sure there is a cloth of some sort to protect the skin from frostbite.

Making hand sanitizer. Though recent research is showing that hand sanitizer is far less effective than previously believed, there are some situations where regular handwashing is difficult. Having some hand sanitizer available is a good idea. However, hand sanitizer is one of those few items that do actually go bad and aren't of much efficacy past their use-by date. And that is because the alcohol evaporates, and it's the alcohol that kills the germs. Your best bet here is to store some aloe vera gel so that you can make your own hand sanitizer as needed. It's really easy.

> **DIY Hand Sanitizer**
>
> 2 tablespoons 91% rubbing alcohol
> 1 tablespoon aloe vera gel or glycerol
>
> Put the alcohol and aloe vera or glycerol in a small squeeze bottle and shake. If you need larger quantities, just keep the same 2:1 ratio. Just remember to keep the container sealed and then replenish it often. Once the alcohol evaporates, the hand sanitizer isn't sanitizing anything.

Starting a fire. Alcohol pads make a great little fire starter.

Cooking. A 91% solution of rubbing alcohol works quite well as a cooking fuel, and instructions abound online for making little stoves that utilize rubbing alcohol as their fuel. Rubbing alcohol is nice in that it can be used indoors without concern for noxious fumes. However, it burns at a lower temperature than other fuels, so it takes longer to cook food.

Sterile saline

Sterile saline is used for irrigating debris out of the eyes and irrigating and washing wounds around the eyes. Grocery stores and pharmacies carry this in the same area as contact lens supplies. However, you can also get small vials of 0.9% sterile saline in three sizes—5 ml, 10 ml, and 15 ml. To help you visualize the amount, 15 ml is a tablespoon. While used primarily by contact lens wearers, these make a great addition to your medical kits. The tiny bottles fit nicely even in small boo-boo kits and IFAKs. While the cap is easily removed, it cannot be replaced, and the vial does not stand up on its own.

Not only are these vials perfect for irrigating foreign matter out of eyes, they are also ideally suited for creating gentle pressure to flush debris out of wounds.

These two reasons alone are sufficient for warranting the purchase of these little vials of sterile saline. But this last point totally seals the deal. They are perfect for making your own (under the direction of a physician) injectable solutions of lidocaine and other medications. They aren't necessarily what you'd want to rely on in a years-long collapse, because the vials don't have a long shelf life. If life gets really hairy before you get a sterile lab established, having these bottles ready to go will save some stress. Also, mixing injectables in these little vials minimizes chances for contamination from other containers, a significant advantage.

It is important to note that these little vials of sterile saline are "not for injection." Sterile saline that is for injection must be tested to show that it is "pyrogen-free," meaning that there are no bacteria in there that could cause an infection. These little vials have not been tested, so they are "not for injection." Using them to produce an injectable solution carries certain risks with it. In a true crisis, you make do with what you have.

If finances allow, sterile water for injection can be ordered through overseas pharmacies like All Day Chemist. Each vial runs about $10.

Sterile saline, as a liquid, will eventually deteriorate. However, these vials should last some time beyond the use-by date that is stamped on the box. As long as there are no particulates and the solution is not cloudy, it should be safe to use.

SUTURES

The plethora of options in sutures makes it difficult for the regular Joe or Jane to figure out what is really wanted for the home medical supply. A suture is absolutely needed if the wound being closed is over a joint or under the skin. It is best if you do not improvise here. In other areas of the body, depending on the location and the time the wound has been open, there are other options, to be covered later.

Sutures are classed by needle type, needle shape, suture material, and size. **Needle type**. A *reverse cutting* needle is usually preferred as it reduces the potential for tearing skin tissue. *Conventional cutting* is what was first invented, but it was observed that it was more likely to weaken and tear the skin. *Tapered* needles are round, like sewing needles, and cause more tissue damage, and increase the pain and scarring.

Needle shape. The most commonly used shapes are 1/2 and 3/8 circle, with the latter being the more common of the two. Other shapes are for specialties that aren't really of concern in a post-apocalyptic world.

Needle size. The image on the suture package indicates the exact shape and size of the needle. The more zeros, the smaller the diameter of the needle and suture material. The size indicates the diameter. 3-0 = 000, 6-0 = 000000, so a 3-0 is larger than a 6-0. The strength of the suture should never be greater than the strength of the tissue. This is because if something is going to give, it should be the suture, not the tissue. Otherwise, you are causing more trauma to the tissue. Example: Don't use a 1-0 suture, a large diameter suture, on a young child or elderly person's skin. In these situations, use 4-0 to 6-0, depending on the location. Fascia, the sheath covering muscles (like on a cut of beef—the very thin, cream-colored sheath covering the meat), is stronger than the muscle it covers and will tolerate a 2-0 to 3-0 suture. Muscle itself will usually tear before 4-0 breaks, but because fascia is usually sutured as well, the 2-0 to 3-0 can be used.

Suture material: The suture material is classed in several different ways, with factors to consider based on the individual patient and location where the suture is to be placed, as well as the supplies you actually have available. You aren't a hospital pharmacy; unless you are really wealthy, you can't possibly stock every possible option. The choices to make with each suture include:

- Absorbable or non-absorbable

    - Absorbable sutures are usually used inside the body, but they are also ideal in someone where the sutures may not be able to be removed due to a chaotic situation or a young child who will remember the trauma of having stitches placed and may not be so cooperative having them removed. Absorbable sutures are broken down and removed by the body.
    - Non-absorbable sutures are usually used outside for skin closure, as well as in patients with a history of reaction to absorbable sutures.
- Monofilament (single ply) or braided (three plies)
    - Monofilament sutures (like fishing line) are less likely to harbor organisms and do not wick any fluid (and possibly bacteria) into the wound. They are less irritating to the skin than many others. Monofilament sutures tie down easily. However, the knots slip more readily and may become weakened if compromised (crushed, crimped, or nicked).
    - Braided sutures are more likely to harbor organisms. They are also stronger and more flexible, thus being easier to work with for some individuals.
- Coated or non-coated. Coated, which usually goes with braided, makes it easier to pull the suture through the tissue. The knots also hold better.
- Material. There is a considerable variety in the choices of materials for sutures.
    - Nylon (Ethilon) is the most common non-absorbable. It is monofilament and less expensive.
    - Polyester (Ethibond) is easier to use than nylon because it is braided and coated and thus holds knots better than nylon.
    - Polypropylene (Prolene) is another non-absorbable monofilament that is easier to use than nylon and less likely to cause a tissue reaction than nylon.

- Polyglactin (Vicryl) is an absorbable, braided suture suitable for general use.
- Polydiaxone is a standard absorbable monofilament suture that retains its strength better and longer than Vicryl.
- Chromic gut is also absorbable but is more likely to cause inflammation than other absorbables.
- Silk is probably the easiest to work with, but because it is braided and not coated, it has a higher chance of harboring organisms. It acts as a very slowly absorbing suture, so it can be used internally and is preferred for ligating blood vessels. Silk is tough, and even silk sewing thread will tolerate autoclaving or other sterilization methods.

There is no one-size-fits-all. Physicians all have their favorite materials to work with, just like the rest of us. As far as what's most commonly used? Needle sizes 2-0, 3-0, and 4-0. Non-absorbable. (Think about it—you're more likely to need stitches for a flesh wound than internal surgery.) Prolene, Vicryl, and Ethilon seem to be the most popular overall. Silk and chromic gut have been around forever, so they've stood the test of time. Get a variety if you can.

Other Wound Closure Options

Here at the Bring Your Own Bandages Clinic, we want you to know that when it comes to wound closure, you have options—options that will fit your budget and desired level of pain and scarring. (All of these options assume that only the skin is involved and that there is no damage to underlying muscles, tendons, bones, etc.)

Do nothing. Yes, this is an option. You do not have to close a long cut, even if you have a big chunk of skin missing. Just keep it clean. Of course, it will take a whole lot longer to heal, and you will have a much bigger scar than if you had closed it. $

Skin glues. You can only get Derma-Bond through a physician. Vet-Bond, the veterinary equivalent of Derma-Bond, is still available without restriction. It is chemically similar to superglue, but much less likely to cause a chemical burn, which is hardly desirable when you're wanting to fix someone. It is ideal for closing smaller wounds on children and facial wounds when minimizing scarring is really a priority. Vet-Bond does not go in the wound; it goes above it. The skin is held together and then the glue is spread on top while the skin continues to be pushed together until the glue dries. $$$

Steri-Strips. These are adhesive strips of tape usually 3-4" long and 1/10-1/2" wide. They are especially valuable for older folks with paper-thin skin and for children on body parts that don't see a lot of action. Do not buy knock-offs, if possible. The adhesive usually is not as strong, and they often have square corners that catch on everything as opposed to the rounded corners of Steri-Strips. If possible, paint on lines of tincture of benzoin where the strips will go to help them adhere better. $$

Staples are best suited to use on the abdomen, back, and scalp. They do not go over joints (too much movement) or on the face (too much scarring). They are used in the field because they are very quick, which is nice if you don't have anesthetic, and because it requires almost no skill to be able to use them. $$$

Duct tape. This can be cut into strips and used just like the Steri-Strips above. However, some people have a reaction to the duct tape adhesive.

Zipstitch. Conventional medicine's answer to the DIY solution above: https://zipstitch.us. It has the medical grade tape and uses tiny zip-ties to close the wound instead of a needle and thread. $$$

Needle and thread. Yes, this is another option. If you're going to go this route, at least get some spools of silk and nylon or fishing line. The risk of infection is going to be higher with this option, and so is the pain. For a more pleasant suturing experience, choose quilting needles instead of yarn needles. $

Hair. If the wound is on the scalp (or really hairy arms or chest), braid or tie hair over the wound to close it up. $

Agave cactus needles and the attached fiber. $

Combat army ants. Find the ants, pick one up and have it bite you with the jaws straddling your wound, then detach the head from its body.

Herbs. Lantana, plantain, and usnea have shown great ability to help speed wound closing. $

As you can see, we the Bring Your Own Bandages Clinic have suggested a number of options that can fit any budget and skill level. It's up to a physician to decide what will work best for your situation.

Which option he chooses for closing a wound depends on a number of factors. What materials are actually available? What is the age and mental status of the patient? Young children can be difficult to work on. Is a screaming toddler going to accept being sutured? After the child has had such a traumatic experience, is it really going to work to have him come back to have sutures removed? Is the wound over a joint? Then a regular suture or needle and thread might be your only effective options. Do you have anesthetic available? How skilled is the physician? How much time is there? Glue is quick, staples are faster. Regardless, use the least invasive method possible.

TAPES

Transpore medical tape is the best. This non-latex all-purpose tape adheres very well, it's clear, and it tears so easily in both directions. If ½" wide is more than you need, it can easily be split into strips 1/8" wide if desired. It's waterproof, yet it also breathes to let sweat out and air in. It is the strongest for adhering to skin. It can be used to prevent chafing and as a butterfly bandage to close minor cuts. Transpore does leave a sticky residue and can irritate sensitive skin. Don't use this for daily bandage changes or securing a SAM splint unless there is no alternative. It's a little rough for frequent bandage changes and will rip the foam off a splint.

Nexcare waterproof tape adheres extremely well to the skin. It's very flexible, making it the tape of choice for areas like under armpits and between fingers and toes. It doesn't stick well to hair, which is good for sensitive skin or daily bandage changes, but not so good if it needs to stick to hairy skin. It is very easy to tear across, but not into lengthwise strips, and it leaves no sticky residue behind.

Paper tape is gentle on the skin. It is not as sticky as the previous two and is inexpensive, so it's what you want for daily dressing changes and sensitive skin. It will not work for situations involving heavy exercise, irregular areas of the body, or blisters or chafing.

Cloth tape, 2-3" wide, has a lot of applications, but the most critical, especially for our purposes, is for taping sprained ankles. A badly sprained ankle can be taped so well and so securely that the patient will be able to walk if necessary. Of course, it is far, far better to rest that ankle and let others do the work, but in some situations, that may not be an option. Ace bandages absolutely will not substitute for good cloth tape and a good taping job.

Duct tape is obviously not designed for medical applications, but it's a favorite for emergency medical kits. Wider rolls are used in splinting limbs and wrapping bandages in place when other tapes just won't work. You can also get mini rolls of duct tape (Duck Tape brand "Ducklings") for smaller applications.

WRAPS

Coban is used for wrapping fingers and limbs and holding bandages in place. Because it is self-adherent, no pins are needed. It is made of non-woven polyester so that it is elastic and conforms well to the body and lets the skin breathe.

Vet Wrap is designed for animals, but there's no good reason not to use it for people, especially when it's so much cheaper than Coban.

9. REUSABLE SUPPLIES

The vast majority of these reusable supplies have the disposable counterparts that are so highly favored in our society. With disposables, there is no concern about whether the item has been properly sterilized, and there's no bother with having to wash, disinfect, and sterilize. With disposables, people always assume that the supply will meet demand.

Until it can't. That's why having at least a small number of reusable supplies is a good idea.

Ace bandages provide support for joints, reduce swelling, and comfortably hold dressings in place.

Eyed suture needles are a good idea, but unfortunately, they are really hard to find. They also aren't a first choice because with the suture material doubled over at the eye, there is more trauma to tissue when the eye passes through. If it's necessary to improvise, a regular sewing needle will do the job. Make sure to have a good supply.

Glass syringes are ideal because they can be sterilized several times. The only risk is to the rubber plunger. Try to get a few syringes because the plunger won't last forever.

Hypodermic needles are also available in reusable options. In fact, many diabetics will reuse their disposable syringes a few times as well, but only on themselves. The reusable hypodermic needles can be easily sterilized. It would also be a good idea to have a means of sharpening the tip of the needle. Try to get a variety of sizes to satisfy different purposes.

Rayon gauze is used just like cotton gauze, but it has a couple of distinct advantages. Rayon gauze can actually be washed and sterilized in an autoclave numerous times before it falls apart. Cotton gauze won't tolerate that kind of abuse. In addition, if a patient is bleeding heavily, rayon gauze can be used to soak up the blood and be wrung out, and then the blood can be re-infused into the patient. Apparently, cotton won't work so well for this purpose. (Also, the blood is being soaked up from within the body, not off the floor.)

Sterile gloves are individually packaged, unlike the exam gloves we store in abundance, and will run about a dollar a pair on a good day. Both the doctor and the assistants need them.

Sterile surgical gowns will be needed because doctors are not loading up on sterile gowns to attend to people outside their own families. Families will need to provide their own. There are a few options to choose from. Basically, you'll need to decide whether you want to get disposable or reusable. You may want to get a few, even if they are reusable. The doctor usually doesn't operate alone. His assistant should have a sterile gown as well.

Sterile towels, whether disposable or reusable, cost about the same initially, but the reusable ones are reusable. The disposable sterile towels will not stand up to repeated autoclaving. Sterile towels will be used much more often than sterile gowns and gloves. Anytime there is any stitching to be done, it's important to cover the surrounding area with sterile towels or drapes to prevent the suture material from coming into contact with contaminants.

SAM SPLINTS

SAM splints are the go-to for dealing with any kind of fracture or joint injury. They are malleable and conform easily to splint any bone or joint. They're washable and reusable. While they are sold in smaller sizes, you don't need to waste your money on the small ones because the 36-inch size can be cut down with trauma shears or even regular scissors to splint the shortest of bones. It can also be fashioned to make a cervical collar for neck injuries. No need to buy a separate C-collar for your medical kit that takes up enormous space and serves no other function. The 36-inch size does it all, except for splinting leg bones in adults. In that case, two 36-inch splints are required, one for each side.

With the instructions for basic configurations printed right on the foam, SAM splints are super easy to use. The foam makes them comfortable as well. Once molded and placed on the body, SAM splints are held in place with strips of cloth, like from a triangle bandage or T-shirt, plastic wrap, duct tape, or medical tape. However, keep in mind that adhesives may remove the foam from the splint.

SAM splints usually come in a rolled-up coil; however, if the splint is unrolled and folded flat, it may fit better in the medical kit.

There are lots of videos that show how to use a SAM splint on various injuries. They're a good idea to watch and become familiar with how to use the splint, but honestly, it's pretty intuitive. The splint must to conform to the body and immobilize the joint or fracture to prevent further injury and pain. When sizing and molding the splint, use your own same body part or the patient's uninjured counterpart to fashion and size the splint, and then apply it to the afflicted bone or joint. This will avoid causing unnecessary pain and perhaps further injury to the patient.

TOURNIQUETS

Tourniquets are still used by physicians today. All the time, like in the operating room. Placing a tourniquet does not mean the patient is going to lose the limb. Even so, it is better to lose a leg than a life.

Having and using a tourniquet can save a life. The first thing to keep in mind is that a tourniquet is only used when all else fails—when up to half an hour of pressure has failed to stop bleeding or when the amount of blood being lost has the potential to be life-threatening. Tourniquets are only used on limbs, never on the abdomen or the neck.

When a tourniquet is placed, the exact time must be noted, and it should be noted in paper notes that the care provider is maintaining. The time must also definitely be indicated on the patient's body with a Sharpie marker. That information will govern the future attending physician's choices in how to handle tourniquet removal.

The two most popular tourniquets for field use are the SOFTT (**S**pecial **O**perations **F**orces **T**actical **T**ourniquet; SOF-T as it's generally pronounced) and the SWAT-T (**S**tretch, **W**rap **A**nd **T**uck **T**ourniquet). The SOF-T is very similar to the CAT (**C**ombat **A**pplication **T**ourniquet), and both are used about the same. However, the SOF-T is made from higher quality materials. If you choose the SOF-T, make absolutely sure it is coming from an American company and made in America. Do not get one that's made in China. The Chinese ones have a reputation for failing in use.

The SOF-T and CAT are used by combat soldiers because they can be applied with one hand, even by the non-dominant hand, and done so very quickly. When blood is spurting out, every second counts. A person can die much more rapidly from the loss of blood than from the loss of oxygen. Every person who carries a weapon should also carry a SOF-T or CAT. You need to practice with it a little bit before using it, but only a little bit. It's not at all difficult.

Like many things in life, the SOF-T and CAT have their pros and cons. They were initially designed for military use, and combat personnel generally have better-developed muscles. They work very well for those people, but if you're dealing with someone with thin arms, like the elderly or young children, they may not work so well, or at all. Likewise, a certain amount of hand strength is required to use the SOF-T and CAT.

For the very young and/or frail, as well as those lacking much hand strength, the SWAT-T tourniquet is an excellent alternative. It basically looks like one of those stretchy rubber exercise bands and comes in orange or black. I prefer orange; the bright color is more visible and helps emergency responders notice it quickly. I think it looks less threatening to children. With the instructions printed right on the tourniquet, it's pretty much idiot-proof. By just reading the instructions on the tourniquet and without any training at all, you can be sure you are getting the right amount of tension for the tourniquet to work. The SWAT-T can also be used to make a sling or as a pressure wrap. In a mass casualty situation, it could even be cut in half to use on two children.

TRIANGLE BANDAGES

These have so many applications. There should probably be at least six or eight in the family medical kit, the one that goes on outings, and there should be more at home.

Now that you have your triangle bandages, what are they used for? Triangle bandages are so versatile that Google will yield a hundred hits, at least, starting at "Five Uses for Triangle Bandages." Here are the most important:

Orthopedic injuries.

- Hold splints in place for fractures to arms and legs
- Stabilize hip injuries and pelvic fractures
- Stabilize a fractured jaw
- Arm sling
- Stabilize a broken arm or wrist
- Stabilize a dislocated shoulder
- Stabilize a sprained ankle

DIY Triangle Bandage

Begin with a freshly laundered (preferably in hot water) old sheet. (You can even use a new sheet if that makes you feel better, but be aware that wives and mothers tend to frown on this sort of thing.)

Cut a 40" square of sheet. Cut the square of fabric in half diagonally to yield two triangle bandages.

Fold them into a small package size, perhaps to fit a snack-size Ziploc bag.

If you iron the bandage at each fold, you'll be able to get it a little more compact, and it helps disinfect the bandage.

Some people assert that the bandage must be boiled to sterilize it. Boiling, as mentioned earlier, does not sterilize, it disinfects. "They" say to put them in sterile bags. The average Ziploc bag is not sterile, it's clean. Clean is good. For what it's worth, none of the commercially available triangle bandages are sterile. They're just clean.

Bleeding

- Hold dressings and gauze in place
- Create a pressure dressing

- Use to apply direct pressure to stop bleeding
- If all else fails, after 30 minutes of constant direct pressure, and if you don't have a real tourniquet, it can be used as a tourniquet. You'll also need a windlass to tighten the tourniquet sufficiently.

Eye injuries

- If one eye is injured, both are usually bandaged, because the eyes track together, (i.e., if one eye moves, the other follows to track the object, even if that eye is bandaged)

Environmental issues

- Fashion an emergency hat for hypothermic patients or to prevent sunburn in balding patients
- Combine with a hand warmer to make an emergency mitten
- Make a cold compress for reducing fever
- Wear as a mask to filter out dust or other pollutants
- A bandana or two *may* serve much the same purpose for some of these uses. However, keep in mind that bandanas are substantially smaller and won't work for everything.

10. IMPROVISATIONAL SUPPLIES

Improvisational supplies are those items that have a different original purpose in life but happen to work very nicely in treating medical conditions. Some of the uses stand to reason; others are really surprising. Along with acquiring all the other medical supplies, be sure to have these on hand as well.

ACTIVATED CHARCOAL

Activated charcoal, also known as activated carbon, is not barbecue charcoal. They are related, like alcohol for drinking and rubbing alcohol are related but are not interchangeable.

Poisoning. Aside from its most common usage in water filters, activated charcoal is used in emergency rooms the world over for treating some kinds of poisoning and drug overdoses. It has application for both internal and external use.

Internally, physicians use activated charcoal to cleanse toxins such as bacteria and most organic poisons from the gastrointestinal tract. It does not work against petroleum, alcohol, acid, lye, or corrosive poisons. Research shows that it will bind enterohemorrhagic *Escherichia coli* O157:H7 while not affecting the beneficial *E. coli* normally found in the body. (And researchers still don't know why that is.)[225]

Overdoses. Doctors specifically use it in emergency rooms to treat overdoses of aspirin, Tylenol, opium, and morphine, among other substances. Activated charcoal is used in doses of 1 gram per kilogram of body weight, so 50-100 grams for adults, and 10-25 grams for children. It must be administered within one to two hours of the time the toxin was ingested to be effective. Plenty of water must be consumed at the same time. To use it internally, mix the powder with clean water and drink it, or use capsules (you're going to need a lot). Activated charcoal may cause constipation and definitely will turn the stool black. It does not enter the bloodstream; therefore, it is of no efficacy in dealing with toxins ingested more than two to three hours before treatment is sought. It cannot be used internally to treat snakebites.[226]

Wound cleaning. Externally, activated charcoal is used to clean out wounds by binding dead tissue, bacteria, and toxins. For more superficial wounds, mix activated charcoal with clean water into a paste and apply to the affected area. For deeper, penetrating wounds, like with a snakebite, mix activated charcoal with more water into a thick juice/thin smoothie consistency and soak the affected area in this. *The activated charcoal has to get into direct contact with the tissue and toxin to be effective*. Leave the plaster on, or let the affected area soak for one to two hours, then wash off the skin and check the wound (it's going to be black, so this may be a little difficult). Repeat the procedure to draw out more toxin. After about four hours, clean it off, and start working with herbs to promote further healing. Charcoal only cleans; it does not help tissue grow and heal.

Contact dermatitis, insect bites, stings. Mix 1/4 teaspoon or one capsule activated charcoal with 1/2 tablespoon water, apply to affected area, and bandage. Repeat every 30 minutes.

Poisonous spider bites. Mix 1/2 teaspoon or one capsule activated charcoal with 1/2 tablespoon water, and apply to a wider area surrounding the bite. Cover with a bandage to prevent staining, and change every two hours. Rinse well between bandage changes.[227]

Gas and bloating. To alleviate gas and bloating associated with foods that normally cause flatulence: take an activated charcoal capsule one hour prior to a meal with one to two full glasses of water.

BAKING SODA

Hopefully, you've already stored baking soda in your food, about 1.5 pounds per person per year. To cover medical and medicinal needs as well, you'll probably want to double that amount. Here are some of the ways baking soda may be used in a grid-down scenario.

Oral hygiene. We've all seen toothpaste tubes proudly proclaiming that they've got baking soda. While most people associate baking soda with whiter teeth (which is true), baking soda also kills bacteria. *Streptococcus mutans*, the bacteria that thrive in the presence of sugar, are totally wiped out by baking soda. One can brush with straight baking soda or make a toothpaste with baking soda and coconut oil (one tablespoon of baking soda mixed with one tablespoon of coconut oil), adding five to ten drops of peppermint essential oil, if desired. To treat canker sores, apply a baking soda paste to the sores, or stir 1 teaspoon of baking soda into ½ cup of water and swish it around in the mouth. The baking soda may cause a burning sensation on the canker sore.

Contact dermatitis, sunburns, splinters. Applying a paste of baking soda and water (about a 3:1 ratio) to calm the itchiness of bug bites and stings has been a home remedy for years. Baking soda is added to bathwater to relieve itchy skin due to poison oak, ivy, or sumac, and other irritants as well as sunburns. Finally, baking soda paste can also be used to help draw out a splinter. Apply the paste, wrap it with gauze or a bandage, and change twice a day. The splinter should come out within a day or two.

Exercise. Taking a teaspoon of baking soda in water before engaging in high-intensity exercise has been shown to reduce muscle pain and fatigue from over-exertion.

Heartburn. This is not for long-term use, but will provide relief while waiting for long-term options to start working. Stir 1 ½ teaspoons into a cup of lukewarm water. Sip this slowly; don't chug it all at once. Use twice per day.

Kidneys. Stir 1/2 teaspoon of baking soda into a glass of lukewarm water. Studies have shown that doing this twice per day can:

- Slow the progression of chronic kidney disease and end-stage renal failure;
- Reduce the incidence of urinary tract infections in women;

- Relieve kidney stones;
- Reduce the inflammation associated with gout (use more often—up to eight times per day).

Disinfectant. Baking soda is a key ingredient in making Dakin's solution (see chapter 8). This solution was developed during World War I as a wound antiseptic. It is used to kill germs and prevent the growth of germs in wounds. It is an excellent solution for irrigating wounds without killing healthy tissue.

CAFFEINE

Caffeine stimulates the central nervous system. It wakes people up and provides a boost of energy. It is also a diuretic, increases acid production in the stomach, increases blood pressure, and may interfere with the absorption of calcium. Some dentists recommend a caffeine drink for their patients after they've received dental work to help metabolize the anesthetic faster and restore feeling to the mouth. A lot of people don't recognize the role these effects play in managing some medical conditions.[228]

Migraines and tension headaches. Caffeine is a vasodilator—it dilates blood vessels. It is a wonder drug in the treatment of migraines and tension headaches. (Caffeine is not effective in treating other kinds of headaches.)[229] That is why drug companies manufacture tablets with aspirin and/or Tylenol and caffeine. It's much less expensive to DIY the combination when needed.

Asthma. Caffeine is administered to improve airway function in individuals with mild to moderate asthma, and in this case very strong coffee is needed.[230] It will enter the bloodstream faster than any tablet, and in an asthma attack, time is of the essence. Caffeine also works for mild to moderate coughing (dry cough) and wheezing because it is a bronchodilator.[231]

Gout. Caffeine (along with cherries, blackberries, other dark berries, and purple grapes) has been shown to lower uric acid levels and is thus useful in treating gout.[232]

Low blood pressure. If someone develops low blood pressure, a physician may advise using caffeine to raise the patient's blood pressure to a more normal level. Blood pressure sometimes drops in older people after they eat, so caffeine is recommended to keep blood pressure in a healthy range.[233]

Premature infants. Caffeine is administered orally or intravenously to slightly premature infants with shortness of breath.[234]

Athletic performance. Studies also show that caffeine may improve athletic performance by increasing physical strength and delaying exhaustion in endurance activities like cycling, running, and soccer. It's not effective for short-term, high-intensity exercise like sprinting or weight-lifting. This might find application in your future, but it works best if caffeine is not consumed regularly.[235]

Caffeine levels in the blood peak one hour after taking it, and the effects last four to six hours. Over-the-counter tablets usually contain 200 mg of caffeine. A cup of coffee contains 150-200 mg. Most cola drinks contain 30-40 mg. Energy drinks contain 60-70 mg. Tea (chai, black, green, white, oolong, jasmine) contains 25-50 mg. Herbal teas contain 0 mg.[236]

Side effects. Most people can consume up to 400 mg of caffeine per day without side effects. Others are more sensitive. In the latter and in those consuming more than 400 mg, the following side effects are possible: restlessness, insomnia, dizziness, headaches, dehydration, anxiety, and abnormal heart rhythm.[237]

Contraindications: Do not use in children under the age of 12 years. Caffeine may affect blood sugar levels in diabetics. Do not operate machinery or drive until you know how caffeine affects you. Caffeine should be avoided by pregnant and nursing women, individuals with sleep disorders, anxiety, insomnia, GERD, ulcers, irregular heart rhythms, and high blood pressure, as well as by individuals taking asthma and heart medications and some antibiotics. (Caffeine is used to treat asthma; however, it may also interfere with some asthma medications.)[238]

COCONUT OIL

Coconut oil is fabulous stuff. It has antibacterial and anti-fungal properties. It promotes healing and exhibits anti-inflammatory and analgesic properties as well. All by itself, it is useful for treating the following:

Ear infections—a couple of drops in the ear

Athlete's foot and other skin fungus—rub some into the affected areas

Skin irritations, including chickenpox, shingles, and eczema—apply liberally to affected areas[239]

Bug bites and stings—apply to affected areas[240]

Nosebleeds—rub inside nose to reduce occurrences

Diaper rash—use instead of diaper rash creams

Burns—apply generously to burn and cover with non-adherent dressing[241]

Wounds—apply generously to wound and bandage[242]

While most readers will accept the idea of using coconut oil to treat the conditions in the first six bullet points on the above list, many are going to dismiss the whole book as quackery upon reading the seventh item, using coconut oil to heal burns. There is solid scientific research backing the use of coconut oil to treat burns; one such address to the article on this research is provided in the endnotes.

In treating and hastening the healing of burns, even partial-thickness burns, coconut oil was spread on the burn and then covered with a non-adherent dressing once a day from the date of the injury until it was completely healed. Coconut oil was also used to treat other wounds. In both instances, it was shown that wounds treated with coconut oil healed much faster than those that did not have coconut oil applied.

Due to coconut oil's antibacterial, anti-fungal, anti-inflammatory, and analgesic properties, it really is the preferred carrier oil for almost everything we are treating when TEOTWAWKI hits. Coconut oil brings an added layer of protection or defense to the table. While coconut oil alone can be used to remedy the following conditions, adding in essential oils ups the game:

Hemorrhoids and **piles**—1 teaspoon coconut oil with 2 drops lavender essential oil

Cold sores—1/4 teaspoon coconut oil with 1 drop oregano essential oil

Thrush—1 teaspoon coconut oil with 2-3 drops peppermint essential oil, swished in the mouth[243]

Wound salve—1 teaspoon coconut oil with two drops each frankincense, lavender, and tea tree oil

Insect repellent 1 tablespoon coconut oil with 2 drops each peppermint, rosemary, and tea tree oil

Perineal tearing prevention—6 weeks before due date, begin massaging perineum with coconut oil to prevent tearing and the need for an episiotomy during childbirth[244]

Head lice. To eliminate head lice, rinse hair well with apple cider vinegar and leave the vinegar in to dry. Then work melted coconut oil into the hair, covering every strand of hair from the roots out, and put on a shower cap. Leave the oil in and shower cap on all day. It will take several hours for the coconut oil to suffocate the lice. Comb the hair with a lice comb to remove eggs and lice. Then shampoo as usual.[245]

Internally, there are a few significant and interesting uses of coconut oil medicinally.

Epilepsy. Coconut oil, as part of a ketogenic diet, has been shown to significantly reduce the incidence of seizures in epileptic children.[246]

Alzheimer's. Coconut oil has been shown to improve brain function in Alzheimer's patients.[247]

Weight loss. Research shows that using coconut oil, a *fat*, actually reduces the number of calories a person desires to consume. Men who ate two tablespoons of coconut oil each day as part of their diet, consumed fewer calories each day. That's significant! When we can no longer afford to eat what we want when we want, and when even just a little bit of hunger can lead to irritation, lack of patience, or worse, any substance that is healthy and makes us feel a little fuller or more satisfied will be more than welcome.[248]

Which kind of coconut oil do you want? For external uses, any coconut oil will work. Cold-pressed and/or "extra-virgin" are preferred with olive oil, but not with coconut oil, at least internally. The heat processing treatment actually boosts the antioxidant properties of coconut oil.

DUCT TAPE

Duct tape belongs in the medical kit along with all the other medical tapes. There are a whole lot of ways to use it in an emergency to substitute for something else. And in some cases, duct tape is the first choice tool for the job. Every medical kit should have a couple of feet or even a whole roll.

Skin

Warts. A clinical study published in the *Journal of the American Medical Association* showed the efficacy of using duct tape to remove warts and calluses, and it was more effective than commercial products. [249]

Blisters. Use duct tape to prevent blisters from forming and protect those that have already formed.

- If you've got a hot spot and are concerned that the friction is going to cause a blister, cover the affected area with duct tape to prevent blister formation.
- If a blister has already formed, cover the blister with a bit of tissue or gauze or paper and then cover the paper with duct tape. Do not permit the duct tape to come into contact with the blister.

Duct Tape Wart/Callus Removal

Cut a small circle of duct tape and apply it over the wart/callus.

Wear the duct tape wart/callus remover for six days, and then remove it.

Soak the affected area in water.

Sand it with an emery board.

Repeat this process until the wart/callus is gone. It may take up to two months.

Splinters can be easily removed by soaking the skin in Epsom salts for 30 minutes to bring the sliver closer to the surface. Dry the skin and apply the duct tape over the splinter. Leave the tape on for 30 minutes, and then slowly peel it away. The splinter should come right out with the tape.

Frostbite. Duct tape can even be used to help prevent frostbite on exposed skin. Simply tear off small strips to cover the nose, cheeks, earlobes, or fingers. It's not fashionable, and certainly not the first choice, but if you've got nothing else, give it a try.

Wounds. Using duct tape as a bandage or to hold a bandage in place is really not the best idea. The adhesive in duct tape is latex-based and may cause a reaction in those with allergies to latex. Even if the individual is not allergic to duct tape, it can cause a reaction and it will definitely hurt when removed from hairy skin. It's always best to use medical tape when it's available, but if it isn't, duct tape will do the job.

Steri-strips. While duct tape is often promoted as being just as good as Steri-strips or butterfly bandages, again it shouldn't be used in this situation unless there really is no other option. The adhesive in duct tape is very effective and there's the risk of damaging tissue further when the tape is removed.

If it's a sizable laceration that needs to be closed, using a duct tape suture will be a better option than placing thin strips of duct tape over the wound. With a duct tape suture, the adhesive is farther removed from the wound. There is also less risk of re-opening the wound when the tape is removed. The tape doesn't actually come into contact with the wound, so there is less chance of contaminating the wound.

Orthopedics

Cracked ribs brace. Duct tape is the tool to have for making a brace for cracked ribs. Have the patient pull on a well-fitted T-shirt and then wrap the tape tight around the shirt to make a sturdy brace.

Splints. Duct tape can be combined with SAM splints, cardboard, Popsicle sticks, or twigs or branches, to fashion splints. If you apply duct tape directly to the SAM splint, you'll remove the foam cushioning. If possible, protect the SAM splint with a layer of paper or cloth.

Ankle sprain. Duct tape can be wrapped around the shoe and ankle to help stabilize the joint. Of course, it is much better for the patient to get off the foot and rest, but if that's not an option and the sprain isn't too severe, this works well.

Pest control

Duct tape does a great job repairing mosquito netting. Strips can also be hung like flypaper to eliminate flies, mosquitoes, and other flying pests.

Disease

Use duct tape to seal off a patient room to prevent the transmission of airborne illnesses. In the event of nuclear radiation, duct tape and plastic can be used to seal off the windows and doors of the home.

Hospitals have started using red duct tape on the floor to mark the area where medical personnel may stand in the room of a patient with a highly contagious disease without having to take protective measures like wearing masks and gloves and washing up. It's actually improved care because doctors can quickly check on a patient more frequently and easily.

Wardrobe malfunctions

Most often wardrobe malfunctions involve needing a shoe repair or possibly some additional insulation that could be provided by wrapping the shoe in duct tape. However, sometimes when a serious injury occurs, clothing needs to be cut away to begin treatment. A careful provider in an austere environment will consider this before cutting away clothing. Removing clothing from an injured patient increases the risk of hypothermia and making a bad situation worse. If you've got duct tape, you can tape the clothing back together. No, it won't be good as new, but it'll suffice to keep the patient warm.

In a really big kit, it's easy to throw in a roll of duct tape, but it will likely be more than is needed. Most medics carry a small duckling (tiny roll of duct tape—check them out on Amazon if you've never seen them—they're pretty cute). The other option, and one that was most often used before ducklings appeared on the scene, was to tear off 2-3 feet of regular duct tape and then roll it up (roll or flat-fold), and put it in a Ziploc bag to keep it clean. If likely to be dealing with children, duct tape is available in fun prints and colors to make a traumatic event a little less scary.

HONEY

Honey is a popular remedy for just about everything right now, and especially for allergies. Here are a few of the ways honey has been used historically and in modern days:

Asthma. Honey was used to treat asthma in the 19th century. Patients were directed to breathe deeply from a jar of honey, and improvement usually occurred within a few minutes. To decrease the number of future episodes, doctors advised drinking 1 teaspoon of honey in 12 ounces of water 3 times per day.[250]

Burns. Honey is an excellent treatment for burns, whether first- or second-degree, and may even be used with third-degree burns when there is no higher care available. After the burned area has been cooled with running water for 15 minutes (not just immersing the wound in water, but *running* water), apply a generous amount of honey. For third-degree burns, make sure this is very thick and covering the entire burn. Cover the honey with cling plastic wrap or a waterproof dressing and tape in place. If the dressing begins to fill with oozing fluid, change the dressing. The worse the burn, the more often the dressing will need to be changed, but make sure to change the dressing at least three times per day. Continue for at least seven to ten days. Do not wash off the honey for at least 20 days (unless the burn has healed). Add more honey as needed, always making sure that there is a thick layer that goes beyond the edges of the burn to prevent infection and promote healing.[251]

Cough. Studies have shown that honey is more effective at quieting a cough in children than any over-the-counter cough syrup. Parents also reported that their children slept better. (However, honey should never, under any circumstance, be given to a child under one year of age.) In addition, it should be noted that the FDA has recommended removing many children's OTC cough syrups from the shelves because of adverse reactions. Fortunately, there is honey, which is safer, more effective, and cheaper. Just a teaspoon or two is all that is needed. And it works for adults as well.

Sore throat. Also, honey tea does a tremendous job soothing sore throats. Just remember, when making the tea, boil the water first, remove from heat, and then add the honey. Boiling the honey itself will reduce or entirely negate many of its medicinal qualities.[252]

Wounds. As far as healing wounds goes, honey works in much the same manner as sugar. Wounds, especially chronic wounds that aren't healing, have an alkaline pH, which provides an ideal breeding ground for bacteria, especially MRSA. Honey is acidic, so it alters the pH and kills the bacteria. Honey may be spread directly on a wound and over the surrounding edges, but it will probably be more comfortable for the patient if the honey is spread on some gauze first and then applied to the wound.[253]

What kind of honey should you use? What is best?

You can buy ridiculously overpriced Manuka or Medihoney if that makes you more comfortable. Manuka is what is most often used in clinical trials. Manuka honey is made by honey bees foraging on the Manuka tree, otherwise known as the tea tree. Tea tree oil is used a lot in treating skin issues. Manuka honey is what has been promoted as the gold standard in medicinal honeys. It costs about as much as the yellow precious metal, at least when wound dressings are made with it or it is packaged as "medical grade."

What do doctors who are teaching others how best to prepare for their own medical issues have to say about Manuka honey? Basically, it's overrated. Most doctors say to use *any* pure, raw honey. The best bet for getting real raw honey is buying from a local beekeeper. An awful lot of grocery store honey is adulterated with high fructose corn syrup, glucose solutions, or even just water. There are numerous tests you can perform at home to determine if your honey is pure or adulterated. The true test, the easy test, is if the honey has crystallized either partially or completely. The fake stuff will never crystallize. The real stuff almost always will eventually. Impatient people put honey in the refrigerator or freezer to test it. Pure honey will crystallize pretty quickly.

Note, again. Honey should never be given to children under the age of 12 months.

MAGGOT THERAPY

As we prepare for interesting times, we come across ideas that make us shudder and say, "I'm not going *there*." *There* varies from person to person. This topic addresses maggot therapy, a practice I have no desire to use, ever. Because we prepare, we will have other options. I'll use sugar or honey. You probably will, too. However, it's important to understand that even practices we find undesirable or distasteful can serve legitimate, medically accepted purposes. We may come across a physician who uses this method for treating a patient. What would you think of that doctor if you didn't know maggot therapy was a legitimate treatment option? In all likelihood, you'd steer clear of the guy, and that might be a mistake. Maggot therapy is what people who didn't store enough sugar or honey or other options will get to use to have their infected wounds cleaned.

Let's check out what maggot therapy really is.

Maggot therapy has actually been around since antiquity, though when Job lamented that "My flesh is clothed with worms and clods of dust; my skin is broken, and become loathsome (Job 7:5)," he might not have understood that the maggots were doing him a great service.[254] Records show that cultures the world over have used maggot therapy for the last thousand years. During the American Civil War, doctors on both sides credited the use of maggots with saving countless lives. However, with advances in the study of germs came the belief that maggots were introducing infection, rather than cleaning it up. Such is actually sometimes the case, particularly when non-sterile maggots are used. The baby (maggots) got thrown out with the bathwater[255], until another war blasted onto the scene.

As often happens during wars with so many casualties to be treated, physicians resort to what actually works to save lives, rather than the newfangled treatments and theories that sound great on paper but don't really work in reality. As a military surgeon in World War I, Dr. William Baer noticed that patients whose wounds were infested with maggots recovered better than those whose wounds were clean. He subsequently used maggots to treat patients in war-torn Europe as well as in his practice at Johns-Hopkins in Boston. In the course of treating patients with maggots, it was found that some patients developed tetanus. That led doctors to begin using sterile flies that they raised themselves.[256]

The practice of using maggots continued into World War II, especially by Americans. However, with the advent of antibiotics, maggot therapy fell out of favor. After all, what would most people want, some little pills or a bunch of maggots?

In the 1980s, however, with increasing cases of antibiotic resistance, maggot therapy was again turned to as a treatment of last resort. Wounds for which maggot therapy is most effective include:

- Burns, partial- and full-thickness
- Pressure ulcers
- Chronic wounds that are not healing

Maggot therapy will not permanently resolve ulcerating skin cancers, but the maggots may remove some tissue. A physician will need to remove the entire cancer and close the wound with sutures.

How would one use maggot therapy in a survival situation? First, one must begin with sterile maggots if at all possible. The green blow fly (*Phaenicia sericata*) and the black blow fly (*Phaenicia regina*) are the most studied and most commonly used. The larvae are placed in the wound, with more used for tissues that are clearly infected and for larger wounds, usually about eight per square centimeter of wound. The wound is then covered with gauze and taped in place, to prevent any escapees. Every one to three days the maggots are washed out with water or sterile saline and replaced with new maggots.[257] Not only do the maggots clean away the dead tissue, they also excrete antimicrobial substances.[258]

However, these highly skilled wound cleaners don't get a lot of respect. Many physicians don't acknowledge or understand the work they do. Why would they? The physicians have no financial incentive to prescribe them (and yes, medical maggots are only available by prescription) because they are so cheap. The maggots are like the lowest castes of society: they're doing a job people don't want to do, doing it much better, and doing it for free. When they're done, they'll be treated like garbage and thrown away. They really do deserve more respect.

PERMETHRIN

Permethrin is the go-to insecticide in a bad situation. It kills bedbugs, fleas, lice, mosquitoes, scabies, and ticks. It is used in medicine and as a pesticide.

Medicinal Uses of Permethrin

Permethrin is available in a few forms, both over-the-counter and by prescription only.

Nix is 1% permethrin lotion for killing lice. It kills both the lice and their eggs. It is sometimes suggested for killing scabies, but is likely not strong enough to eradicate them completely.

RID shampoo kills lice but not their eggs, so the treatment needs to be repeated a week later.

Elimite, a 5% permethrin cream, is available by prescription only and is used for treating scabies. It is applied from head to toe, including the hairline, under finger- and toenails, and between toes and fingers. In babies, it is also applied to the scalp, but this is usually not necessary in adults. The cream is left on for 8-14 hours and then washed off in the shower. One treatment is usually effective.

Insecticidal Uses of Permethrin

Permethrin is an extremely effective insecticide. It kills and repels mosquitoes, ticks, lice, scabies, fleas, and livestock parasites. Due to resistance, it is becoming less efficacious in killing bed bugs. Unfortunately, permethrin also kills bees, so it should not be used on gardens, though it is often used in commercial agriculture.

When sprayed on clothing, permethrin will kill and repel ticks and mosquitoes for six weeks or six washes.

Permethrin may also be sprayed on dogs to repel fleas and ticks. If possible, their fur should be fluffed up before spraying, and permethrin should be sprayed all over, avoiding the genitals and eyes. Permethrin is toxic to cats.

Purchase options, in addition to the medicinal use options above, include the following:

- **0.5% Sawyer Premium Permethrin Insect Repellent**; each bottle treats clothing and gear and dogs.
- **10% permethrin from Martin's Multi-Purpose Insecticide.**
- **13.3% permethrin from Martin's Multi-Purpose Insecticide.**
- **36.8% permethrin from Control Solutions Inc.**

Each bottle contains directions for mixing your own solutions. One teaspoon plus water to make 12.5 ounces of a 0.5% solution; 1 tablespoon plus water to make 37.5 ounces of a 0.5% solution (like the Sawyer brand, used for clothing, tents, and dogs).

Permethrin appears to be safe for use in pregnancy and for babies over the age of two months; however, breastfeeding should be discontinued during treatment.

Cautions: Permethrin may cause an allergic reaction in individuals who are sensitive to ragweed. Side effects include a rash or irritation at the area of use.

PLACEBOS

Remember that episode on *M*A*S*H* where the 4077th, as they are treating the casualties of a recent battle, runs out of morphine? Hawkeye and BJ have patients in excruciating pain with nothing to give them and no prospects of supplies coming in anytime soon. As caring physicians desiring to alleviate their pain, in response to this crisis they resort to the unthinkable. Quackery. They give them sugar pills. Miraculously, the placebo works on everybody, even Klinger, who is merely bothered by the heat.

The placebo effect is real. All physicians know it, but they can't explain it.

In 2018, a rather lengthy article on the placebo effect appeared in the *New York Times Magazine*. Now, the *NYT* is not something generally cited for anything scientific, but this topic is too intriguing to ignore, and the *NYT* is where the article appeared. The address for the article is provided in the endnotes. What follows is an abstract of that article.

"What If the Placebo Effect Isn't a Trick?"

> Placebos work best in individuals with chronic, stress-related conditions, especially if administered by someone they trust. Though the placebo effect is real, many physicians do not acknowledge it or utilize it because they do not understand it and do not know which patients are likely to benefit. Placebos have been shown to be effective in treating migraines, irritable bowel syndrome, PTSD, depression, Parkinson's, and back pain. Researchers are beginning to study why the placebo effect works better for some people and some disorders than others. The placebo is part of every clinical trial, but is not studied itself because there is no money in it. The doctor-patient relationship is fundamental to understanding how placebos work and in helping them to be effective. There is some evidence to suggest that the placebo effect is a biological response to the act of caring—and the more caring, the better the response. An enzyme called COMT affects the body's response to pain and painkillers. COMT levels are also significant in individuals with Parkinson's, depression, and schizophrenia, people who have also exhibited a strong response to the placebo effect. MRI studies demonstrate a consistent pattern of brain activation in response to a placebo.[259]

So why should we include placebos in our kit? A placebo is a tool, and as supplies are exhausted, it may become a very valuable tool. But the most important take-away is that in difficult situations, a truly caring caregiver may be the very best medicine on the path to recovery.

SUGAR

Sugar, regular white granulated sugar, has a clinically researched and proven medical use. The studies came about because an African physician working in a hospital in the UK noticed several patients for whom conventional drug therapy had failed to treat acute and chronic exuding wounds. He wondered why the treatment he had seen his tribal doctor grandfather use in Africa was not being employed here. Didn't everybody know about using sugar to treat such wounds? It took a bit of doing, but that African doctor eventually got permission to conduct a limited trial in the hospital where he worked on patients for whom every other treatment had failed. And miracles happened.[260]

Apparently, such knowledge had been long forgotten in first-world countries where people can afford expensive drug therapies. Unfortunately, some of those very expensive antibiotic therapies are failing the fight against MRSA. Sugar, however, has been shown to work. And it is easy to use.

With a wound, such as a diabetic ulcer on the legs or feet or a burn or cut, apply sugar to it. If the fluid in the wound immediately soaks up the sugar, apply more until some dry sugar remains on top. Cover with a non-adherent bandage and secure in place. Change the dressing every other day. Do not wash away or remove the old sugar when changing the dressing; that will also remove the very delicate new tissue that is forming. Just add more sugar on top. Keep doing this until the wound is healed.

In the case of a large wound, put a ring of petroleum jelly around the edges to better contain the sugar.

Why does sugar work? First, sugar draws fluid in the tissue out, keeping it dry and better able to heal. Second, it creates an acidic environment which is very hostile to bacteria. Third, it also helps relieve pain, contributing to a greater sense of well-being in the patient and less stress in the body.*

SUGARDYNE

Sugardyne is another means of treating wounds that happens to be more effective than conventional pharmaceuticals, less expensive, more natural, and it's easy to make.

Using granulated sugar to treat open wounds and burns was just covered. However, there are cases where using sugar alone is a little more difficult due to the location of the injury. This is where sugardyne comes in.

Sugardyne is prepared in two different ways. The most common method of making sugardyne is to mix approximately two parts sugar to one part Betadine. Start with the sugar first, and gradually add in the iodine. Mix it very well. You want to achieve a consistency of peanut butter or very thick honey. This combination of ingredients has been more thoroughly researched than the following method.[261] Another way of preparing sugardyne is to mix three parts powdered sugar with one part oil, such as olive or coconut (and no iodine). It should be mixed very well before applying to a wound.[262]

Both sugardyne mixtures can be packed into wounds and bandaged in place. The dressing will need to be changed daily, and in some cases, even more often than that. Both mixtures may be made up as needed, but they are also completely stable and can be stored in a closed container for future use.[263]

Note that while iodine alone should never be used in a wound, the iodine in sugardyne does not harm the raw and wounded skin and is perfectly safe to use. Sugardyne is an ideal treatment for burns, even serious ones. Sugar is a natural anesthetic and antibiotic. It is effective against both Gram-positive and Gram-negative bacteria. Sugardyne is also an effective treatment for

---

* This research was conducted using granulated sugar in the UK. In the United States, well over 90% of sugar beets are grown with Roundup. Pure cane sugar may be a better choice.)

human bites, brown recluse bites, frostbite, and shotgun blasts. It is not effective against allergic dermatitis, including poison oak, ivy, or sumac.[264]

Sugardyne does nothing to control bleeding. All bleeding must be totally stopped before applying sugardyne.[265]

Contraindications: Do not use sugardyne made with Betadine in individuals allergic to iodine.

11. TOOLS AND EQUIPMENT

Beyond the expendable and reusable supplies and medications, there are several essential tools that will make caring for family members much easier, more effective, and less painful.

DIAGNOSTIC

Blood pressure cuff (sphygmomanometer). The blood pressure cuff is instrumental in diagnosing so many conditions and offering appropriate care. Without critical care equipment, a doctor has one hand tied behind his back. There are hundreds of options on Amazon. An aneroid cuff—non-digital and non-battery, is the only way to go. Get something of quality here, probably around the $20-25 range.

Otoscope. This instrument must seriously be considered for all young families. While ear infections are not life-threatening, they are extremely painful to all, but more especially to infants and young children who can't express themselves. Parents will really want to know whether their child has an ear infection or if there is something more serious going on. An otoscope is easy to use and makes determining whether an ear is infected simple as well.

Pulse oximeter. This simple clip-on device provides rapid information on what's going on with a patient by showing the pulse rate and measuring the amount of oxygen in the blood. It is especially valuable in cases of pneumonia and coronavirus, as well as some chronic conditions. Unfortunately, there is no non-digital option for this instrument.

The pulse oximeter is clipped onto a finger, toe, or ear, and after a few seconds, it yields a reading. The amount of oxygen in the blood in a healthy person ranges from 95 to 100%. A level of less than 94% suggests the need for supplemental oxygen. Anything less than 90% indicates respiratory disease and is cause for grave concern.

Pulse oximeters for personal use can be purchased in drugstores or on Amazon. I'd recommend looking to the latter for reviews. Those designed for home use are relatively inexpensive, running around $20.

Do you really want one? If someone in your family suffers from heart failure, chronic bronchitis, sleep apnea, or COPD, they've probably already got one. It is nice for measuring oxygen levels in cases of allergic reactions or for those with mild asthma. People with moderate to severe asthma should definitely have their own. In the case of pneumonia and other serious respiratory infections, every family should really consider having their own. Without a laboratory, determining the oxygen levels is very difficult. Being able to tell a doctor what the level is will help him decide what actions to take.

Factors that interfere with accurate reading:

- Bright light (shield device from bright light when taking a reading)
- Shivering
- Low blood pressure
- Vasoconstriction (if the patient is cold the blood may be restricted to fingers and toes)
- Carbon monoxide poisoning (may give a false high reading in smoke inhalation patients)
- Nail polish (the light can't get through) [266]

Pulse oximeters aren't used all that often, so they might not be at the top of the list for equipment to acquire. Honestly, SAM splints, otoscopes, and tweezers are going to be used a whole lot more, but they can be really helpful devices.

Stethoscope. The stethoscope is most often used for listening to the lungs and heart, though doctors will also use it for listening to the abdomen and monitoring the heartbeat of a fetus. There are thousands of options on

Amazon. You don't want to go ultra-cheap, but you don't need super expensive either. My husband purchased a very expensive, sensitive one that he could use with his nearly deaf mother in case her hearing aids got lost or the batteries failed (a less expensive model would have worked just fine).

Thermometer. The thermometer has to be extremely accurate. Changes in body temperature can be diagnostic for some illnesses. Some fevers rise in the morning, afternoon, or evening. It's critical to be able to chart temperatures and spot trends. Even being off a couple of tenths can throw diagnosis off and hinder treatment. Digital thermometers are so nice, so easy, so tempting. But in general, they don't have a great reputation for accuracy from one minute to the next and they need batteries. Glass thermometers are where the action is. They'll still be working in a hundred years and after a dozen electromagnetic pulses. They take a little practice to use, but it's not rocket science. Just remember that the bulb of the thermometer must go under the patient's tongue and remain there for three to five minutes before reading. If the patient is too young or unconscious, use a rectal thermometer.

Ear thermometers are the worst for accuracy. Armpit temperatures are unreliable. Forehead scanners? Let's not even go there. It's got to be an oral or rectal thermometer, not both. Perhaps consider getting both.

Wind-up watch with a second hand

The second hand is needed for being able to calculate accurate heart and respiration rates. This is going to be the hardest item to find, but not impossible. There are only a few options on Amazon at best. A pawnshop might have something. Obviously, relying on batteries isn't the best idea. Good luck. Make sure you know how it works, and that it works, and then put it with the medical supplies reserved for true TEOTWAWKI.

LIGHTING

All medical kits must contain means of providing light. Good lighting is critical to being able to provide good medical care. Make sure there are several options. Murphy's Law dictates that medical emergencies will not happen on a bright, sunny day with light reflecting into exactly what you need to see.

For all items, purchase LED options if at all possible. LEDs provide more light with far less energy draw. Some headlamps and penlights are rechargeable with a USB. Combine those with a BioLite Camp Stove or similar with a USB recharger (we've actually tried this, and it works) or some kind of solar recharger for long-term sustainability.

Hand-powered flashlight. While these are popular for regular emergencies, they are not a great idea for a primary or even secondary choice in the medical kit. One person who could be helping in other ways has to be dedicated to providing light in the medical emergency. That person has to be close to the patient and is going to be in the way of the caregiver. Other options are much better.

Credit card magnifier. This is extremely helpful for magnifying slivers or other debris in wounds and in reading pill bottles and other fine print. Some of these also have a built-in light feature.

Chemical light sticks. Just like most children only get sick at night and on weekends, most emergencies where we really need a lot of good light will happen at night and the power will be out. A single headlamp won't provide enough illumination, so it is chemical light sticks to the rescue. They're lightweight and easy to move around without the risk of flame or fumes from a lantern. White light is best. Plan on at least half a dozen per incident.

Headlamps. These allow for a high intensity, focused light while keeping both hands free. No matter what, if you only have one fixed source for light to examine a wound and clean thoroughly, your head is going to block that light. When lighting is inadequate and when you really need to have good, strong light to see clearly, you've got to have a headlamp. Headlamps run the gamut in price and quality; Streamlight has a good reputation. Possibly consider one that is rechargeable with a USB to use with a solar or rocket stove USB recharging port.

Penlights. Penlights are used for pupil checks, exploring around a dressing without pulling the whole thing off, or cleaning out a wound. If the care provider can peek under the dressing without removing it, time and resources are conserved. Penlights also allow patients to be checked on in the dark, without disturbing the patient's sleep. They're helpful in checking in a patient's mouth or ears (though not as nice as an otoscope) and for looking for the ever-dreadful foreign-body-in-nose in a two-year-old.

With potential concussion patients, medical personnel are checking whether the pupils are equally reactive—if they dilate at the same speed and to the same extent. (About 10% of the population has pupils that normally differ in size. If this applies to you or your family, make sure anyone attending to you or them knows this. It should also be very clearly stated on the top page of your medical records.)

Penlights for checking pupils are a much lower intensity than other penlights. For your patients' comfort, try to have a lower intensity light as well. For convenience when checking patients, some penlights have a pupil gauge and a ruler. Many penlights on the market, especially those marketed for outdoor adventure, are too powerful for pupil checks. A two-power option with a USB charger or replaceable batteries would be ideal. The low-power option for checking pupils should be 15 lumens or less.

Extra batteries and rechargers. Make sure you can power every light you have. Store batteries separately from the devices they power and avoid extremes in heat.

PRESSURE CANNER

A pressure canner may also be used as an autoclave for sterilizing medical instruments. As such, you may want additional racks or space to accommodate larger items. The procedure for sterilizing instruments is covered in chapter 4.

TREATMENT

Before getting into specifics here, let's make sure we're all on the same page regarding the understanding of minor surgery. True minor surgery involves only cutting and stitching. Anesthetic, if any, is only local. No respiratory assistance is required. Minor surgery pertains to medical issues such as lacerations, abscesses, and ingrown toenails.

As with any job, having the right tools makes the task easier, faster, and more pleasant for all. You can sometimes improvise a tool, if necessary. I have been known to improvise a flathead screwdriver for a Phillips on occasion. It usually doesn't work as well. I've also been known to improvise a butter knife for a flathead screwdriver, and it doesn't work as well, either. However, both of them save me a trip to the garage. I also only make these substitutions for little, temporary jobs, but if I want to do the job right, I get the right tool.

When you're dealing with medical issues with your family, you want the right tools for yourself or the doctor doing the work for you. You don't want the absolute cheapest instruments, but you don't need surgical suite quality, either.

Ideally, you'd find a doctor to help you out with specific purchases. Most pre-assembled kits marketed towards the preparedness community will cost more than what you'd pay by assembling your own. Instruments are most often made in China or India. Noteworthy, however, is that the Indians have been producing some very nice quality tools—better than the Chinese of late.

Instruments

As far as the actual instruments go, this is what most doctors have and use:

- Hemostats (look like clamps)
    - Mosquito, curved (2)
    - Kelly, straight (2)
    - Hagar needle driver (also known as a needle holder), 5", (1). These look like clamps but are not. They are strictly for holding the suture needle.

- Scissors
  - Bandage scissors (1)
  - Metzenbaum (tissue) scissors, curved, 6" (1)
  - Suture scissors. These have a curved, blunt blade on the bottom to prevent injuring the patient. (1)
  - Trauma shears for cutting away clothing (1)
- Scalpels
  - Disposable units or the handles (#3 scalpel handle) with replacement blades
  - Scalpel blades, at least a dozen each of #10, #11, and #15
- Forceps (tweezers to non-doctors)
  - Splinter forceps, ultra-fine tip with tip protector (1)
  - Smooth pick-ups, holding dressings (1)
  - Toothed pick-ups (Adson's forceps/tissue forceps. Especially useful in pulling the skin together so that skin staples can be well placed.)

Ask a doctor, and he'll reply that these instruments are not really interchangeable. They're the bare basics for most minor surgeries. When a patient needs minor surgery, it's best to have everything necessary for the job to be done well and safely, without introducing infection.

And finally, a couple of other items for cleaning wounds:

- Baby brush. The soft little baby brushes that are sent home from the hospital are ideal for gently cleaning out debris from abrasions.
- Razors. If the laceration is within a hairy part of the body, the skin needs to be shaved clean before suturing begins. Otherwise, the risk of contaminating the underlying tissue is too great.

Trauma shears

These will cut through clothing, tape, seat belts, and skin if you're not careful.

Klever Kutter

This is a light-weight, less expensive, more compact alternative to trauma shears. Not actually designed for medical use, it's marketed as "the safest disposable box cutter on the market today." I've actually started carrying one in my pocket instead of a pocket knife.

The Klever Kutter makes removing the bandages easier and safer. With the curved edges and recessed blade, there are no concerns about injuring a wiggly child or uncooperative patient. The Klever Kutter cuts away tape and bandages quite well. It is easily used by lefties and fits nicely into emergency medical kits.

Tweezerman tweezers

Quality tweezers are essential for removing slivers and dirt from a wound. Make sure to select tweezers that come to a point, not a slant.

There will always be more tools and equipment to buy. Be sure to purchase what is needed to care for the illnesses most likely to occur in your family, especially anything pertaining to chronic conditions that are already known.

12. SUPPLY ACQUISITION

The previous chapters have covered a sizable number of medical supplies a family would be well-served to store. Most are general use items that everyone should have, but some are a bit more specialized. Unfortunately, a lot of people are limited by a budget. We can't buy everything. We have to make choices. So how do we prioritize our acquisitions?

PRIORITIZING THE ACQUISITION OF SUPPLIES

The first priority for everyone must be solid hygiene and sanitation practices. And the first and foremost of these is washing hands well. Make sure you have plenty of soap for washing hands, in addition to detergent for dishes and laundry.

The second priority must be a healthy, well-balanced diet. Nutritious food with sufficient calories will build and maintain healthier bodies. There is no substitute for good food. Variety in the diet will help maintain morale and be more likely to provide essential vitamins and minerals as well as micronutrients.

As far as actual medical supplies go, factors to consider include:

Personal medical history. What conditions do you already have? Store what you know you need. If you require maintenance medications, get them now. While building up a supply using insurance may be difficult or impossible, purchasing pharmaceuticals from overseas pharmacies is relatively simple and usually pretty inexpensive. Check into possible alternatives. Diabetics will have a hard time building a supply of insulin if they're using bottles that retail at $600 or more, three per month, but they can make do with the cheap stuff from Walmart for $25 each. Some people will be able to use alternative medicine to manage. Research your options and plan accordingly.

Family medical history. Next look at what conditions run in your family and which might be an issue to consider. My husband's brother is allergic to bee stings, but he's the only one of the eight siblings with that problem. We have one nephew among the twenty-four nieces and nephews with severe environmental and food allergies (but he's the oldest and his house is just about as sterile as can be, even now with three younger siblings—studies show that children need a little dirt, dust, and dander to build strong immune systems). If we were more concerned about anaphylactic reactions within our immediate family or if we had more disposable income for preparing for far less likely emergencies, we would probably have an Epi-pen.

Migraines run on both sides of our family, and so far, one daughter is affected by them. However, they could kick in for the rest of us at any time, so we have strong pain relievers for that. I have the same body type as my paternal grandmother. She had hyperemesis gravidarum (it's much worse than the normal morning sickness) when pregnant with my father, had her gallbladder removed, and often had adhesive tape on her left thumbnail to protect that nail from catching and splitting more. I have also experienced all of these, and based on that, I anticipate developing arthritis in my knees at around the age of 65, just like she did. I'm also taking measures to try to prevent that from happening, but in the meantime, I prepare for the worst. If chronic conditions run in your family, acquire medicines or supplies that could be helpful.

In addition, look at what your extended family members are prone to. We've had zero broken bones among the extended family on both sides. We're pretty careful people and not really accident-prone, so we're less concerned about trauma. We stock some supplies for these kinds of injuries, but not a lot. However, my husband is really a bleeder, so we stock a lot of gauze. My husband and son have a lot of issues with stomach acid and ulcers, so we have a pretty hefty supply of those medications as well.

Stage of life. How old are you? What is your family composition? If I had infants and small children, I'd seriously consider having an otoscope to check for ear infections. I'd probably stock more amoxicillin and Keflex, and I'd contemplate buying strep throat test strips. Any woman of child-bearing age should have several pregnancy tests, not for satisfying one's curiosity, but for ruling out pregnancy when medications need to be administered or for diagnosing illnesses. Individuals over the age of 60 and those on some stomach medications should seriously consider stockpiling vitamin B12 (see chapter 5).

Geographical location. Where do you live? What diseases are endemic to your area? Here in the high desert, we have very little concern about mosquitoes. We have absolutely no worries about malaria, so we don't store those medications. If I lived in Florida or Louisiana, it would be an entirely different matter. Ticks are an extreme rarity here. If we had more ticks, I'd store a lot more doxycycline so that it could be taken prophylactically anytime a tick attached to anyone. If we lived in a northern latitude with little sunshine, we'd store more vitamin D.

Everyday life. What do people go to emergency departments and urgent care centers for now?[267]

Having the supplies to manage these common problems means you'll be prepared to handle about 95% of the medical issues in your family. Cold remedies and antibiotics, regular over-the-counter pain relievers, sutures and tapes, splints, and oral numbing gels should be in every medical stockpile. Based on my family's history, we should probably have more sutures and Steri-Strips than anything else. Knowing what I know now, I could have dealt with all those minor lacerations at home.

Top Ten Reasons for Going to the ER or Urgent Care:

Chest pain
Abdominal pain
Upper respiratory infections
Minor cuts and lacerations
Broken bones and sprains
headache
Foreign objects in the body
Toothaches
Skin infections
Back pain

Survivalist writers suggest that medical preparedness is all about having tourniquets, chest decompression needles, and QuikClot. The reality is that minor issues sideline a lot of people, but that doesn't have to include us. Look at what is most realistic for you based on your family medical history, your ages, and climate, and start there. After you cover your known medical conditions and what you are more likely to encounter based on your family history, then move on to the common issues. When those needs are satisfied, then consider the stuff of Hollywood.

An understanding of the most commonly used medications and the most common reasons why people seek emergency care will not only help fill in holes in your supplies, but will also provide the reassurance that you're on the right track and preparing well.

Reports from care providers in austere environments suggest that approximately 90% of the medications being dispensed are over-the-counter. They're the common pharmaceuticals that we can all acquire without restriction. People already know where the pain is and most likely already

Most Common Reasons for Seeking Non-Emergency Medical Care

Upper respiratory tract infections, including sinusitis, pneumonia, influenza, ear infections, strep throat

Viral infections and fever

Asthma

Allergies, hay fever, and anaphylaxis

Gastrointestinal pain and infections—gastroenteritis, food poisoning, appendicitis, vomiting, diarrhea

Chest pain

Urinary tract infections, kidney stones

Burns, mostly second-degree

Open wounds—bites, lacerations, abrasions

Skin infections, rashes

Sprains and minor fractures

Dislocations and major fractures

Dental abscesses

Pregnancy, miscarriage, contraception, and STDs

Mental health issues

Fainting

have the medication on hand, so why are they going to see a doctor?[268]

Much of it all boils down to the fact that we need a little reassurance. The patient got stressed that some illness or injury was more serious than it actually was. What's great about this is that you're not treating the public. You aren't even treating your own family, except for the issues you have the confidence and skill to manage. Think about what happens when your children come to you for a scratch or scrape or bruise. They're usually looking for comfort, care, and sympathy. Someone to wash the wound, put the Band-Aid on, and cuddle and reassure. Adults may not necessarily need the cuddling, but when they've injured themselves enough to ask for assistance, it's because something really hurts. They need to be reassured regarding the proper treatment and course of action.

The above constituted approximately 95% of all visits. Most of these are managed with over-the-counter medications and compassion.

The most commonly prescribed or recommended over-the-counter drugs for non-chronic conditions include:

- Pain relievers (Tylenol, hydrocodone, morphine)
- Antibiotics (amoxicillin, Augmentin, Zithromax)
- Antihistamines (Benadryl, Zantac, Zyrtec)
- Anti-diarrheals (Imodium)
- Anti-fungals (nystatin, Diflucan)
- Prilosec
- Throat lozenges
- Hydrocortisone cream
- Asthma inhalers[269]

One clinician reported that, according to his records, 90% of visits were managed with over-the-counter medications. Eight percent required antibiotics. The remaining 2% were actual traumas, half of which were minor and could be treated on-site, and the other half requiring evacuation to a hospital. Basically, with the supplies on this list, a doctor will be able to handle most problems.

It also bears repeating that proper handwashing and sanitation will prevent many of these illnesses, as will safe food handling methods. Taking care of these little things will mean there are far fewer big issues to manage.

SOURCES FOR PURCHASING SUPPLIES

As has been previously mentioned, so very many of our medical supplies come from China. And when people start panicking about being unable to get whatever, the prices on those items skyrocket.

So, how does one acquire antibiotics?

Ideally, you have a good relationship with a family physician who understands the need to prepare. These are getting harder and harder to find. If you're looking for a new physician who will share your ideas about preparing and be willing to help you (after you have established a good relationship), off-grid medicine doctors suggest that the best chances are with an older physician who maintains paper, not electronic, records.

> Do not try to build your antibiotic supply by not taking the full course of antibiotic therapy when it is prescribed. One reason for the rise in antibiotic resistance is that people do not finish the course of treatment, so the harmful bacteria making them sick are not wiped out. Superbugs develop resistance and emerge.)

Sometimes a physician will prescribe an antibiotic just in case. Like you take your child in to see him with what is probably only a bad sore throat, but it could be strep. If the child is not feeling better in a day or two, he gives you a prescription to fill. (Make sure to get pills instead of syrups--pills have a much longer shelf life.) Or you are planning to travel and ask for a prescription or two to deal with diseases you might encounter and wish to avoid ruining your trip with a case of traveler's diarrhea.

Here are some other options for procuring medicines and supplies:

Foreign pharmacies. AllDayChemist.com has been my supplier for ten years. I recently read, however, that India is halting shipment of pharmaceuticals out of their country. Whether truth or rumor, I don't know. And what is rumor this moment may be truth tomorrow. Other overseas pharmacies may still be filling orders, but with so many raw materials coming from China, no one knows how long this will continue. Those who live near the border might consider making a trip south or north.

Fish antibiotics. Fish antibiotics are not made out of fish, and they are not fed to fish, especially in the same dosages that are used for people. They are theoretically designed to be added to aquariums to treat specific bacterial infections in fish. Although you cannot purchase antibiotics for people or non-aquarian pets in the US without a prescription, for some reason, we still have a loophole in this country that allows these very same antibiotics to be sold over-the-counter "for aquarium use." Most of these fish antibiotics are of the same quality and dosage as antibiotics for people. It is illegal to sell these medications to treat infections in people or pets other than fish. The FDA has been cracking down on retailers, especially those marketing these products to people who clearly are not obtaining them to keep their pet fish healthy.

As far as the following online options go, I have no experience with any of them.

- ThomasLabs.com
- Kraftdrug.com
- Chewy.com
- Walmartpetrx.com
- CampingSurvival.com

For all other over-the-counter supplies, here are some suggestions:

Amazon. Like it or not, Amazon has just about everything except antibiotics. Amazon Prime Pantry has even better prices on bulk bottles of medications than Amazon, Costco, and Sam's. It might be worth it to take advantage of a free trial to do your ordering.

Costco and Sam's Club generally offer the best prices for over-the-counter medications in bulk—antihistamines, pain relievers, etc., as well as supplements, gloves, and so on.

Dollar stores aren't my favorite place, just because I think there are better prices elsewhere. But if you are only preparing for yourself, or really need only small amounts, it can make sense to shop there.

Ranch and feed stores carry a surprising variety of veterinary supplies marketed to ranchers and hobby farmers. It's often the same stuff used in medicine, without the hefty price tag. Selection varies substantially from one store to the next. In addition to fish antibiotics and other medications, you can also find bandages, wraps, gauze, and insecticides.

Prepper stores. If you've got one of these in your community, it can be a great place to stock up on medical supplies. Ours purchases medical supplies in bulk and then sells items singly. This can be a fabulous way to go for individuals and couples.

ShopMedVet.com is *the* place to go for bulk buying of everything except pharmaceuticals. They have the best selection of everything you need to stock your medical kits and phenomenal prices.

SECTION 3—ILLNESS AND DISEASE

13. SUPPLIES FOR DERMATOLOGIC ISSUES

BLEEDING

When you encounter someone who is bleeding, time is of the essence. A person can die from blood loss a lot faster than from a lack of oxygen. When you come across someone who is bleeding, you need to determine immediately whether the bleeding is life-threatening.

- Is all or part of a limb gone?
- Is blood spurting out of a wound?
- Is blood pooling on the ground?
- Is blood soaking clothing or bandages?

If the answer is "yes" to any of the above, and if it is a limb that is bleeding, a tourniquet may need to be applied. However, tourniquets are used only as a last resort, when bleeding can't be stopped after 30 minutes of constant, direct pressure. Tourniquets should be applied two to three inches above the wound, and never above a joint, so go a little higher if you have to. Directions are not noted here because it will vary according by type of tourniquet. A correctly placed tourniquet is going to hurt a lot. The patient will not be happy. The exact time the tourniquet was placed must be noted on the patient's body using a Sharpie marker and in paper notes.

Now, let's assume the bleeding is not so severe, because in most situations you are not going to encounter life-threatening bleeding. Most of the time, it's going to be much less serious. Stopping the bleeding is basic first aid. It doesn't take medical school.

Work with whatever supplies you have. Fortunately, we all have the most important supply with us all the time--direct pressure. Direct pressure will stop the vast majority of bleeding. It may take more than a minute or two or even ten, especially if the person is on blood thinners or the wound is a substantial one. What is used in addition to direct pressure? Many preppers favor using sanitary pads and tampons for bleeding. But any woman will tell you that those products do absolutely nothing to stop bleeding. They only soak up blood. Direct, firm, constant pressure must be applied. Hemostatic agents like QuikClot or Celox powder or gauze work quite well to *help* stop bleeding, but it is the direct pressure that is essential. Pouring QuikClot on a spurting blood vessel is a complete waste.

Deep wounds are a little trickier. After determining exactly where the blood is coming from, hemostatic gauze or even clean strips of fabric can be utilized to pack into a deep wound. Continue applying pressure as you pack in the gauze or fabric strips. Maybe a triangle bandage or bandana or other clothing can be used to aid in creating that direct pressure. Also, keep the patient nice and warm. Cold blood does not clot well. Warm blood clots much better.

A note regarding gloves: Wearing gloves is much more for your protection from the victim's blood rather than protecting him from your germs. If gloves are not available, have the patient, if possible, apply pressure himself, or enlist his family or associates in applying pressure. It gives them something to do to help and frees you to gather supplies and work more easily.

ABRASIONS

Using iodine, rubbing alcohol, peroxide, or whiskey to clean a wound makes for good TV drama. Tough guys wince or swear, children whimper and cry. In reality, it makes for dead tissue which then has the potential to get infected and create a whole other host of problems. On top of that, it is a waste of what may be very precious disinfecting agents. So let's learn to clean a wound properly.

Assume your teenage boy has come to you with a really nasty road rash. It's kind of sizable and extremely dirty--sand, mud, organic matter--all kinds of grossness. And it's bleeding a bit. What do you do first?

Stop the bleeding. Right. Now it may be hard to tell whether the bleeding has actually been stopped with all that gunk in the abrasion, so you may have to use some water to wash it out so you can see better. If you've washed it out and you now see that it's still bleeding--oozing out and pooling, then go back to applying pressure to stop the bleed. Only once the bleeding has completely stopped do you go on to the next step.

Now it's time to debride the wound, i.e., remove all the dirt, dead tissue, gunk, bacteria, etc. Clean water--it doesn't have to be sterile--is all you need. Tap water, bottled water, a clean, clear mountain stream. Boiled water. Saline solution, sterile or not. It all works. Never use iodine, rubbing alcohol, peroxide, or any alcohol used for drinking. That only works on TV, and you are not on TV. All of those will kill healthy tissue (because those disinfecting agents are being used to kill living things like bacteria) and make it dead tissue that can create an infection. And then you'll need to clean it out properly, waste supplies, and maybe even need to start using some antibiotics. Just do it right the first time.

You may need a whole liter of water, even for a small injury. It's not an exaggeration. And yeah, that's not how they do it on TV. Back to our teenage boy with the nasty road rash. You're not simply pouring water from a bottle or using a washcloth. You're going to need to create some pressure to dislodge that debris in the wound. A large syringe (without the needle), like around 60 ml, is the best option. A curved tip might be nice. Or you can use a perineal bottle (usually simplified to peri bottle), the bottles given to new mothers in the hospital to rinse with every time they use the toilet. Both of those will create nice, gentle pressure for removing debris. You don't want a fire hose that is going to do more damage. Don't be surprised if you need to refill a few times.

If the wound is substantial, or if it has some larger contaminants that irrigation alone can't dislodge, you'll need some tools. Doctors call them forceps. The rest of us call them tweezers. Tweezerman point tweezers are the way to go. Uncle Bill's sliver gripper tweezers are also nice. This is not an item you want to go cheap on.

Once you have thoroughly debrided and irrigated the abrasion so that there are no contaminants or dead tissue left inside the abrasion, it's time to clean *around* the wound. Using a disinfecting solution (Hibiclens, Betadine, benzalkonium chloride, rubbing alcohol, peroxide--just one--they're listed in order of preference), starting at the edge of the wound and being very careful not to touch inside the wound, wipe in a circular motion around the wound and work your way out, like two to three inches.

After the area around the wound is dry, finish up treatment with a bandage or gauze (possibly spread with triple antibiotic) and tape to protect the wound from getting contaminated and infected.

This is probably where the doctor would stop, and hopefully it's all that is needed. But what if things have really and truly fallen apart? What if it's only you providing care? What if you missed something? What if there is no triple antibiotic to spread on the bandage? You might consider covering the wound with sugar, granulated pure cane sugar. It's a natural antibiotic and provides some pain relief as well.

LACERATIONS

A *laceration* is doctor-speak for a cut or tear in the skin. A laceration may involve underlying tissue, including large arteries and veins, tendons, nerves, muscles, or the abdominal cavity. You want a real doctor for the latter, even if it means traveling a significant distance in a dangerous situation.

Assuming that the bleeding has already stopped, the first thing a physician will do is to wash out the wound, exactly as outlined for abrasions. As the wound is being washed out, the caregiver will look to be sure that there is no damage to underlying tissues. If there is, your job is done. Tape sterile gauze over the wound and send the patient for professional help.

Once you're sure that the underlying tissue hasn't been damaged and the wound is thoroughly cleaned, it's time to clean around the outside of the wound, the same as for abrasions.

The above two measures should be taken, no matter what. But now decisions need to be made. The first is, how long has the wound been open to the environment? If it has been more than six hours, then it is covered with gauze taped in place. This is because the opportunity for bacteria to collect and multiply has been too great; closing the wound at this point risks trapping bacteria inside and significantly increasing chances of infection. If the wound is to the face or neck, the window for closure is twelve hours because the face and neck have a greater blood circulation, which fights infection and promotes healing. If the wound is to a hand or foot, it does not get closed. There is too little blood flow, there are too many bacteria, and there are too many structures to be really adversely affected by a bacterial infection. All of these wounds that do not get closed initially should be closed five days later, assuming there is no sign of infection.

Now you've washed and cleaned the wound properly and determined that it should be closed. And yes, the wound really should be closed to hasten tissue healing, decrease opportunities for infection, and reduce scarring. At this point, tissue scissors or a scalpel should be used to remove uneven edges or flaps of skin. Smooth edges heal better with less scarring.

The goal, ideally, is to bring the edges together perfectly. The patient would like this to be done as painlessly and with the least amount of scarring as possible. Steri-strips and skin glue (Vet-Bond is the same as Derma-Bond, without the hefty price tag or having to go through a doctor to get it) are quite effective at holding the skin together until it's healed. They require less skill and inflict far less pain, for sure. Scarring may be less, assuming the strips or glue were well placed to begin with, and there won't be any additional scars created by the sutures or staples. And they may work better than sutures or staples because the tissue is not being further injured by the suture needle or staples, both of which can actually introduce bacteria.

Unfortunately, Steri-strips and glue can't be used everywhere, especially for more extensive wounds or areas of the body under tension, due either to the size of the injury or the actual location. Sutures are stronger and more secure than strips or glue. If the injury is over a joint, sutures are best. Even staples shouldn't go over a joint. If so much skin has been lost that the edges of the skin are under some tension, that's another time sutures are going to be the best choice.

How long are the sutures or staples left in place? It's a balancing act. Sutures and staples should be removed as quickly as possible to minimize scarring, but not so soon that the wound is at risk of re-opening. On the face, in wounds without tension, sutures can be removed in three to five days (remember, better blood flow means faster healing). For the rest of the body, it's usually 10-14 days. But this can vary substantially. Is the patient already weakened from other conditions like age, illness, or malnutrition? Was there substantial tissue loss such that there's a lot of tension and the skin hasn't stretched and relaxed to accommodate it yet?

Suturing and gluing and taping and stapling are not exact sciences, like just about anything with medicine. It's called *practice* for a reason. Have the supplies, have the books, have the desire to learn, and maybe some pain meds and hope you never need any of it.

THE BASICS OF SUTURING

Let's begin by going in a bit of reverse order by listing the wounds that *do not* get sutured and closed until later. These wounds may be too contaminated, even after thorough cleansing and irrigation, and the risk for infection is too high. These wounds are not closed until usually five days later, and the terms doctors use to refer to them are *secondary intention* and *delayed closure*.

Puncture wounds have penetrated deeper into the tissue. They probably carried a lot of bacteria and contaminants in with them. They must be irrigated and cleaned out as well as possible. However, it can be incredibly challenging to clean them out. Puncture wounds do not get sutured because the risk of trapping bacteria and contaminants is too high. If there is no sign of infection after the fifth day, then the wound may be sutured.

Bites, animal or human, carry too many bacteria. Even if the bite isn't very deep, the wound does not get closed until the fifth day, and only then if there are no signs of infection.

Wounds open longer than 6 hours (12 hours on face) do not get closed. This is because bacteria have had the opportunity to establish a good foothold, and closing may trap bacteria within the wound. Just thoroughly clean and dress, leaving the wound open. Change the dressings every 48 hours. If there are no signs of infection by the fifth day, the wound may be closed.

Wounds to the hands and feet, due to the numerous tendons and ligaments, have way too many opportunities for something to go wrong and infection to set in.

All other wounds get closed. When it happens right after the injury, within the acceptable time frame for safe closure, it's called *primary intention*.

Ideally, you've got some sterile gloves to use for doing your work. But if those need to be saved for a more intense situation, non-sterile gloves washed with Hibiclens or Betadine will suffice. As far as the patient is concerned, the care provider doesn't need to don a mask, goggles, or gown, as long as the provider isn't coughing or sneezing into the wound or allowing the wound or suture to come into contact with non-sterile clothing. However, these personal protection items are recommended for the care provider's safety, to protect from accidental sprays of fluid from the patient.

After cleaning out a wound by irrigating with clean water and then cleaning around a wound with disinfectant, a *fenestrated drape* (sterile sheet with a hole to expose the wound) is placed over the wound. This prevents the suture material from coming into contact with contaminated clothing or other objects and dragging bacteria into the wound.

The goal of the suture is to *approximate the* skin tissue. (That's doctor-speak for fitting the skin edges together like you put a puzzle together.) Jagged edges or flaps of skin will not heal well and may actually cause more scarring, so these need to be trimmed with a scalpel or tissue scissors. For the best healing result with minimal scarring and risk of infection, the sutures should bring the skin tissue together without any puckering or gathering up of the skin. Each passage of the suture needle should be through the skin, but not into underlying subcutaneous fat or other tissues. As skin is not of a uniform thickness over the body, the depth of the sutures will vary by location on the body. For example, skin on the face and the back of the hands is quite thin. It is much thicker on the back and soles of the feet.

There are numerous types of suture stitches, and it would be a good idea to learn a few of the most common. *Interrupted sutures* are single stitches that pass through each side of the wound and are then knotted and cut. They are good for irregular edges, and if the wound happens to get infected, one or two may be removed to allow the infection to drain while leaving the others in place. A *running* suture (whip stitch) can be quickly put in place, with knots only at the beginning and end. Square knots with an additional throw or two are the most commonly used for suturing. Do not use a granny knot. It will slip, and then you're back at square one.

Keep the wound dry and protected from contamination.

Suturing is a skill that needs to be seen repeatedly and practiced even more repeatedly, with real instruments and suture materials. That's the only way. Numerous videos online show you how. Most instructional videos feature suture boards or pigs' feet, which is a bit of an unnecessary expense, especially in the beginning. Banana skins are great for beginners. They have a bit of depth to them and clearly show the spacing of your stitches so you can improve your technique.

FIRST-DEGREE BURNS

Most everyone has experienced first-degree, or superficial, burns. The most commonly seen are sunburns, followed by those due to excessive heat (like brief exposure to hot water, hot pans or utensils, mechanical devices), and then chemical burns.

Treatment for all of these burns is the same:

- Cool the burn with running cool water, not immersing the burned area in a bowl or basin of water alone. You need running water to carry the heat away and prevent further injury. Let the water run for 10-15 minutes.
- The skin usually remains intact, so no antibacterial creams are used.
- Usually no dressing is applied.
- Offer Advil for pain. Topical options include aloe vera gel or zinc oxide. A drop or two of lavender essential oil is very effective on small burns.
- For sunburns, aloe vera gel with lidocaine is very soothing.
- To reduce irritation, wear light, cool clothing.

There may be superficial peeling about a week later, but there will be no scarring. In more serious burns, when the amount of skin burned is calculated, the area of first-degree burns is not included in the calculation.

All of the above applies to individuals one year of age and older. However, sunburns are an entirely different matter in babies under one year of age. A sunburn, even if it appears mild, is much more serious in a baby. Baby skin is extremely sensitive, and sunburns can occur in as little as ten minutes, even on a cloudy day. Keeping a child in the shade may not be adequate. Any sunburn in a baby is reason to see a physician immediately.

But if that is not an option:

- Cool the baby in a cool bath with baking soda or oatmeal. Pat the skin dry. Do not rub.

- Also, apply a clean, soft washcloth dipped in cool water several times per day.
- Make sure not to chill the baby.
- Let the baby nurse as much as he wants and offer water in a bottle as well.
- Apply aloe vera gel.
- Dress the baby in loose clothing.

Keep in mind that the higher the altitude, the thinner the atmosphere, and the more the sun's rays penetrate. Researchers used to say that the atmosphere thinned 4% for every 1,000 feet above sea level. Some assert that that number is now closer to 8% per 1,000 feet. Regardless of which number it is, when in the mountains, one needs to be much more careful in the sun. Even staying in the shade is not adequate protection. Sunlight can reflect off water, snow, sand, and pavement.

SECOND-DEGREE BURNS

Unlike first-degree burns, there is a huge range in the severity of second-degree burns. Anything with a blister qualifies as second degree, but a smaller burn, for example, due to contact with a curling iron or hot skillet, is managed much differently than a blistering sunburn from spending a day at the beach without sunscreen. Likewise, treating a substantial second-degree sunburn in an infant is a whole lot different than treating the same in an adult. Location is also important in determining the approach to treatment. A smaller burn on the face, hands, feet, or genitalia (like from driving with hot coffee) needs greater attention and care than something similar on an arm or leg, due to the risks of infection, scarring, disability, or proximity to delicate, vital structures.

In a functioning medical system, patients with second-degree burns covering more than 10% of the body would be referred to a specialized burn unit. Assuming that no higher care is available, how does one calculate the total body surface area has been burned? And why is it important?

It's called the "Rule of Nines." The palm of the patient is considered to be about 1% of the total body surface area. For the rest of the body, the rule of nines works pretty well.[270]

Rule of Nines	
Head and neck	9%
Each arm	9%
Chest	18% (2x9)
Back	18%
Each leg	18%
Genitals	1%

It is important to be able to calculate because in a patient with burns covering more than 10% of the body, dehydration is a real concern. The patient needs to be rehydrated with an oral rehydration solution (ORS). (The formula for calculating the amount of ORS is called the Parkland Formula and is covered in the following section on third-degree burns.)

Even with "only" second degree burns, the patient will need intensive care, particularly with regard to fluid loss. Dehydration and renal failure can easily happen here. Keep the patient very well hydrated.

Second-degree burns, sometimes called partial thickness burns, may occur in numerous ways:

- Serious sunburn
- Hot liquids
- Steam
- Hot skillets

The skin will be quite red and very painful. It may blister immediately, or the blisters may appear sometime later. The pain can last for days to weeks.

Regardless of how you plan to manage treatment of the patient, the following must be done:

- As with first degree burns, place the affected body part under cool (not icy), running water for 15-20 minutes, without giving the patient hypothermia.
- As the body part is under running water, remove all jewelry from the afflicted limb(s), even if the burn is higher up on the arm or leg. Swelling on a burned limb can be far worse than one might imagine.

The primary concern with second-degree burns is the potential for infection. Blisters should be left intact if at all possible. Blistered skin rarely develops an infection unless the blister is opened. Grossly enlarged blisters that you just know are going to burst may be nicked at the lower edge with a sterile needle or scalpel to decompress them. Do not remove the skin. [271] It is normal for blister fluid to re-accumulate.[272]

All decompressed blisters and areas where the skin that has sloughed or peeled should be covered with a non-stick dressing like Telfa. Any creams or ointments should not be applied directly to the skin to avoid inflicting pain and damage, but rather should be applied to the non-stick dressing. Antibacterial ointment or cream such as bacitracin is available over-the-counter. Silvadene is available by prescription only and is generally reserved for more extensive burns.[273]

Change the dressing daily to inspect for signs of infection. If the site has become infected, the burn may present with expanding areas of pinkness around the edges. Other signs include bad odor, pus, increased pain and warmth of the site, fever, and red streaks.

Conventional Treatments

In addition to the antibiotic ointment and Silvadene mentioned previously, Advil may be taken for pain. Other options for topical relief include benzocaine and lidocaine ointments or burn gels. When shopping around, keep in mind that some burn gels only contain 1/2% lidocaine, while others contain 4-5%. Make sure you're getting the maximum pain relief possible.

If infection develops, most doctors would prescribe Keflex, Augmentin, or erythromycin as first choices. Second line options would be doxycycline, Cipro, or Levaquin. Treatment would be continued for two days beyond resolution of the infection. In order to conserve the supply of antibiotics, bacitracin, Silvadene, and/or honey might also be recommended.[274]

Alternative Treatments

When it comes to alternative treatments for burns and pain management, options abound, many more than can possibly be included here. The following are those most applicable in a post-disaster scenario.

Aloe vera. Good for first and second-degree burns. If you have a plant, cut off a leaf, open it up, remove the gel, and apply it to the burn four to six times per day.[275]

Baking soda. Add 1/4 cup to a warm bath and soak for 15 minutes or more.[276]

Black tea

- Soak 3 tea bags in cool water for 5 minutes. Dip cotton compresses or gauze in the tea and apply to the burn area.
- Steep 4 tea bags and 2 cups fresh mint leaves in 4 cups boiling water. Strain the liquid into a jar and let cool. Dip cotton compresses or gauze in the tea and apply to the burn area.
- If the patient has to be mobile, use 3 wet tea bags that have cooled down. Wrap with gauze and tape in place.[277]

Essential oils

- Lavender oil may be applied without dilution.[278]
- Tea tree oil should be diluted in a little water before applying to the skin.[279]

Vinegar, any kind

- Dip a clean cloth into a 50-50 dilution of vinegar and cool water and apply to the burn. When the compress feels warm, re-soak and re-apply as often as desired.
- For a burn on the trunk of the body, soak a cotton t-shirt in the same solution.[280]

Honey. More clinical research has been conducted with using honey for burn treatment than with any other alternative treatment. Research studies demonstrated that honey-treated wounds healed more quickly with less bacteria. Over-hyped Medihoney or Manuka honey are not necessary. Regular raw, unprocessed honey will work just as well. Right after cooling the skin as above, apply a thick layer of honey all over the burn. Then cover it with cling plastic wrap. Change the dressing if fluid begins to ooze out, and regardless, change it at least three times per day for seven to ten days. Do not remove or wash off the honey for three weeks, unless healing is complete before that time. Add more honey often and fill in depressed areas as needed. Do not leave any burned skin exposed to the air.[281]

Note: Deep partial burns over joints will require physical therapy in the form of gentle stretches, five to six times per day for six months to a year.

Also, when dealing with hot liquids, cooking, or working with machinery, have a supply of clean cool water, preferably running, available for burn treatment. If running water is not an option, at least have some basins to pour water back and forth in case of an accident.

THIRD-DEGREE BURNS

Third-degree burns are full-thickness burns. There is no skin left, and no skin cells to re-grow new skin. These burns penetrate all the way into subcutaneous tissue and even muscles and bones. Naturally, there is going to be nerve damage. The edges of the remaining skin may appear black, brown, yellow, or white.[282] That affected area of the body may appear sunken if a lot of tissue has been lost. It is a bad sign when a substantial burn is not painful, as this suggests a very deep injury.[283]

The immediate treatment is the same as for second-degree burns: Cool the burn with cool running water for 15 minutes and remove all jewelry and constrictive clothing above and below the burn. In a functioning society, most third-degree burns are treated at burn centers.

Before getting into treatment options, let's take a look at the numbers you need to know.

- Use the rule of nines (covered above) to calculate how much of the body has been burned. Basically, the palm of the hand is 1% of the body surface. The head and neck and each arm are 9%. The chest, back, and each leg are 18% (2x9). The genitals are 1%.
- If the burn covers more than 10% of the body, the patient may go into shock. *This is a life-threatening situation.*
- If the burn covers more than 30% of the body, it is probably going to be fatal.
- If the burn covers more than 40% of the body, it is definitely going to be fatal. There won't be the resources to manage it.[284]

The treatment goals are to keep the burn clean and to prevent infection, dehydration, and shock. Accept the reality that there is going to be significant scarring.

Treatment for the burn itself is not complicated. After the burn has been cooled under running cool water for at least 15-20 minutes (but without causing hypothermia), apply honey generously all over the burned area and beyond the edges. Always maintain a thick layer of honey that extends beyond the edges of the burn. Cover the honey with plastic wrap or waterproof dressings. If and when the dressing begins to fill with fluid, change the dressing. More severe and extensive burns will necessitate more frequent changes. Regardless of the amount of fluid oozing, change the dressing at least three times per day. Continue this process for at least 7-10 days, and up to 20 days. Do not remove or wash off the honey for the first 20 days, unless healing is complete. Throughout this process, watch for any signs of infection.[285]

A substantial burn is going to cause dehydration, and as stated previously, even with a burn covering only 10% of the body, there is a significant risk of dehydration and shock. The patient must somehow increase fluid intake. The Parkland formula is what medical personnel use to calculate the volume of fluid to be administered in the first 24 hours following a burn: 3 ml/kg times the percent of body surface area burned.

If a patient weighs 50 kg (about 110 pounds) with 10% of the body burned, that is 3 ml multiplied by 50 kg multiplied by 10, or 1500 ml.

One-half of this amount must be administered in the first eight hours. The other half is given over the next 16 hours. After 24 hours, the amount of fluid administered is based upon urine output and other signs of perfusion. The goal in urine output is at least 50 ml per hour in an adult. If the urine output is less than this, give more fluids. If there is low blood pressure or other signs of shock, administer more fluids.[286]

Burn patients need a lot of additional protein and calories. Those with burns covering less than 20% of the body can manage by eating and drinking more, but normal eating will likely not be sufficient for those with burns covering more than 20% of the body.

Survival and Austere Medicine, 3rd Edition provides details on skin grafting for dealing with burns covering 5-10% of the body surface. That book is a free download and covers some conditions that other grid-down medicine books omit.

There's not a lot more that can be done for a burn patient. The pain is going to be substantial. The likelihood of infection is high, as is the demand for supplies. Keep in mind that large burns to limbs may not heal and the disability may be to such an extent that amputation is preferable.

TETANUS

Tetanus has been a reportable disease in the US since 1947, and cases of tetanus have decreased every year since reporting began. Annually, we have about 30 cases in the US. With only a few dozen cases each year, the vast majority of physicians in the US will not have any experience treating tetanus. Tetanus is actually much more of a third world disease with about 500,000 cases each year.[287] However, as decreasing numbers of people are immunized each year, those numbers in the US may start rising soon. Fortunately, tetanus is not contagious.

Causes

There are numerous ways for people to contract tetanus. The most common are:

- Animal bites, especially from dogs and pigs
- Gunshot and knife wounds
- Barbed wire
- Puncture wounds from thorns, splinters, nails, etc.

Tetanus can develop any time the skin is compromised, including from burns, lacerations, and crush injuries. Punctures just happen to be of greatest concern because the bacteria that cause tetanus, *Clostridium tetani*, are anaerobic bacteria. They thrive in the absence of oxygen, which is exactly what happens with puncture wounds. The wounds are deep, the oxygen supply is poor, and the bacteria grow. When these Gram-negative spores invade, they mature, become active, and start producing the tetanospasmin toxin that attacks nerves connected to muscles.

Prevention

The very best prevention is to be fully immunized as a child and to receive boosters every 10 years as an adult. In addition, wearing shoes when outdoors and long sleeves and gloves when working in the yard offer further protection.

Prophylaxis

Prophylactic measures should be taken with every wound, no matter how "trivial." Indeed, with many cases of tetanus, the patient has no idea how he became host to the bacteria. Even small splinters or a little prick from a thorn can become life-threatening.

Each and every wound must be cleaned thoroughly, no matter how small it is. Some physicians may prescribe further prophylactic treatment of taking an antibiotic such as penicillin, ampicillin, or metronidazole, to kill any *Clostridium* bacteria that may have entered the body.[288]

Signs and symptoms

It may take up to two weeks for the first symptoms of tetanus to appear. These symptoms include sore muscles, especially near the site of the injury, weakness, irritability, difficulty and discomfort in swallowing, and then lockjaw.[289]

As there are no lab tests to detect tetanus, diagnosis is made based on the signs and symptoms. An initial test a doctor may perform when examining a patient suspected of having tetanus is to test the knee reflexes. When the doctor taps the knee, a little bit of a response is normal. However, a significant kick up suggests tetanus (or meningitis, or poisoning).[290] To further differentiate from meningitis or poisoning, there is the spatula test. Touch the back of the throat with a spatula or other soft-tipped instrument. If the patient gags, it is highly unlikely that the patient has tetanus. If the patient experiences involuntary contraction of the jaw muscles and thus bites down on the spatula, there is a greater than 90% chance the patient has tetanus.[291]

As the disease progresses, the muscle spasms spread from the local area of injury and the jaw to the rest of the body. During this period, bright light, loud noises, and moving or touching the patient may trigger sudden spasms, which may be strong enough to dislocate or break bones. Accordingly, the patient must be protected as much as possible from these stimuli.[292] If the muscles that govern the movement of the diaphragm become affected, the patient's ability to breathe diminishes, and the patient may suffocate if mechanical ventilation is not available. Other symptoms include fever, high blood pressure, and irregular heartbeat.

Treatment

There is no cure for tetanus. Treatment lies in supportive care, the best methods of which may be impossible in a grid-down situation.

First, find the source of the infection, open it up, and clean it out. Bear in mind, that if the cause was a minor splinter or thorn prick, there may not be a wound to clean out. If available, a doctor will likely administer 1 million units penicillin IV, (preferred), or tetracycline.[293]

If intravenous antibiotics are not available, metronidazole, 375-500 mg 2x per day, or doxycycline, 100 mg 2x per day, may be prescribed.[294] These antibiotics are not killing the toxin; they are killing the bacteria. The bacteria cease reproducing, so they stopping making the toxin. There is nothing that will hasten removing the toxin that has bound to the nerves.[295]

In addition to antibiotics, valium (10-20 mg to start), diazepam, or phenobarbital may be administered to reduce spasms.[296] Magnesium sulfate, some beta blockers, or morphine might also be used to regulate involuntary muscle contractions.[297]

The patient may also require intravenous fluids.

Outcome

The mortality rate for tetanus cases ranges from 20 to 75%, depending on age. There is a 50% mortality rate for all tetanus patients treated in hospitals, 75% mortality in patients over the age of 60, and an 18% mortality rate for younger patients, except for newborns. Their mortality rate is much higher, and that is with modern hospital care.[298]

Newborns contract tetanus when dirty instruments are used to cut the umbilical cord, when the cord is not cut close to the body, or when the cut umbilical stump is kept tightly covered and not dry. When the mother is fully immunized, newborns are protected from tetanus. In newborns, the first signs of tetanus appear three to ten days after birth. The umbilical area is usually dirty or infected, and the baby usually cries continuously and is unable to suck.[299] If the baby stops nursing in the period from 5-15 days after birth, suspect tetanus. Nasogastric tubes are often inserted to feed the babies.

SHINGLES

According to the Centers for Disease Control, one in three Americans will suffer from shingles at least once. Those at risk of developing shingles are those who have had chickenpox. That's about 99% of people born before 1980. While children as young as nine have been afflicted with shingles, it generally affects only those over the age of fifty, and the risk increases with age. It more commonly occurs in individuals with lowered immune function, especially due to stress and chronic diseases. TEOTWAWKI might qualify as stressful, so it would be a good idea to learn a bit more about shingles now so that we can prepare for it.

Shingles (*Herpes zoster*) is an infection caused by the chickenpox virus. Interestingly, the virus is not contagious in that it cannot cause shingles in another person; however, it is contagious to those who have not had chickenpox or been vaccinated against the disease. Like with chickenpox, the patient is contagious until the blisters scab over. But in contrast to chickenpox, covering the blisters generally prevents spreading the disease to others at risk.

Risk factors

The greatest risk factors for developing shingles include:

- Over 60 years
- Female
- Caucasian
- History of immune disease
- Family history
- Injury
- Poor gut health
- Stress
- Taking drugs that affect the immune system[300]

Prevention

The best preventative measure would involve never getting chickenpox in the first place. It's a little late for most of us. There are two shingles vaccines. The first, Zostavax, only decreased the risk of developing shingles by half and the risk of the subsequent neuropathy by two-thirds.[301] The new vaccine, Shingrix, which came out in 2019, appears to be 97% effective.[302] Beyond this, the best bets for preventing shingles are maintaining good health and avoiding stress.

Symptoms

Before the shingles rash appears, many patients report feeling an itchiness or tingling sensation and can even feel it moving through the body. The first sign is a line or patch of painful blisters that suddenly appears, most often on the face, neck, chest, or back, and usually only on one side of the body. The pain of these blisters may be excruciating. Other possible symptoms include fever, enlarged lymph nodes, stomach upset, loss of appetite, and chills. Ear and lower back pain may also occur. The blisters last two to three weeks then disappear, but the pain may last much longer. Rare complications include encephalitis, pneumonia, hearing problems, and death.[303]

The greatest complication and fear concerns the onset of what's called post-herpetic neuralgia. About 10% of people will develop this extremely debilitating, burning or stabbing pain at the site of the blisters as the nerves are damaged. Healing may take up to a year, and the older the individual, the longer it takes.[304]

Conventional treatment

Antivirals such as acyclovir, valacyclovir, or famciclovir may be effective, but must be started within two to three days from the first appearance of the blisters to be effective.[305] That's going to require a trip to urgent care or the emergency room for most people, and that's in good times. These antivirals are available by prescription only in the US. However, they can be pretty easily obtained through overseas pharmacies.

While the pain of shingles can be extremely debilitating, it is not life-threatening. Some off-grid physicians recommend saving any antivirals you have stashed for more serious illnesses or more serious cases of shingles. However, if the eye or the area around it is affected, that patient should be treated with an antiviral to prevent permanent damage to the cornea and resulting blindness.[306]

To reduce irritating the blisters and shedding the virus, place bandages over the rash to prevent clothes from rubbing against them. Aspirin, Tylenol, Advil, and Aleve may all be taken for pain relief. Creams with lidocaine or capsaicin (but this latter may also exacerbate the pain) may be used for topical relief. Some have used cold packs, oatmeal baths, and calamine lotion.[307] A physician may prescribe a low-dose antidepressant like amitriptyline or if the patient is really in pain, and really lucky, an opioid.

Alternative treatments

A few herbs have been reported as effective in the treatment of shingles. St. John's wort is quite beneficial, internally and externally, especially when combined with a creosote bush (*Larrea tridentata*) tincture or infusion.[308] Lemon balm tea, three to five cups per day, may be taken while symptoms persist. Lemon balm tincture may also be used in a dosage of 1/4 teaspoon three to six times per day. This is also good for preventing recurrences. The tincture and the infusion may also be applied topically for relief from the pain.[309]

The following supplements have been shown to be helpful in healing and preventing future outbreaks: vitamin B12, L-lysine, L-carnitine, alpha-lipoic acid, and inositol. Consuming fruit as a regular part of the diet is also important. Nuts, dark chocolate, and L-arginine supplements should be avoided.[310]

14. BITES AND VECTOR-BORNE ILLNESSES

While basic hygiene and common sense will prevent many bites and the potential resulting diseases, there are other measures to take that will go a long way towards preventing getting bitten in the first place, whether from bugs that are barely visible or the family pet.

INSECTS AND ARTHROPODS

Bedbugs

Is there anything that can give a person the creepy-crawlies as well as the mere thought of having bedbugs? If it really did happen, how would you handle it? They can go months without feeding, if necessary. They can just chill in the seams of your mattress or in the wallpaper or in the furniture. How do you get rid of them?

It's not easy. Try finding their nests; they like to hang out in families and are often found with individuals of varying ages. In addition to the usual mattresses and furniture, bedbugs also live in linens and backpacks. They retreat into cracks in the walls and electrical outlets. The college-educated ones hang out in books. Unless their daytime accommodations can be located, it will be tough to eliminate them. When there are a lot of bedbugs, they may emit an odor that smells like rotting raspberries.

What do they look like? The eggs are difficult to see, pearl-white and the size of a pinhead. The brown adults are the size of an apple seed. Then there are the five nymph stages as the bedbug hatches from the egg and matures.

Once a bedbug has been identified, it's time to take immediate action to prevent an infestation. Clothes and linens need to be washed in hot, soapy water above 125°F. A hot dryer will also suffice.[311] Alternatively, in far northern latitudes in the winter, four to seven days of temperatures that don't get above 0°F may also work. Traditional pesticides like Malathion and those in the pyrethroid family like permethrin may kill them. Unfortunately, bedbugs are developing some resistance to permethrin, so it's wise to have an alternative in this situation. Diatomaceous earth is another option. Several treatments will probably be needed, just to be on the safe side. Vacuuming may help, if there is electricity.

Bedbug Repellent #1

1 cup water
10 drops eucalyptus essential oil
10 drops lavender essential oil
10 drops rosemary essential oil

Put the above in a spray bottle and shake well before using.

Bedbug Repellent #2

1 cup water
20 drops juniper berry essential oil
15 drops peppermint essential oil

Put the above in a spray bottle and shake well before using.

As far as disease management goes, bedbugs at least have a bright spot: they do not cause any illnesses in and of themselves, though they may carry other disease-causing organisms. In that respect they aren't as bad as body lice or fleas. They don't live in clothing seams, unlike body lice, or on your body, like fleas. They take their meals while you sleep and then go back to their daytime homes.

Identification. Bedbug bites look a lot like mosquito bites, but they usually have a pattern to them, unlike mosquitoes. They take a bite, or a whole breakfast, walk on for a little bit to digest, then stop for a bite of lunch, walk on to digest, then stop for a bite of dinner, and maybe a little dessert later on before retreating until tomorrow, or next week. It often looks like there are lines of bites on the body. Bedbug bites are also distinguished from fleas in that fleas normally bite around the ankle and usually have a central red spot. As bedbugs prefer open-air dining, or taking their bites from exposed areas of skin, most bites are on the face, neck and arms. Wearing pajamas may help in this case.

Prevention. As far as repelling the little beasts goes, Native Americans used juniper boughs to deter bed bugs with some efficacy. Other natural repellents include mint, black cohosh, bay leaves, and tobacco.

Keeping your environment and belongings clean and tidy at home and when away is of paramount importance in preventing an infestation. Ideally, you have to keep from bringing them home with you. Don't put suitcases and backpacks on the floor in hotels—the best place for them is the bathtub. The same goes for clothing—don't leave it on the floor. Keep areas around the bed clean and free of clutter. Once bedbugs invade, they're difficult to eradicate.

Treatment. Benadryl is administered for the allergic symptoms and itching, and hydrocortisone cream helps reduce the inflammation. That's it for treatment.[312]

Scabies

Unfortunately, while scabies is commonly found among the unwashed masses, it is very easily spread to all, even the very most hygienic and sanitary of people. There are numerous reports of transmissions to health care providers in hospitals. Compounding the problem is that many physicians aren't able to recognize a scabies infestation and the afflicted individual continues to suffer while spreading the buggers everywhere.

What exactly is scabies? It rhymes with *rabies* and is about as pleasant to consider. Scabies is a skin infection caused by the tiny burrowing mite *Sarcoptes scabiei*. The eight-legged mites reproduce on skin, but generally only the female burrows into the skin, where she lays eggs and lives. For months if permitted. Most infestations involve ten to fifteen scabies mites, though if untreated the infestation may quickly escalate into Norwegian scabies, with *millions* of mites involved. Worldwide, it's estimated that between 100 and 300 million people are affected at any given time.

Transmission. Scabies is highly contagious; Norwegian scabies is even more so. Both are transmitted by direct physical skin contact or by infested linens, clothing, or furniture. Because it is so contagious, usually the whole group of people living together are treated when one individual is infected. Infestations also occur in schools and hospitals. While scabies is most often passed to family members in the home, it is also spread easily in daycare centers, rehab centers, sports facilities, prisons, and public transportation. Though it is not really a sexually transmitted disease, it is often found in sexually active teens and young adults.

Signs and symptoms. For a first time occurrence, the symptoms may take two to six weeks to appear. During this incubation period, it's being spread to the rest of the family, who will also take two to six weeks to exhibit symptoms. What are the signs and symptoms of scabies? Nothing more than an itchy red rash on the skin. An itching so intense that its victims will do anything to get rid of it. An itching so intense that the sufferers cannot even sleep at night. Indeed, that is the biggest clue that the rash is scabies—the itching is worse at night. The itching is actually an allergic response to scabies' bites, eggs, and waste. In repeat infestations, the body has already been sensitized, so the response is much more rapid—in as little as 24 hours.

The scabies rash looks like tiny bites, pimples, hives or bumps under the skin. Sometimes the burrow tracks of the mites can actually be observed. A magnifying glass may help you see the mites going in and out of their burrows in the skin. Sounds lovely, doesn't it? The most common places for the scabies to burrow are where it's likely to be a little warmer and moister: wrist, arm, genitals (especially in males), breasts, armpits, elbows, waist, buttocks, and the areas between the fingers and toes. In babies and toddlers, scabies also burrow into the palms of their hands and soles of their feet.

One of the chief complaints of those afflicted with scabies is that physicians do not understand how intense the itching is and that a lot of treatments are ineffective. Furthermore, the intense scratching of the afflicted areas creates sores which can then become infected (impetigo) and require antibiotics to treat.

Norwegian scabies, or crusted scabies, is a much more serious form of scabies found most often in the immunocompromised (rheumatoid arthritis,

HIV, AIDS, chemotherapy) and elderly, where thick crusts of skin containing thousands of mites develop. It is extremely contagious. Noteworthy is that itching may be minimal or absent.

Scabies is often confused, even by physicians, with psoriasis. How are they differentiated? In psoriasis, lesions may or may not itch, they appear in patches, and they may cause the skin to flake or scale. In contrast, scabies lesions are intensely itchy and do not cause the skin to flake or scale.

Conventional treatment. There are no approved over-the-counter medications for treating scabies.

Conventional medications commonly prescribed to kill scabies include:

- 5% Permethrin cream (Elimite) is applied to the entire body and left on the skin for 8-10 hours. Permethrin cream is safe for individuals aged two months and older, including pregnant women.
- 25% Benzyl benzoate lotion
- 1% Lindane lotion is only for people who can't use other medications and children over the age of ten years. It is not for use in pregnant women or anyone who weighs less than 110 pounds. It may cause seizures. It is not a first choice treatment.
- 10% Sulfur ointment
- 10% Crotamiton cream is not for children, people over the age of 65, or pregnant or nursing women.
- Ivermectin is a veterinary medication. It is not for use in pregnant women or children under 33 pounds. It is not approved by the FDA for treating scabies, though it has been shown to be effective. The CDC recommends a dosage of 200 micrograms per kilogram of body weight in a single dose, followed by another dose two weeks later. Oral ivermectin has a greater risk of side effects than permethrin and usually does not work better. It is only used when topical medications have failed or the patient cannot tolerate them.

- Sulfur in petroleum jelly is one of the earliest known treatments for scabies. It is not FDA approved, but it is safe for pregnant women and children. It does not smell good.

Alternative treatments. What many patients do not realize is that even when the mites are killed, the itching may continue for several weeks afterward. After all, as noted above, the itching is due to biting, but it is also an allergic reaction to eggs and waste, which do not magically disappear from under the skin. The usual course is that the itching intensifies for the first week after treatment, and then gradually tapers off to no itching by the fourth week after treatment. Physicians often suggest antihistamines to reduce itching and help with sleep. Other methods of reducing the itching include:

- A bath with cool water and oatmeal
- Calamine lotion
- Paper towels dipped in rubbing alcohol and applied to the skin (limited usage for small areas of treatment)

The following are home remedies that scabies patients reported using. No claim is made as to efficacy or safety. Many of these sufferers had already tried conventional prescribed treatments, without finding any relief. However, as noted above, it takes time for the itching to subside even after the scabies have been killed, so patients may have improved even without these treatments.

- Vinegar
    - Apple cider vinegar bath
    - Full strength apple cider vinegar and salt soak (will burn, but only for a little while)
- Ivermectin and 10% permethrin
- Diatomaceous earth
    - Diatomaceous earth and baking soda mixed with water into a liquid paste applied all over the body twice, one week between applications

    - Diatomaceous earth and olive oil paste
- Essential oils
    - Neem oil bath daily for six weeks
    - Rosemary essential oil and tea tree oil
    - Witch hazel and tea tree oil
    - 1:1 Tea tree oil and olive oil to dab on affected areas
- Lysol
    - Lysol and Ben-Gay (with or without Vicks Vaporub)
    - Hot water and Lysol
- A hot bath with one to two cups of salt each night for a week
- Japanese honeysuckle (*Lonicera japonica*) leaves prepared as an infusion and used as an external wash

No matter what method of treatment is used, all bedding, towels, clothes, stuffed animals, any personal items that could harbor the mites need to be washed in water as hot as possible, but at least above 120°F. Items that cannot be washed need to be strictly avoided for at least three days.[313]

Lice

There are three kinds of lice; they have some things in common but other aspects that are unique to each.

Head lice are what most people are familiar with. They're about the size of a small sesame seed. While they do not typically carry disease, scratching can compromise the skin and introduce infections. Children are less bothered by lice; the bites don't cause them to itch like they do in adults, so they can become pretty infested before anyone notices. Unfortunately, lice are pretty easily passed from one child to another, whether it's just in playing together or sharing combs and brushes. If you happen to notice something suspicious and wonder whether it's lice or dandruff, here's a quick and foolproof test: Dandruff will flake and shake off; lice will not. If you're still unsure, and there is a black light available, nits (lice eggs) will fluoresce as blue dots attached to the hair near the scalp (the mature lice do not fluoresce).[314]

Body lice appear very similar to head lice, but they generally confine themselves to the body. They differ from head lice and pubic lice in that they live in and lay eggs on bedding and/or clothing, especially the seams, and only come out to feed. Body lice are larger than head lice and can live only one to two days off the host.[315] They cause severe itching in an area of infestation, with small red, swollen bumps or welts often found at the base of the neck or torso where they feed. Unlike head lice, body lice can spread diseases like typhus and trench fever. Left unchecked, they can actually bleed a person to death.[316]

Pubic lice (crabs) are difficult to see because of their smaller size and their preferred habitat, pubic hair. However, while pubic hair is home base, they're open to checking out new locations like mustache or armpit hair or eyelashes and eyebrows. They spread primarily through sexual intimacy and are considered a sexually-transmitted disease (STD) that is not prevented by using condoms. Pubic lice do not transmit other STDs. They can also be spread through sharing hairbrushes, towels, or clothing. They cause severe itching.

Prevention. The best prevention option, beyond strict hygiene and keeping clothes clean, especially when working among people who have lice, is to use permethrin. Permethrin kills lice, but not the eggs. However, it is long-lasting and will thus kill any newly hatched lice. Permethrin is available commercially in sporting goods stores where camping equipment is sold. It comes in spray bottles to easily apply it to clothing and gear and lasts several weeks.

Regardless of which treatment options are selected, all linens must be washed in hot water—at least 130°F. Burning would be better, if it's an option. Items that cannot be washed should be placed in plastic bags for two weeks (head and pubic lice) to five weeks (body lice). Combs and brushes should be soaked in alcohol or hot water (130°F) for an hour.[317]

Physicians often recommend Benadryl to relieve the itching.

Conventional treatments. For all lice, treatment options include the following over-the-counter commercial products:

- RID
  - Active ingredients are piperonyl butoxide and pyrethrum extract
  - Designed only for head lice, but physicians recommend it for pubic and body lice as well
  - Kills lice only, not eggs, so retreatment is required in seven days
  - Not for individuals allergic to ragweed
- Nix
  - Permethrin-based
  - Like RID, it is designed only for head lice, but physicians recommend it for pubic and body lice as well
  - Kills both lice and their eggs

Alternative treatments:

- Mix salt, vinegar, tea tree oil, and neem oil and apply daily for three weeks for head lice.[318]
- Apply witch hazel and tea tree oil after showering daily for three weeks for head and pubic lice.[319]
- Bathe daily with 1/2 cup each borax and hydrogen peroxide for three weeks.[320]
- Smother lice and nits with olive or coconut oil, and then use a nit comb to remove lice and nits. This will take a very long time and must be repeated three times per week for one month.
- Combine 20 drops of tea tree oil and 2 drops of lavender essential oil with 2 tablespoons of olive or coconut oil. Work thoroughly into hair at the scalp and cover with a shower cap. Leave this on for at least eight hours. A 2010 clinical trial in Australia demonstrated this was much more effective than commercial treatments.

- Shave the whole body and follow this with several hot baths.

Mosquitoes

Mosquitoes and the diseases they transmit truly are not much of a threat in the United States, even in more tropical locations. Air-conditioning, functioning sanitation systems, and municipal spraying programs for killing mosquitoes have kept mosquito populations in check.

There are dozens of diseases transmitted by mosquitoes; most are found only in third-world tropical countries. The illnesses are managed quite differently. As an ounce of prevention is worth a pound of cure, the first topic to be covered is preventing bites.

Bite Prevention

Use mosquito repellents. In the US, the Environmental Protection Agency advises using only EPA-approved repellents. EPA-approved repellents display an EPA registration number and must contain at least one of the active ingredients listed below. No number, no approved active ingredient=not approved. The higher the content of the active ingredients, the longer lasting each application and the more effective.

- DEET
- Picaridin
- Oil of lemon eucalyptus (not for children under 3 years)
- IR3535
- 2-Undecanone
- Para-methane-diol[321]

Apply repellents properly. If using sunscreen and mosquito repellent, apply the sunscreen first. Mosquito repellent should only be applied to exposed skin, not under clothing. Do not use on babies younger than two months. Instead, cover babies well with clothing and protect them with mosquito netting over cribs and strollers.[322]

Experiment now. If using natural or DIY repellents, try them out now to determine whether they are effective for you, and whether they will actually repel the mosquitoes in your area. Some natural repellents may be species-specific in their efficacy.

Treat clothing and gear. Permethrin treatment, even if it is not done professionally, lasts through several washings. Do not apply permethrin to the skin.[323]

Wear light-colored clothing. Cover the skin as much as possible. Clothing with a tight weave, especially those made with synthetic fibers and anything with an SPF rating, can prevent mosquitoes from biting through.[324]

Essential Oils Insect Repellent

1/2 cup apple cider vinegar
1/2 cup rubbing alcohol
50 drops total of at least three of the following essential oils:

Catnip
Citronella
Clove
Eucalyptus
Lavender
Lemongrass
Peppermint
Spearmint

Combine all ingredients in a small spray bottle. Use as needed.

Lotion Bar Insect Repellent

The same herbs and oils listed above can also be used to make insect repellent lotion bars. Let the herbs infuse in 1/2 cup of olive oil in a dark place for a month. Strain to remove the herbs. In a double boiler melt 1/2 cup of coconut oil and 1/2 cup of beeswax. Stir in the infused olive oil and pour into molds. When hardened, remove from molds and use as lotion.

Mosquito-proof the home.

- Mosquitoes generally stay within one to three miles from where they hatched.
- Remove standing water from around the house and any debris where they can lodge.
- Inside the home, keep a few fans running. Have you ever noticed that mosquitoes disappear when the wind comes up? Mosquitoes can't fly well in the wind. Use a fan to your advantage and bring that wind indoors.
- Repair all window and door screens.[325]

Some people are just genetically prone to attract mosquitoes, and there's nothing that can be done to change that. However, taking the above steps will go a long way towards preventing bites and the resulting discomfort. If we can prevent bites now when they're only an annoyance, we'll be better prepared to prevent them when they could be transmitting disease.

Fresh Herbs Insect Repellent

1 cup water
2 tablespoons peppermint or spearmint, finely chopped
6 tablespoons catnip (the best choice), lavender, and/or citronella, finely chopped
1 cup rubbing alcohol

Bring the water to a boil in a small saucepan. Remove from heat, add herbs, cover, and cool completely. Strain to remove the herbs. Add rubbing alcohol to the infused water. Pour into a spray bottle and store in the refrigerator. Use as needed.

Dried Herbs Insect Repellent

1 tablespoon catnip
1 tablespoon peppermint or spearmint
1 tablespoon lavender
1 tablespoon rosemary
1 tablespoon thyme
1 cup apple cider vinegar
1 cup water

Put herbs in a one pint canning jar. Add vinegar, place lid on jar, and shake well to combine. Store in a cool, dark place for three weeks, and shake daily. Strain out and discard the herbs. Pour remaining liquid into a spray bottle and add water. Store in the refrigerator and use as needed.

DIY Insect Repellent

Recipes for homemade mosquito repellent abound. The herbal options are likely to be more sustainable in the long-term. The fresh herbs option can be made and ready to use within an hour, if necessary. The essential oils recipe is another option.

Bear in mind that while the DIY options can work every bit as well as commercial repellents, *they do not last as long.* Homemade sprays will need to be reapplied frequently, perhaps even hourly.

Ticks

Unlike lice and bedbugs, which are insects, ticks are in the same family as spiders and scabies. Fortunately for us all, ticks do not reproduce as prolifically as lice, bedbugs, and scabies, and they're generally a lot easier to find—if you go looking for them. Ticks don't jump like fleas do, and they don't drop down from trees like spiders. Ticks in the larval stages prefer hanging out in leaf litter, just waiting for you to brush by so they can hitch a ride and see the world. Once on you, they crawl wherever their heart leads them—and their favorite hang-outs are behind the knees, between the legs, in the belly button and around the waist, in your hair, behind the ears, and under the arms.[326] Adult ticks are more commonly found on game trails, and all stages like chilling in a shady wood pile.

Prevention. When it comes to tick bites, prevention is far better than the cure. Prevent ticks from getting to your body by wearing long pants, and for the best protection, tucking pant legs into thick socks and wearing high top boots as well.[327]

> **Essential Oil Tick Repellent**
>
> 9 drops citronella essential oil
> 6 drops tea tree oil
> 6 drops peppermint oil
> 1 tablespoon carrier oil
>
> Combine and apply to exposed skin before going outdoors. Reapply often.

Stinking it up a bit (from the tick's point of view) will make you even more unappealing. DEET and picaridin work well. Permethrin is quite effective in treating clothing. Permethrin treats not only clothes, but also footwear and camping gear—and it remains effective through several washings.[328]

While being aware of places you're most likely to encounter ticks and preventing them from getting on you is essential, don't forget to check pets frequently. It's quite possible for a dog or cat to pick up hitchhikers outside and then drop them off in the house.

Studies show that taking a shower within two hours of getting home from an outdoor excursion substantially reduces the incidence of tick bites.[329] All clothing should be immediately washed in hot water (cold or warm water will not kill ticks) if possible, or at the very least placed in a dryer with a hot temperature setting for ten or more minutes.

Removing ticks. Even with the most diligent efforts, ticks will sometimes find their way to a meal on you. Fortunately, most diseases are not transmitted until 24 hours after the tick attaches. That's why early detection and removal are critical. The best bet for removing the whole tick is to grab it with tweezers and pull straight up, not at an angle. Pulling at an angle increases the chances of the mouth parts breaking off. However, if that happens, it's ok. The important thing is that disease transmission has been halted. With the tick parts still in your skin, there will probably be a bit of a reaction, as well as some inflammation and irritation. Disinfect the area by washing with soap and water and using Betadine or triple antibiotic.[330]

Signs and symptoms. If disease happens to have been transmitted, it can take up to thirty days for symptoms to appear. A health care provider must always be informed of any recent tick bites. The most common symptoms, especially for Lyme disease, include a rash and influenza-like complaints, especially fever and a general achy feeling.

The geography of ticks. The CDC has generated several geographic distribution maps[331] for the most common species of ticks in the United States. Check them out to see which ticks are most common in your location and for any further specific actions to take for protection.

> **Tick Tubes**
>
> What you'll need:
>
> Cardboard toilet paper or paper towel tubes (cut paper towel tubes into two or three pieces)
> Cotton balls (or dryer lint)
> Permethrin
>
> Dilute permethrin with water so that it is a 7-7.5% solution. How much water is needed depends on the concentration of permethrin. If you are using 36.8% permethrin, about one part permethrin to five parts water will yield a 7.5% solution.
>
> Spray the cotton balls well with the permethrin solution and then let them dry. Now stuff the cardboard tubes with the permethrin cotton balls. Place the tubes in discreet areas around the perimeter of the yard. Mice will take the cotton balls to build their nests. The ticks, which reproduce in mice nests, are killed on contact with permethrin. The mice remain unharmed.
>
> Permethrin also kills beneficial insects like bees and butterflies, so it's not something to be used indiscriminately around the yard.

Tick-Borne Bacterial Diseases

Ticks spread pain and suffering in a much wider variety of ways than lice and scabies. Their bites can transmit bacteria, viruses, and other parasites. Some species of ticks may carry more than one kind of disease.

Signs and symptoms. The common signs and symptoms are headache, rash, muscle and joint pain, and altered mental status.

Prophylaxis. If you have the resources, every patient presenting with a tick bite in a high risk area may be given doxycycline in a 200-mg single dose.[332] The CDC only recommends this practice if the bite occurs in an area endemic for Lyme disease. They advise against this prophylactic treatment for other tick-borne diseases.

Treatment. Even today, if a patient indicates he has been bitten by a tick, and he displays signs and symptoms consistent with a tick-borne disease (and which are common to many illnesses), a physician will start him on a course of antibiotics immediately. Blood test results take time, and at least one of these tick-borne illnesses can quickly become fatal. If a patient reports flu-like symptoms after a tick bite, antibiotics are automatically administered.[333]

Regardless of whether a tick-borne disease is identified sooner or later, antibiotics are still used. Those identified later may need a longer course of therapy, up to four weeks, and there is the possibility of suffering the consequences for life.

The treatment for most tick-borne diseases that are bacterial in origin is the same—doxycycline. Physicians typically prescribe doxycycline at 100 mg, 2x per day, 10-14 days. Amoxicillin is another option, 500 mg, 3x per day, 14 days.[334]

Lyme disease. Lyme disease mimics many other illnesses with rashes, headaches, and muscle and joint aches, and has a very long incubation period—up to 30 days. If a patient recalls being bitten by a tick that helps with diagnosis, but most patients—over 60%—do not recall being bitten. Remember, a tick doesn't latch on and stay on. It attaches for a very long feeding and then falls off. Early signs include a characteristic bullseye rash around the site of the bite. There may be meningitis or inflammation of heart muscle, neither of which is going to be easily diagnosed in an austere environment. Later symptoms include severe arthritis involving many joints or chronic meningitis—headaches, problems in thinking clearly, and sleepiness.

The ticks that carry Lyme disease are found all over the US, but most infections occur in the Northeast and North Central US.[335]

Rocky Mountain spotted fever. The ticks carrying this disease are found throughout the US, but most frequently identified in Arizona, Oklahoma, Missouri, Arkansas, Tennessee, and North Carolina. The incubation period is three to twelve days. Early signs (one to four days) include a high fever, severe headache, gastrointestinal symptoms (nausea, vomiting, anorexia), and edema around the eyes and on the back of the hands. Later signs include altered mental status, cerebral edema, pulmonary edema and respiratory distress, necrosis (tissue death requiring amputation), and kidney failure. If there is any suspicion of RMSF, begin treatment immediately. Delay may be fatal.[336]

The rash associated with RMSF begins two to five days after the onset of symptoms. The small, flat, pink, non-itchy spots first appear on the wrists, forearms, and ankles and sometimes spread to the trunk, palms and soles. About 10% of patients never develop a rash and the decision to begin treatment should not be based on the presence of a rash. Later, the rash turns red to purple. This is a sign of severe progression of the disease and treatment should have already begun.[337]

Rickettsiosis. The ticks that carry this disease are found in the southeast and Mid-Atlantic US, as well as southern Arizona. The incubation period is two to ten days. The disease is less severe than RMSF, but the symptoms and treatment are the same.[338]

Ehrlichiosis. The ticks that carry this disease are found in the southeast and south-central US. In addition to the symptoms of RMSF, other symptoms include chills and diarrhea. The incubation period is 5-14 days.[339]

Anaplasmosis The ticks that carry this disease are found in the Upper Midwest and Northeastern US. Additional symptoms and incubation period, as well as the treatment, are the same as for ehrlichiosis. There is the possibility of co-infection with Lyme disease.[340]

Tick-borne relapsing fever. The ticks that carry this disease are found primarily in the western US. Most cases occur when people sleep in rustic cabins, whether in the summer when ticks are most active or in the winter when fires are heating cabins and ticks nesting in walls and woodwork are activated. The incubation period is about seven days. The febrile periods last three days, followed by a seven-day break, then another three-day fever, and so on. The symptoms are headache, myalgia, chills, nausea, and vomiting. The usual antibiotics are tetracycline or erythromycin, both in the same dosages: 500 mg, 4x per day, 10 days.[341]

Tick-Borne Viral Diseases

In addition to the bacterial diseases caused by tick bites, it's probably a good idea to consider the viruses that tick bites can spread as well. Though generally not so serious as the bacterial tick-borne diseases, the viral diseases ticks transmit may also cause substantial harm, even death. Without advanced medical care and lab facilities available, these viral tick-borne diseases are going to be particularly difficult to identify and treat. In most cases treatment is only supportive and often a patient will never know what it was that made him sick.

Colorado tick fever. This rare viral disease transmitted by the bites of infected Rocky Mountain wood ticks (*Dermacentor andersoni)* cannot be transmitted from person to person (except in the case of a blood transfusion). These ticks are only found in the Rocky Mountains of North America at elevations of 4,000 to 10,000 and are most active March through August. Onset of symptoms from the time of the tick bite ranges from one to fourteen days. The most common symptoms are fever, headache, chills, fatigue, body aches, and exhaustion. Some patients may experience sore throat, stomachache, vomiting, rash, or a stiff neck. Like some other tick-borne illnesses, the patient may experience several days of illness, followed by a recovery period, and then followed again by more fever and illness.[342]

Heartland and Bourbon virus. Heartland viral disease afflicts people mainly in Missouri and Tennessee between the months of May and September. It is believed to be caused by the bites of lone star ticks. The symptoms are very similar to another tick-borne disease, ehrlichiosis, and include fever, headache, body aches, fatigue, and various stomach problems. Bourbon virus was first identified in Bourbon County, Kansas, and since then other cases have been found in Missouri and Oklahoma. These very rare diseases cause joint and muscle pain, rashes, fever, and fatigue.

There are no specific medications for treating these diseases. Most patients recover completely within a few days. Supportive care for reducing pain and fever and increasing fluid intake may be desired.[343]

Powassan viral disease and Powassan encephalitis. This is a serious viral disease spread by blacklegged (*Ixodes scapularis*) or groundhog (*Ixodes cookei*) ticks. Fortunately, there is no person to person transmission of this disease. Most cases of this disease occur in the northeastern US and Great Lakes areas from April through October. The incubation period ranges from one week to one month. More serious symptoms include dementia, muscle weakness, seizures, and even death. As there is no medicine to treat this disease, most treatment is supportive and may include hospitalization and IV fluids.

Bee and Wasp Stings

When a bee stings, she loses her stinger. (Female honey bees are the only insects to lose their stingers and die. Most other species of bees and male bees do not have stingers.) She may escape and fly a little distance, but death is imminent. When that sting happens, the bee sends out pheromones in the process. That pheromone is a banana-like scent telling all the other bees in the vicinity that an attack is underway and beckoning all to join in the fight as noble kamikazes.[344]

A victim may experience multiple stings, but they are from different bees. This is why it is critical to teach everyone to leave the vicinity where they were stung immediately.

For most of us, bee and wasp stings are merely an annoyance and the pain resolves without complications. For 3% of the population, however, even a single bee sting is life-threatening, and nearly 100 people die from these stings in the US each year. Individuals with a known allergy to bee or wasp stings should carry an Epi-pen at all times when outdoors.

Six tips to reduce the risk of getting stung

Wear light-colored clothing

Avoid perfume, cologne, scented toiletries, and especially anything banana-scented

Wear clean clothes and bathe daily (sweat makes bees mad)

Cover as much skin as possible

Avoid flowering plants

Don't swat at flying insects

Treatment. Unfortunately, these life-threatening anaphylactic reactions aren't always known. The first bee sting a person has rarely causes an anaphylactic response. It's a subsequent sting that becomes problematic. Anaphylactic reactions usually develop within the first hour of a sting. If someone is suspected to be developing an anaphylactic response, there are a few options if there is no Epi-pen nor medical facilities immediately available. The first choice is Benadryl liquid or chewable, if they're available, as these get into the bloodstream faster. Other options are H2 blockers like Zantac or Pepcid. Primatene Mist and oral steroids like prednisone may also help.[345] The patient will probably need intramuscular injections of epinephrine, antihistamines, and steroids in the hospital.

After being stung and removing to a safe distance, remove the stinger as quickly as possible. Using a fingernail to scrape it out is the preferred method. Tweezers may actually squeeze any venom remaining in the stinger into the patient. The longer the stinger remains in the body, the greater the chances for a worse reaction.[346] Next, wash the area surrounding the sting thoroughly with soap and water. Ice packs and lidocaine or benzocaine anesthetic ointments will reduce swelling and provide topical relief.

Several hours after the sting it is common to develop a local hypersensitivity reaction. This is not an infection and the goal is to provide symptomatic relief.

In addition to the cold packs and anesthetic ointments used right after a sting, any of the following remedies may be used:

- Benadryl. An oral medication will offer the best relief, but is not for children under the age of six without first consulting a doctor. Benadryl cream or spray may be used in children over the age of two years.[347]
- Tylenol or Advil for pain
- Antibiotic ointment to prevent infection
- Essential oils—lavender, helichrysum, tea tree, peppermint, 1-2 drops on the site, 3x per day[348]

- Baking soda paste[349]
- Activated charcoal paste
- Plantain leaf poultice

A physician may also treat a severe local reaction with oral steroids like prednisone if available. Individuals who have a severe reaction, even anaphylaxis, with bee stings and who wish to be better prepared may consider working with an allergist to reduce their sensitivity.

Wasp stings are similar to bee stings, but at the same time, entirely different. Unlike bees, wasps do not die when they sting. Because they have smooth stingers rather than barbed stingers like bees, they can continue to sting away as long as they wish. Bee venom is acidic; wasp venom is alkaline. The theory behind a baking soda paste is that the base neutralizes the acid of a bee sting to provide relief. Based on that, a baking soda paste would not work with a wasp sting. However, because the venom is injected quickly and spreads rapidly, the venom isn't available to chemically react with the baking soda. Because wasp venom is close to neutral anyway, it's not likely that the pain from the sting is due to the alkalinity of the venom.

Spider Bites

Frequently, what a patient believes to be a spider bite is not actually a bite at all. The fact is that most spiders have fangs too small or fragile to break through human skin. That little raised red mark with what looks like a central puncture to it is often a MRSA infection. If it gets bigger, antibiotics may be required. (Penicillin-family antibiotics are useless in this situation. The drugs of choice here would be trimethoprim-sulfamethoxazole or doxycycline.)[350]

Fortunately, when a spider bites, it doesn't usually break the skin. However, if you do happen to get bitten by a spider, kill it and take it to the doctor for positive identification. Lots of people overreact and mistakenly believe they have been bitten by a black widow or brown recluse, when in fact it was just a common non-venomous spider.

Unfortunately, most people fail to catch the spider.

Common Spider Bites. Most spider bites are not cause for concern and rate right up there with mosquito bites. How people react to them varies greatly, whether it's a non-venomous spider or a black widow.

The following are common natural treatments for spider bites. They may also be used for black widow and brown recluse bites *when there is no other option*.

After cleaning the bite site with soap and water, do any of the following to alleviate pain and swelling, singly or in combination:

- Elevate the affected body part
- Apply ice
- Apply a baking soda paste in a 3:1 ratio of baking soda to water several times per day
- Lavender essential oil, a few drops applied with or without dilution in a carrier oil directly on the bite site
- Apply an aspirin paste (grind up aspirin and make a paste as with baking soda)
- Wintergreen essential oil, a few drops diluted in carrier oil and applied to the bite site
- Raw peeled and shredded potato poultice, with potato shreds placed in between layers of gauze and replaced when potatoes dry out
- Apply witch hazel
- Apply aloe vera gel
- Activated charcoal poultice, applied for 1-2 hours, 2x per day

Black Widow Bites. With a functioning medical system black widow bites are cause for a quick trip to the ER, during which time any of the above remedies may be applied to relieve the pain. They are not a substitute for competent medical care.

Black widows are found mainly in the southwestern United States. They're more active at night and like to hang out in garages, sheds, and barns—any place nice and dark. Most black widows are a glossy black color. Southern black widows have the infamous red hourglass pattern on the abdomen; this hourglass may be absent or harder to see in other subspecies.[351]

Black widow venom, a neurotoxin, is potent stuff and hits the central nervous system hard, but the reaction varies considerably from person to person. The bite site itself is a raised red bump, and with the naked eye one may be able to identify the two punctures. Intense pain is the first symptom, which occurs pretty quickly after being bitten. According to one patient, the pain initially was that of an ant bite, then it progressed pretty quickly to a bee sting, and within 20-30 minutes it was at the level of "SHOOT ME NOW!" The pain may spread from the bite site to the back and abdomen.

As the reaction of patients varies widely, they may experience any of the following symptoms:

- Weakness
- Shakiness
- Fainting
- Chest pain
- Breathing difficulties
- Muscle cramps at the bite site or all over the body
- Abdominal pain
- Profuse sweating and salivation
- Nausea and vomiting
- Disorientation or mental confusion
- Increase in heart rate
- Increase in blood pressure[352]

Black widow bites are much more serious in children, seniors, and those with compromised immune systems, but fortunately are rarely fatal. Physical health and the age of the patient have the most significant effect on the course of illness and the outcome.

Tylenol and Advil are often recommended for pain. Narcotics used to be prescribed, but they're a lot harder to come by in the current environment.

Benadryl may help alleviate inflammation and itching. Hot and cold compresses may also be used. An activated charcoal poultice for removing the toxin from the body is highly recommended, as is taking capsules internally. A warm bath may help alleviate muscle cramps.

Brown Recluse Bites. The brown recluse spider, also called the violin spider because of the violin-shaped pattern on its back, is most commonly found in the warm, dry climates of the southern Midwest and South. It inhabits dark, quiet areas like basements and closets and areas behind furniture. The initial bite is usually painless, but within eight hours any or all of the following symptoms may manifest:

- Burning, itching, pain and/or redness at the bite site
- Red or purple ring or target pattern around the site
- Fluid-filled blister at the bite that may become an ulcer[353]
- Additional possible symptoms include:
- Headache
- Fever
- Chills
- Nausea and vomiting

More rarely, symptoms may include:

- Coma
- Jaundice
- Blood in urine
- Kidney failure
- Seizures

Like black widow bites, brown recluse bites are rarely fatal, but they are much more serious in children, seniors, and those with compromised immune systems. All of the above methods for dealing with common spider bites may be employed with brown recluse bites. However, just as with black widow bites, *none of these is a substitute for competent medical care when it is available.*

When there is no higher medical care anywhere, there are two alternative treatment options that have shown positive results.

- Apply a poultice of *Echinacea angustifolia* or *Echinacea purpurea* (the former is much stronger) to the bite. Change the poultice 2-3 times each day. An echinacea tincture may also be taken internally, 4-8 ml of a 1:4 tincture, 2-3 times each day.
- Apply a poultice of activated charcoal moistened with lavender essential oil. Change this poultice every two to three hours. Activated charcoal may also be taken internally. Be aware that it will turn the stool black.[354]

VENOMOUS SNAKEBITES

The numerous species of venomous snakes in the continental US inject their victims with either a neurotoxin (coral snakes) or hemotoxin (everything else, with the exception of the Mojave rattler, which has both kinds of toxin). All snakes are most active in warmer temperatures and seasons, so that is when bites occur. Unlike what is shown on TV, especially the old westerns, many snakes are active at night and they hide in logs, under rocks, and in old structures. Especially in contrast to what's on TV, a snake doesn't always leave the scene of the crime. It may still have venom to inject. If the snake didn't flee the scene, the victim and everyone else should. If possible, killing the snake for positive identification is an idea. Just be aware that a dead snake is not necessarily harmless; it can still bite for up to 90 minutes after the head has been severed from the body. Be careful, though: a lot of people are actually bitten while trying to kill snakes.

Rattlesnake bites are generally the most dangerous in the US. There is a wide range of toxicity among the species of rattlesnakes. Recent research has shown that as far as rattlesnakes are concerned, the larger the snake, the more toxic the venom.[355] (FYI, poisons are absorbed through the digestive tract or the skin; venom enters the blood directly.)[356]

Venomous snakes have hollow fangs through which they deliver their venom; however, not every bite is envenomating. That is, about 25-30% of bites are actually *dry*.[357] No venom, no ill effects. Another 30-40% of bites are considered lightly envenomating because the snake either didn't inject much or some was lost in the air before or after the bite.[358] With rattlesnakes only, denim for some reason reduces the amount of venom injected by about 60%.[359] Even full envenomation does not necessarily equal death. Beyond that, a lot will depend on the age and size of the patient. Younger children are more at risk than older children and adults.

Before going any further, how do you know that the snakebite was from a poisonous snake? Look at the bite mark pattern. Bites from venomous snakes will leave two distinct punctures from the fangs, and possibly two rows of little marks made by the other teeth. Conversely, bites for non-venomous snakes will leave two distinct rows of teeth marks for the bottom teeth, and four rows for the top teeth.[360]

Now, how do you know whether the snakebite was envenomating? The first clue is that there is a burning pain at the site almost immediately. Within a few minutes, swelling begins and starts traveling up the affected limb. Pit viper bites (rattlesnake, cottonmouth, copperhead) may cause bruising and blisters at the bite site. The afflicted area may become numb. The lips or face may also become numb, and some bite victims will say they have a metallic or odd taste in their mouths. A severe bite may cause spontaneous bleeding from the nose or gums. The extremities may become numb or start tingling 30-90 minutes later, followed shortly thereafter by nausea, vomiting, and/or fainting. During this time the swelling and discoloration of the afflicted limb continues to spread.[361]

Coral snakes have a different type of toxin, a neurotoxin, and thus affect the body in a totally different manner. Symptom onset is much later, from four to six hours and up to twelve hours after the bite. Coral snake venom causes mental and nerve changes such as muscle twitching, mental confusion, and slurred speech. As the venom spreads, the central nervous system is affected, and there may be problems with swallowing and breathing, and even complete paralysis.[362] Coral snakes are distinguished from non-venomous king snakes by the following ditty: "red touches yellow, you're a dead fellow; red touches black, you're ok jack" or something along those lines. As long as you're in North America. It's not necessarily true elsewhere.

Some of the distinguishing characteristics of each of the families of venomous snakes:

Copperheads have the least potent venom and thus the lowest mortality rate. Supposedly they are not aggressive, but they account for the highest number of bites. Their bites result in localized tissue destruction.

Cottonmouth (water moccasin) venom is next in potency. They become aggressive when provoked. Unlike other non-venomous water snakes, they swim on top of the water.

Rattlesnakes are next in potency, but it varies widely among the species. Pygmy rattlers are much less toxic than Mojave rattlers, which are more often deadly. Most snakebite deaths in the US are attributed to Eastern and Western diamondback rattlesnakes. Numerous species of rattlesnakes are found throughout the continental US. The bite causes toxicity throughout the body as well as an ugly wound.

Coral snakes possess the most potent venom but are the least aggressive, and death from their bites is rare.[363]

Bites from non-venomous snakes and non-envenomating bites are still cause for concern. They are puncture wounds, and there is always the potential for infection as with any other puncture wound. However, they are less likely to cause infection than cat, dog, or human bites, so antibiotics are not routinely prescribed in this situation.[364]

Conventional treatment

The treatment, always, is to get to a hospital for antivenin, also known as antivenom . Nobody carries it in a medical kit or an ambulance because about

10% of people treated with antivenin will have an allergic reaction to it and need to be at a hospital to be treated for the reaction to the antivenin.[365]

Lacking hospitals and antivenin, how does one go about treating a venomous snakebite in an austere environment?

- Keep the patient calm
- Remove all jewelry and any potentially constricting clothing immediately
- Immobilize the limb below the heart. The venom moves in the lymph. Any movement at all moves the toxin into the body faster
- Clean the wound thoroughly, irrigating copiously to remove venom that is not deep in the bite
- Use a Sharpie to outline the edge of the swelling and do this frequently to track progression
- Complete bed rest for at least 24-48 hours[366]

What about using a Sawyer extractor? They're very popular among outdoor enthusiasts and survivalists. The doctors and authors of off-grid medicine books all pretty much agree: the Sawyer extractor does nothing.[367] So what about claims from people who have used them and didn't suffer the ill effects of a snakebite? Remember that 25-30% of bites are non-envenomating. Another 30-40% are only lightly envenomating. That's what worked. However, if you've already got one, and if someone is bitten, it can still be used. While doing other things to manage the patient and the bite, give the extractor to someone else to use on the patient. The patient will calm down because he feels something is being done. That's the first thing that needs to happen for treatment.

That's it in the conventional world of medicine, if you don't get to a hospital where antivenin can be administered. There is nothing

Snakebite DON'TS

Don't cut the bite and attempt to suck out the venom

Don't numb with ice

Don't give the patient alcohol or caffeine

Don't apply a tourniquet

Don't use a stun gun

more you can do beyond offering OTC pain meds and antibiotics if infection sets in. Recovery may take weeks to months.

Alternative treatment

However, in the alternative medicine world, there is a lot more that can be done. At least it has been done with animals, with excellent results. The treatments below have only been used with snakebites in animals and with poisonous spider bites in people. No one has gone on record using these treatments for snakebites in people. In a functioning society with advanced medical care, snakebite victims are always sent to a hospital. The potential consequences of doing otherwise in a litigious society such as ours are too significant.

Activated charcoal. If the wound is open enough and fresh enough (less than 30 minutes have passed), make a poultice or plaster with water. If possible, make a little bath in a basin or small tub to soak the limb in. Bear in mind that the activated charcoal has to get to the afflicted tissue to be effective. It will not work through intact skin. Do this for 30-60 minutes. Once a day for the next five to seven days, give the patient one capsule (00 size, or ½ teaspoon) of activated charcoal, two hours before or after any herbs that are taken internally.[368]

Echinacea angustifolia, pallida,* and/or *purpurea are all used. The herbalists disagree on which is more potent. I suspect it could have something to do with the climate the herbs are grown in. Regardless of which you use, apply a plaster or poultice immediately and change it every two to four hours. Also administer the *Echinacea* tincture internally. Recommendations vary from one tablespoon three times per day for an adult to one tablespoon every two to four hours for the first day, then twice per day for a week.[369]

Milk thistle seed, **plantain**, **Joe Pye weed,** and **nettles** are all recommended for additional support to the body.[370]

Dandelion root, echinacea root, plantain, and **mallow** in equal parts topically and internally every four hours should also be used. If the herbs are fresh, grind them up and apply. If they are dried, mix them up with a little water for a poultice. Change the poultice every four hours. Take the tea (or a tincture of these herbs) internally every two to four hours the first day, then twice per day for a week. This formula may not work for coral snake bites.[371]

DOMESTIC ANIMAL BITES

Dog and cat bites happen all the time now. Knowing how to treat bites and being prepared to do so is a fundamental skill no one should lack. As always, an ounce of prevention is worth a pound of cure. Children should be taught from a very young age to stay away from an animal that is eating, but also one that is playing too roughly. Everyone should avoid an animal that is angry, aggressive, or ill.

Bites in general

Treatment. All animal bites should be cleaned thoroughly with clean, soapy tap water, sterile water, or saline. Use a blunt tip syringe or bulb syringe to irrigate underlying tissues. Taking eight to ten minutes to do this would not be excessive. Your best bet is to wash away all bacteria and any remaining tooth fragments to prevent infection. Jagged edges of skin may need to be trimmed away for better healing.

Lacerations, where the skin is torn, are managed differently than punctures. In general, lacerations may be closed. Punctures are usually not closed until five days after the injury, when there is no sign of infection.

Animal bites to the hands do not get closed by any means. All are considered grossly contaminated, even after immediate and thorough cleaning, and are extremely prone to infection. That bacteria must not get trapped in the wound by closing it. If the bite is on the arm or hand, all jewelry must be removed, even if it's far away from the bite. The same goes for anklets and toe rings with bites on the lower extremities. A bite to the face or neck may be closed if it occurred less than twelve hours previous.

If no infection has set in five days after the bite occurred, then the wound may be closed.

Dog Bites

Dog bites account for about 85% of domestic animal bite wounds. Of these, about 20% will be serious enough to warrant professional medical attention. Dog bites involve the hands about two-thirds of the time and the face the remaining one-third. Children ages five to nine years are most at risk. Statistics show that the biting dog is known to the child 70% of the time, and half the time the children say the attack was unprovoked.[372]

The bacteria most commonly found in dog bites are *Streptococcus viridans*, *Bacteroides*, and *Staphylococcus aureus*; *Pasteurella multocida* is also sometimes found.[373]

Treatment. Prophylactic treatment for dog bites most often prescribed by physicians is Augmentin, 250-500 mg, 3x per day, 3-5 days. This preventative treatment begins immediately after the dog bite, before any signs of infection are observed. It is to prevent an infection from developing. Alternative prophylactic antibiotic regimens include:

- Penicillin, 500 mg, 4x per day, 3-5 days
- Amoxicillin, 500 mg, 3x per day, 3-5 days
- Doxycycline, 50-100 mg, 2x per day, 3-5 days (but not for children under the age of nine, or pregnant or nursing women)
- Erythromycin, 250-500 mg, 3-4x per day, 3-5 days
- Do not use Keflex[374]

With an established infection, the same antibiotics are prescribed for seven to ten days.

Cat Bites and Scratches

Everything about cat bites also applies to cat scratches, though most scratches are superficial and do not cause any trouble. If the scratch is deeper, treat it like a bite. Cat bites account for about 15% of domestic animal bites, and most victims are adult women. It's usually the hands that are affected, and statistics indicate that the cat is usually provoked into biting.[375]

Physicians always take a cat bite seriously. Most cats carry the *Pasteurella multocida* bacteria, and every cat bite should be considered infected. Cat bites on the back of the hand are particularly troubling because the infection can quickly spread to underlying tendons.[376]

Treatment. Prophylactic treatment for cat bites is highly recommended. It is not being wasteful or careless with resources. The antibiotic choices are the same as for dog bites. Just as for dogs, prophylactic treatment is administered for three to five days. If any sign of infection is present, antibiotics are administered for seven to ten days.[377]

RABIES

Human cases of rabies are rare in the US, with generally only two to three occurrences per year, most of which are contracted overseas.[378] However, more than 50,000 people worldwide die from rabies each year, and most of these cases are due to bites from unvaccinated dogs. In developed countries wildlife exposure is the most common cause of rabies deaths. With modern medicine available, *any* encounter with a bat warrants receiving the rabies vaccination. The most insignificant of scratches can be fatal.

Vaccination is required by law for veterinarians and veterinary office workers. It is recommended for cave explorers and those traveling to rabies-endemic regions.[379] Pre-exposure immunization is over $500 and is usually not covered by insurance. At the very least, make sure your pets are vaccinated for their protection and especially for yours.

What can we do?

Prevention

Strange behavior and excessive salivation are signs of rabies. In addition, nocturnal animals will appear during the day, and most will show aggressive behavior. Rabies, an exclusively mammalian disease, is most commonly spread by raccoons, skunks, bats, opossums, coyotes, foxes, and dogs. There has never been a documented case of rabies transmission to humans in the US from cows, squirrels, rabbits, rats, sheep, or horses.[380]

If there is any concern that an animal has rabies, that animal should be isolated and observed for at least a week. A biting animal with rabies usually dies within five to seven days. As rabid animals are only contagious the last few days before dying, observe the animal. If it doesn't die within ten days, it doesn't have rabies.[381] Any unvaccinated pet or animal whose vaccination has lapsed that has been bitten or otherwise attacked by another animal should be isolated for at least seven to eight weeks. In most cases, if rabies is going to manifest, it will happen during this period. However, keep in mind that sometimes rabies symptoms can take up to two years to develop.[382]

Prophylaxis

In people, signs of rabies usually appear one to three months after initial exposure. However, the signs may take up to two years to appear. The first course of action whenever someone has been bitten or scratched by an animal suspected of having rabies (and any bat contact at all) is to seek medical attention and the life-saving prophylactic rabies vaccines, currently a course of five shots administered over a two-week period.[383] That will likely not be an option in a disaster.

Is there anything that can be done?

Studies suggest that vigorous scrubbing and irrigation of the wound may reduce the risk of transmission. While washing and scrubbing with soap is good, benzalkonium chloride is best as it has demonstrated some efficacy against the rabies virus.[384] Antibacterials, including iodine, have zero efficacy against viruses. The caregiver must don gloves to protect himself, and then the wound should be irrigated with a syringe and scrubbed vigorously for at least 10 minutes to flush out the virus, saliva, debris, and bacteria.[385] Do not close the wound, but keep it bandaged to prevent infection.[386]

Signs and symptoms. Early symptoms of rabies include fever, headache, over-sensitivity to light and sound, difficulty swallowing, and (in animals) a fear of water. Once the sickness has begun, there is no known treatment to save a person's life.

15. COMMUNICABLE DISEASES

There are numerous communicable diseases to prepare for. Americans regularly vaccinate for the most common ones—measles, mumps, rubella, diphtheria, pertussis, polio, etc. Those who forgo the vaccinations need to know how to treat these diseases. It's difficult, because there is very little practical information on identifying these diseases and the protocols for treating them without modern medicine. The vast majority of doctors have never even seen patients with these illnesses, so they may be at a loss as well. This chapter will only address those communicable diseases for which we don't have readily available vaccines, which can be fatal, and which do not have to be fatal if antibiotics are available.

CHOLERA

Untreated cholera in large outbreaks has a mortality rate of about 60%. That's pretty significant, especially because when cholera is managed the mortality rate drops to 2%. That's a lot better, but still pretty frightening. What if it's *your* family? How is it treated? How is it identified?

Cholera is extremely rare in the US, with an average of ten cases per year. The overwhelming majority of physicians here have never even seen a case. What does it take to change the number of cases? Not much.

According to the CDC, Haiti had not experienced a cholera epidemic in at least 100 years when they were devastated by an earthquake in January 2010. With crowded conditions and poor sanitation, an epidemic was inevitable. Of the 91,000 cases of cholera, over 43,000 were hospitalized. That's a lot of hospital beds. For the fatalities, the time from onset of symptoms to death averaged eight hours.[387]

Transmission. Absent a laboratory for identifying the *Vibrio cholerae* bacteria, diagnosis will have to be based on the symptoms. Cholera is not transmitted by casual person-to-person contact, but generally through water (most often) or food (rarely) contaminated with the feces of infected individuals. Cholera is a human disease; animals are not affected by it. In addition, persons infected with cholera may have no symptoms, only mild symptoms, or it may be fatal. Death comes from dehydration due to diarrhea, vomiting, and electrolyte loss.[388]

Risk factors. Those at greater risk for developing cholera (beyond what happens with poor sanitation and hygiene) are:

- Children, especially two- to four-year-olds
- Individuals taking proton-pump inhibitors (reduced gastric acidity)
- People with blood type O (doctors don't know why)
- Immunocompromised and malnourished individuals[389]

Signs and symptoms. Lacking laboratory equipment for definitive diagnosis, one needs to know the symptoms of cholera to distinguish it from other diarrheal diseases and provide effective treatment.

- Profuse diarrhea and vomiting of clear liquid
- Diarrhea that looks like "rice water" and may smell like fish
- Skin turning a bluish-gray color
- Typical signs of dehydration—sunken eyes, dry mouth, clammy skin, wrinkled hands and feet
- Seizures or coma in children

Conventional Treatment. Physicians generally administer antibiotics to moderate and severely ill patients:

- Doxycycline, 1 dose of 300 mg OR
- Zithromax, 1 dose of 1 gram OR
- Cipro, 1 dose of 1 gram OR
- Tetracycline or erythromycin, 500 mg, 4x per day, 3 days

Do NOT administer anti-diarrheal medicines like Imodium. Cholera needs to get *out* of the body; Imodium works by keeping waste *in*.[390]

Whereas just a few decades ago there were no reports of antibiotic resistance among cholera bacteria, now there are many strains resistant to most antibiotics. Even though the above antibiotics were effective in Haiti, there is no guarantee they would work in an outbreak today.

Alternative Treatments. There are clinical studies showing that berberine (available on Amazon if you don't want to make your own) combined very well with tetracycline to reduce diarrhea due to cholera and enterotoxigenic *E. coli* infections.[391] One of the berberines is Japanese barberry. Other berberines are Oregon grape, goldenseal, and phellodendron (not to be confused with philodendron, an entirely different plant).

PNEUMONIC PLAGUE

Bubonic plague rears its head rather frequently among rodents and occasionally makes the jump to people, as has been occurring in Los Angeles. As long as the form of plague remains bubonic, the rest of the country can breathe easily.

But sooner or later in situations where public health attitudes are lackadaisical, the bubonic form will give rise to its much deadlier cousin. When pneumonic plague appears at the party, it will make COVID-19 look like a walk in the park. Think of pneumonic plague as a very gregarious party animal bacteria. It shows up in the lungs and finds itself all alone. So it breaks down the barriers and invites every single pathogen in, and they all work together to completely trash the lungs. Even with the best antibiotic treatment from the time symptoms first appear, a lot of people will die. This is the pneumonic form. Airborne.[394] Like our friend COVID-19.

Pneumonic plague looks like a lot of other illnesses—pneumonia, influenza, etc. If a nice middle class person living in a nice middle class neighborhood fifty or a hundred miles from the outbreak comes down with flu-like symptoms, what is he going to think? Influenza or pneumonic plague?

Normalcy bias alert—most people are going to go with influenza, until it's too late. So it spreads further.

Of course there are antibiotics to treat bubonic and pneumonic plague. These drugs and modern medical care work wonders if the dosages are correct, if administered at the first signs of illness, and if the patient gets hospital care....

Will there be enough antibiotics to go around? Think about how much hydroxychloroquine is manufactured in the US and how difficult it was doctors to get it for their patients. What will happen in a pandemic that spreads more easily and has a higher mortality rate?

There is precious little information on pneumonic plague in off-grid medicine references. Antibiotics may work if they are started in time, but that's a pretty big *if* in the early stages of an epidemic. Once people figure out that pneumonic plague is in the neighborhood, proper treatment will be initiated sooner and prophylactic measures can be taken.

Signs and symptoms. In addition to the general influenza- and pneumonia-like symptoms that a patient exhibits, within one to three days of exposure the patient will begin coughing up blood and develop chest pain and shortness of breath. Left untreated, that individual will probably die within 48 hours. What do you do if you suspect plague is in the air?

Treatment. First off, institute strict quarantine for all exposed individuals and isolate the ill people and the caregiver(s). *Everyone* gets face masks and gloves.[392] The following are the standard treatment protocols:

- Prophylactic treatment (for those who have been exposed to pneumonic plague, but are not sick)
    - Doxycycline, 100 mg every 12 hours for the first day, then 100 mg per day, 7 days, OR
    - Cipro, 500 mg, every 12 hours, 7 days[393]
- For sick individuals, any one of the following options
    - Cipro, 500-750 mg, every 12 hours, 14 days

- Doxycycline, 100 mg, every 12 hours the first day, then 100 mg per day, 10 days[394]
- Minocycline, 100 mg every 12 hours the first day, then 100 mg per day, 10 days[395]
- Levaquin, 500 mg per day, 10-14 days
- Moxifloxacin, 400 mg per day, 10-14 days[396]

Most sources state that the antibiotics are taken for 10-14 days or until 2 days after the fever subsides.

Ninety-five years ago Los Angeles experienced an outbreak of pneumonic plague. It was a time when the threat was taken seriously, quarantine measures were implemented, and public health officers scoured affected neighborhoods for contacts and suspected illnesses. People were generally cooperative, and yet government officials still had their petty disagreements about managing the situation. Public health services received only half the amount of money requested to eradicate the plague and the rats. Money that should have been spent where people were living was instead funneled to the harbor areas, because shutting down the ports due to plague would have caused substantial economic losses. Local government instituted a news blackout for Los Angeles and refused to let the public know it was plague and called it instead "a strange malady" and "malignant pneumonia." Fortunately, other California cities reported more accurately. The whole situation was poorly managed. With the current political climate, one shouldn't expect it to be any better managed next time.[397]

TUBERCULOSIS

There are approximately one billion people in the world with tuberculosis, about one-seventh of the planet's population. According to the Centers for Disease Control, just over 9,000 people were diagnosed with active tuberculosis in 2018 in the US. It is estimated that 13,000,000 people in the US have latent tuberculosis. The states with the highest incidence of the disease are Alaska, Hawaii, California, New York, Minnesota, Texas, Florida, Massachusetts, and Maryland. In the US, tuberculosis is more common among black, Hispanic, Asian, homeless, and incarcerated populations. It is most common in people between the ages of 15 and 35 years.

Signs and symptoms. Latent tuberculosis causes no symptoms. Most of the estimated 13,000,000 people in the US who have the latent form are completely unaware. In a long-term collapse, many of these will convert to the active form, when they actually start exhibiting the common early symptoms:

- Chronic coughing that lasts for more than three weeks, and which is often worse just after waking up
- Low fever in the afternoon
- Night sweats
- Chest pain
- Chronic weight loss and fatigue

As the disease progresses, the following symptoms appear:

- Blood in the sputum
- Pale, waxy skin
- Hoarseness

The course of the disease progresses differently in younger children. Signs in them include:

- Weight loss
- Frequent fever
- Pale skin

Clinical diagnosis with laboratory tests probably won't be an option in a collapsed society. Before the advent of antibiotics, patients were sent to tuberculosis sanatoriums for treatment and hopeful recovery. They were fed good food rich in vitamins, minerals, and protein. And they spent a lot of time resting and sleeping, all of which is critical to recovery.

Because tuberculosis is very contagious, especially among family members, extra precautions need to be taken. The patient with tuberculosis should sleep in a separate room and wear a face mask. Tuberculosis is an airborne disease; however, it is most frequently transmitted to people in close contact with the patient.

Conventional treatment involves the use of at least two different antibiotics that can take *over a year* to cure. Unfortunately, most families will not have stocked enough antibiotics to treat a case of tuberculosis. And using up the antibiotics to only possibly cure one person will mean that others will die of simple infections that could have been easily treated. Hard decisions will have to be made. That's the reality of it.

Alternative treatment may be more realistic in a long-term situation. While some of the herbs recommended for use singly and in formulas are found in the wild, others with a track record in tuberculosis treatment do not grow naturally in this country. Seeds need to be procured in advance and practice gained in growing the plants.

Stephen Buhner recommends the following three formulas to be used concurrently for treating tuberculosis in his book *Herbal Antibiotics*:

- *Cryptolepis* and sida tincture, in equal proportions: 1 teaspoon to 1 tablespoon, 3-6x per day, depending on the severity of the disease.
- Piperine: 20 mg, 2x per day, first dose in the morning 1/2 hour before taking other formulas. Second dose at 4PM.
- *Lomatium*, licorice, and *Rhodiola* tincture, equal parts, 1 teaspoon 3x per day.

Other herbs that have been used historically by cultures around the world to treat tuberculosis include:

- *Artemisia annua, Artemisia tridentata*[398]
- Oregon grape and Japanese barberry
- Japanese honeysuckle
- Juniper
- Peppermint

- *Echinacea* (some sources recommend *Echinacea* for TB and some advise against it), and
- *Usnea*

There's nothing anywhere on how to use these herbs or how long to continue treatment. One of the problems in treating tuberculosis today is that the antibiotic regimen needs to be strictly observed for about a year. That's really hard to do when life is good and normal. A year is a long time to be taking pills. And it's difficult to remember when a patient no longer feels sick. One Chinese study showed that usnea resolved symptoms in most patients in two months. That's all I could find regarding the duration of treatment. Using the herbs for at least four months would probably be a good idea.

To be sure, tuberculosis is going to be tough to defeat. It's often a death sentence. It will likely kill many in our future in the US. These herbal treatments may make a difference, especially when combined with good food and rest.

TULAREMIA

Tularemia is a bacterial disease associated with rodents, rabbits, and hares. Usually confined to rural areas, it occurs throughout the United States, except Hawaii, though most cases occur in the south central and western states. The mortality rate without treatment is 33%; with treatment it is less than 2%.[399]

Prevention. As with any disease, prevention is always the best way to go. To prevent tularemia, take the following preventative measures, only one of which is unique to this disease:

- Use insect repellent. Most cases of tularemia are transmitted by tick and deer fly bites. Use DEET or something similar on the skin and permethrin on clothes.
- Wash hands often when handling sick animals or carcasses, especially rabbits and hares.
- Cook food thoroughly and make sure your water is pure.

- Note any changes in pet rabbits, rodents, and hares.

Signs and symptoms. Tularemia is unique in that the bacteria responsible for the disease can be transmitted in numerous ways. Diagnosis is much more difficult because the signs and symptoms vary depending on how the person was infected and where the bacteria choose to set up house. The incubation period is generally 3-5 days, but may range from 1 to 14 days.[400] Tularemia manifests in the following forms:

- **Ulceroglandular**. 75% of tularemia cases are ulceroglandular and result from a tick or deer fly bite or the handling of infected animals or carcasses. There is a single lesion at the bite site with a central eschar. The lesion looks like other bug bites—swollen and raised, and the eschar is the actual site of the bite with the dead tissue and scab spreading out. However, if there are multiple bites, the disease may be misdiagnosed as chickenpox or herpes simplex. There is prominent lymphadenopathy (swollen glands). The first cases identified in the United States were in Utah, and the disease, *Francisella tularensis*, is named for the Utah man who first researched it, Edward Francis.[401]
- **Glandular**. This is the most common form in children. There is regional lymphadenopathy. Swollen and painful glands may need draining. The bite may have healed over or may have been overlooked.
- **Oropharyngeal**. This form presents with a fever, severe sore throat, mouth ulcers, exudative pharyngitis, and tonsillitis. It arises from ingesting contaminated food or water. There is prominent lymphadenopathy around the neck, ears, and jaws.
- **Oculoglandular**. This form is marked by eye pain, including photophobia, excessive tearing, conjunctivitis, and small ulcers of the cornea. It may result from airborne bacteria, a splash of contaminated water, or rubbing the eyes with contaminated hands. There is prominent lymphadenopathy around the neck, ears, and jaws.

- **Intestinal**. This is a rare form of tularemia marked by intestinal pain, vomiting, and diarrhea. It arises due to eating undercooked, contaminated food or drinking contaminated water.
- **Pneumonic or pulmonary**. This form occurs due to inhalation or spread from ulceroglandular or typhoidal forms. Farmers, sheep shearers, landscapers, and lab workers are at greater risk for this form of the disease. Symptoms are very similar to pneumonic plague and influenza, including chest pain, dry cough, and shortness of breath. Untreated, this form has a 30-60% mortality rate.
- **Typhoidal**. This form is difficult to diagnose. There is little if any lymphadenopathy. Symptoms are not specific and may include a high fever, nausea, vomiting, diarrhea, abdominal pain, cough, and pneumonia.[402]

Fortunately, there is no documented transmission of tularemia from person to person, so the patient does not need to be isolated. However, and of significance to those with dogs, our pets can transmit it to us. Dogs in rural areas often supplement their diet with rabbits and hares. Sick animals are easier to catch. The dogs may contract tularemia and pass it to us.

The CDC classifies tularemia as a Category A bioweapon. It's right up there with anthrax, smallpox, plague, and botulism. It is easily disseminated and very few bacteria are needed to cause illness.[403]

Treatment. Tularemia is generally treated with gentamicin or streptomycin, both of which are intramuscularly or intravenously administered, and neither of which is commonly available to preparedness-minded individuals. In the absence of these medications, physicians may prescribe doxycycline 100 mg or Cipro 500 mg, both every 12 hours for 10-14 days. Unfortunately, there's a good chance for relapse with both of these drugs.[404]

TYPHOID FEVER

Typhoid fever isn't a concern for us; there are only a few hundred documented cases each year in the US, and the vast majority of those are contracted by travelers visiting Africa and Southeast Asia.[405] What if municipal water systems fail? What happens if people are relegated to getting their water directly from rivers, streams, or shallow wells? Yes, typhoid will rear its ugly head.

Typhoid fever, also known simply as typhoid, is a bacterial infection with *Salmonella enterica* serotype Typhi bacteria that is spread through food or water contaminated with feces. Only people can get it; animals do not and they do not transmit it (other than flies carrying it from feces to food).[406]

Most typhoid cases occur in poverty-stricken areas of Southeast Asia and Africa, with children more likely to be stricken. There were over 160,000 deaths from typhoid worldwide in 2013. Typhoid has a 20% mortality rate untreated, or about 2% if treated. Children under the age of four years have the highest mortality rate. Historically, in the United States, more men died of typhoid in the Civil War and Spanish-American War than died of battle wounds.[407]

Prevention. Typhoid is best prevented using good sanitation and hygiene practices, including thorough handwashing, good latrine and waste management, as well as chlorination of drinking water. Typhoid vaccines, which are effective for about three years, are usually recommended for people traveling to high-risk areas.

Signs and symptoms. Symptoms begin 6-30 days after exposure, and the course of the disease ranges from mild to severe and fatal. Without proper treatment, symptoms may continue for weeks to months.[408]

- First week: It begins like a cold or flu. The patient often reports a headache and sore throat. The fever rises and falls, gradually edging higher each day (104°F). The pulse is often quite slow in relation to the fever. There may be abdominal pain and a dry cough. One-fourth of patients have nosebleeds. Take the pulse and temperature every 30 minutes. If the pulse decreases as the fever increases, typhoid is most likely the cause.[409] There may be vomiting, diarrhea, or constipation.

- Second week: The patient is too fatigued to rise from bed, the high fever and slow pulse continue, and delirium may occur. About 25% of patients develop a rose-colored rash of flat spots on the trunk of the body that fade with pressure, there may be constipation or diarrhea, and the liver and spleen become enlarged and tender. For the first and second week, the fever rises higher in the afternoon.[410]
- Third week: If there are no complications, the symptoms slowly fade away. Complications in more serious cases include intestinal hemorrhage and perforation, pneumonia, bronchitis, encephalitis, and neuropsychiatric symptoms like picking at imaginary objects on bed linens and muttering.[411]

The course of the disease may persist for weeks or months. Unique to typhoid is the fact that about 3% of patients become chronic carriers like the infamous Typhoid Mary, who was responsible for at least 53 more cases and 3 deaths until she was permanently isolated. The patient must remain in bed, resting, until the fever is completely gone.

Definitive diagnosis requires laboratory tests.

Conventional treatment. Dosing regimens for Cipro and amoxicillin come from the CDC and the health department of Fiji. The CDC indicates that Zithromax, ampicillin, and TMP-SMZ may also be used, but no dosing protocols are provided.

Cipro has recently been the antibiotic of choice; amoxicillin and chloramphenicol have 5-15% relapse rates. Unfortunately, the bacteria causing typhoid fever are becoming increasingly resistant to Cipro, especially in India. Zithromax and Rocephin are other options.[412]

Alternative treatment. Herbs shown to be effective in treating typhoid include *Echinacea angustifolia* and pomegranate peel.

Typhoid dosing protocols by age		
	Cipro	Amoxicillin
Adults and children 12+ years	500 mg/2x per day/5 days	75-100 mg/kg per day/ 14 days
Children 8-11 years	250 mg/2x per day/5 days	
Children 2-7 years	125 mg/2x per day/5 days	
Children under 2 years	7.5 mg/kg/2x per day/5 days	

TYPHUS

There are three kinds of typhus:

- Scrub typhus, which occurs only in the Asia-Pacific region, and thus will not be addressed here
- Murine (or endemic) typhus, caused by Gram-negative *Rickettsia prowazekii* bacteria, which are flea-borne, usually from fleas found on rats
- Epidemic (or louse-borne) typhus, caused by *Rickettsia typhi* bacteria, which are transmitted primarily by body lice

Murine Typhus

This form of typhus occurs worldwide, but mainly in tropical and subtropical areas where rats and their fleas are present. It is actually transmitted by the feces of the fleas usually found on rats, in areas with poor sanitation and lots of rats. Murine typhus can also come from fleas on mice, cats, opossums, and rarely, dogs. People contract it when they inhale the flea feces, or more commonly through scratched or otherwise compromised skin. Most cases occur spring to early fall, and in the US are usually found in Texas, California, and Hawaii. This includes the October 2018 outbreak in Los Angeles.[413]

Epidemic or Louse-Borne Typhus

As the body louse carries the bacteria that causes typhus, the same conditions that are favorable for acquiring body lice favor the transmission of typhus—crowded, unsanitary conditions such as occur with war, famine, refugee camps, prisons, and homelessness. Transmission occurs when people come in contact with the feces of the body lice or crush the body lice, through cuts or injured skin, or inhalation, the same as with murine typhus. As the bacteria remain viable for up to one hundred days and body lice proliferate rapidly, this disease can quickly reach epidemic proportions.[414] Consider these few gems from history:

- In a siege of the Moors during the War of Grenada, the Spanish lost 3,000 men in battle, and 17,000 to typhus.
- Typhus is estimated to have killed more than 10% of Germans during the Thirty Years' War.
- In 1812, during Napoleon's retreat from Russia, more of his men died from typhus than from battle with the Russians.
- During a famine that occurred between 1816 and 1819 in Ireland, including a period known as The Year without a Summer, more than 100,000 Irish died of typhus.
- During World War I, more than 150,000 died of typhus in Yugoslavia alone.[415]

Typhus is first mentioned in historical records in the 1400s, and almost all historical references to typhus are considered to be epidemic typhus. In the United States, almost all cases of epidemic typhus occur east of the Mississippi.

Prevention. Beyond maintaining strict hygiene and sanitary conditions, permethrin is what will save lives. Permethrin kills lice and does so for a long time. It is often applied to clothing and will remain effective through numerous washings. It is also ideal for applying to items that cannot easily be washed, like mattresses. Do not apply permethrin to the skin. Any washable items suspected of harboring body lice must be washed in water that is at least 140°F to kill lice. Items that cannot be washed should be encapsulated in plastic bags for at least five weeks. Burning is also a good idea.

Signs and symptoms. The symptoms of both kinds of typhus are very similar, but as epidemic typhus is the disease to be most concerned with, that's where the focus is for diagnosis.

One to two weeks after being infected, the illness begins with the sudden onset of a high fever. Other flu-like symptoms, especially rapid breathing and headache, follow. Five to nine days after the initial onset of symptoms, a rash begins, usually on the trunk, and then spreading to the limbs, but sparing (and this is key in diagnosis) the face, palms of the hands, and soles of the feet. Other symptoms in the second and third weeks include sensitivity to light in the eyes and an altered mental state.[416]

Treatment. Even today, with advanced medicine, diagnostic tests take time and if an individual is suspected of having typhus, treatment begins immediately while awaiting test results to confirm the diagnosis. The treatment is the same, whether it is murine or epidemic typhus: doxycycline. The dosage recommended for adults is 100 mg twice per day until at least 3 days after the fever subsides, usually 7-10 days in all. For children under 100 pounds, the dosage is 2.2 mg/kg twice per day. Prophylactic treatment with a single dose of doxycycline in individuals exposed to typhus but who have not developed symptoms, may be effective.[417]

Alternative treatment. Unlike other communicable diseases, there is no alternative or herbal treatment for typhus. Without treatment—doxycycline—most patients die. In wartime outbreaks, many of the typhus fatalities were actually among those nursing the ill and wounded.

YELLOW FEVER

We don't hear much about yellow fever; it's been a really long time since the United States experienced an epidemic. The epidemic of 1793 in Philadelphia (at that time, the capital of the United States) prompted George Washington and the rest of the government to flee. At that time, 9% of the population died due to yellow fever. In yellow fever we have another example of where starvation and disease kill more than war itself—more men died of yellow fever than in the battles of the Spanish-American War in 1898. It was rightly considered one of the most dangerous diseases in the world during the eighteenth and nineteenth centuries.[418]

Yellow fever remains a concern today in Africa and South America. In 2013, there were 127,000 severe cases, mostly in Africa, and 45,000 people died. Interestingly, yellow fever has been researched as a potential biological weapon.[419]

Signs and symptoms. Yellow fever is a viral disease so named because of the jaundice (yellowing of the skin and eyeballs) that occurs in the most serious cases. Once bitten, the incubation period is generally three to six days. Most people are sick for three to five days and experience the following symptoms:

- Fever
- Chills
- Loss of appetite
- Muscle pain
- Back pain
- Headache[420]

Those symptoms alone make diagnosing yellow fever rather difficult. It looks like a whole host of other diseases, including malaria and other viral hemorrhagic fevers. However, in about 15% of patients, after a one-day respite, the fever returns, the pain resumes, and liver damage begins, as evidenced by jaundice. Bleeding in the mouth, eyes, and gastrointestinal tract is common, and kidney failure and delirium may occur as well. Among those who develop jaundice, 20-50% will die. Jaundice is the key to realizing that the patient has yellow fever, and there's a good chance many others will fall victim.[421]

If the patient has recently arrived from an area where the *Aedes aegypti* mosquitoes (the most common vectors for yellow fever) live and breed, the outbreak may be contained. The *Aedes aegypti* mosquito, the most common vector for yellow fever, unlike most other mosquitoes, feeds during the day.[422]

Conventional Treatment. Treatment of yellow fever is strictly supportive. Because it is a viral disease, antibiotics are not effective. There is a vaccine for yellow fever, and some countries require it for travel.

Alternative Treatment. Antiviral herbs that have been historically used and found to be effective include elder, ginger, and licorice. Unfortunately, information on dosages or frequency could not be located.[423]

Caution. Aspirin and other anticoagulants should not be administered to a person with yellow fever.

OTHER MOSQUITO-BORNE DISEASES

Chikungunya. Most cases occur in Africa and Asia, with almost all cases among Americans originating in those visiting foreign countries. While the CDC distribution map suggests that Chikungunya is found in the US, there was only one case in the American Caribbean islands in 2013. There was one locally acquired case in Texas in 2015. There were twelve locally acquired cases in Florida in 2014. The rest of the cases in the US were from travelers. Most people who become infected will develop symptoms three to seven days after being bitten. The symptoms are very similar to dengue and Zika, with the most common symptoms being fever and joint pain. Other symptoms include headache, muscle swelling, and a rash. Most patients feel better within seven days, but for some, the joint pain persists for months. Chikungunya is not often fatal, but the symptoms can be disabling and severe. There is no vaccine to prevent the disease nor medicine to treat it. Those most at risk for developing a severe case of the disease are newborns, those over 65, and those with high blood pressure, diabetes, or heart disease. The CDC advises Tylenol for pain and fever and warns against using aspirin.[424]

Dengue. This tropical disease very rarely occurs in the US. Local outbreaks have occurred in Hawaii, Texas, and Florida. However, the mosquitoes carrying dengue range over much of the US, so the potential for outbreaks elsewhere is great. Dengue is found in over 100 countries, and 40% of the world's population lives in areas at high risk for dengue. About 25% of individuals infected with dengue will become sick, and the disease can range from mild to severe. About 5% of individuals will develop severe dengue. Those most at risk for severe dengue are people who have had dengue in the past, infants, and pregnant women. Symptoms of dengue include fever plus any of the following: nausea, vomiting, rash, aches and pains, especially behind the eye, and muscle and joint pain. There is no vaccine and no medications beyond supportive care. Warning signs of severe dengue usually begin 24-48 hours after the fever has subsided and include belly pain and tenderness, vomiting (at least 3 times in 24 hours), bleeding from the nose or gums, vomiting blood or blood in the stool, and feeling tired, restless or irritable. Severe dengue is a medical emergency.[425]

West Nile. This virus is transmitted to horses, people, and birds. Unlike many of the other mosquito-borne diseases, West Nile virus (WNV) actually occurs in most of the US. It usually causes no symptoms in 80% of the people bitten; however, 20% will develop a fever with other symptoms of body aches, rash, nausea, vomiting, joint pain, headache, and/or diarrhea. Severe illness with WNV can occur at any age, but the elderly are most at risk. There have been 42,000+ cases of WNV in the US in the past 20 years. Of these, 19,000 experienced neurological symptoms. Just under 10% of these people died. WNV is most commonly spread through mosquito bites, though it may also occur through blood transfusion or from mother to baby during pregnancy or through breast milk. In about 1 in 150 patients, WNV can become life-threatening within a few hours and require hospitalization. The development of encephalitis or meningitis includes the following symptoms: high fever, headache, neck stiffness, stupor, disorientation, tremors, coma, vision loss, numbness, and paralysis. About 10% of those who develop encephalitis or meningitis symptoms die. Some effects to the central nervous system may be permanent.[426]

Zika. Most people bitten by mosquitoes carrying the Zika virus have no symptoms or only a mild form of the illness. However, others have more serious cases and in pregnant women there is the threat of microcephaly developing in the unborn child. Local transmissions of Zika virus occurred in Florida and Texas in 2016 and 2017. The most common symptoms are fever, rash, joint pain, conjunctivitis, headache, and muscle pain, which can last several days to a week, and which are very similar to dengue and Chikungunya. While most people do not become very ill, there are a few fatal cases. The treatment is rest and fluids to prevent dehydration. The CDC advises Tylenol for pain and fever and warns against taking aspirin. Take the usual precautions when dealing with any bodily fluids.[427]

16. RESPIRATORY TRACT ISSUES

Upper respiratory infections (URIs) are the most common reason parents take children to see a doctor. Influenza and pneumonia are leading causes of death in the elderly. Having the right medications on hand will generally be a nicety for children, and others will be essential to survival for elders.

COLDS, INFLUENZA, AND COLD-LIKE ILLNESSES

Colds don't get much press in off-grid medicine books. We've all had colds, our children have had them, and while they can make us miserable, they always come to an end without any long-lasting effects. Colds are caused by all kinds of constantly mutating viruses, and as such, no antivirals have ever been developed for them and antibiotics are of no efficacy. When physicians recommend medications to their patients, Sudafed (real Sudafed--pseudoephedrine) and Afrin top the list. Even most bad colds are no match for those two. Using these medications can also be diagnostic; they will relieve cold symptoms but will do nothing against influenza.

So how else do you differentiate between a cold and influenza? And is it important?

The chart at right can help distinguish between the two. On the one hand, it shouldn't matter whether we have a cold or influenza; perhaps one blessing to come from the COVID-19 pandemic is that people will learn social distancing, become responsible, and stay home when they are sick.

Distinguishing between a cold and influenza

Signs and symptoms	Cold	Influenza
Nasal congestion	Common	Uncommon
Sore throat	Common	Uncommon
Aches and pains	Common	Severe
Cough	Mild	Severe
Fatigue	Mild	Severe
Fever	Uncommon, low	Common, high
Headache	Uncommon	Common

On the other hand, if an illness is influenza, we can take greater protective measures than we otherwise might, and we can monitor a patient more closely if influenza is involved. Antivirals may lessen the duration and severity of influenza if treatment is initiated within 48 hours of the onset of symptoms. With influenza, generally the greatest concern, especially in the elderly, is watching for and preventing the development of a secondary infection with pneumonia.

However, most upper respiratory infections are just garden variety colds. In addition to Sudafed and Afrin, other medications can alleviate the symptoms and make a patient feel better—Tylenol for aches and pains, lozenges for a sore throat, Mucinex for coughs.

But what about those times when a cold is not a cold? The following infections all start out looking just like other colds with the usual symptoms—runny nose or congestion, cough, low fever, etc. And most of the time, that is all they are and parents are never the wiser.

Respiratory syncytial virus can be very serious and even fatal in infants, especially those who are premature or immunocompromised. It can also be serious in the elderly.

Infectious mononucleosis puts COVID-19 to shame with its nearly six-week incubation period.[428] In children under the age of 12, mono is generally an asymptomatic infection, and everyone over the age of 30 is presumed to have already experienced mono. But in a teenager, it can be an entirely different infection with a much worse outcome. Symptoms begin like a normal cold with a sore throat, fever, and fatigue, but last well beyond a few days. The course of the illness can actually last for weeks to months. While over 90% of patients will recover without any special treatment, some will develop secondary infections, including strep and respiratory infections.[429] In addition, some will develop abdominal tenderness, indicating enlargement of the liver or spleen. During this period all contact sports and similar activities must be avoided to reduce the risk of rupturing those organs.[430]

Whooping cough is another illness that begins like a normal cold, with a fever, runny nose, and cough.[431] The whooping begins two weeks later, where the child coughs repeatedly without breathing, until a plug of mucus is expelled, and the air rushes back into the lungs with a very audible whoop. While coughing, the lips and nails may turn blue due to the lack of oxygen, and after the whoop the child may vomit. Whooping cough can last more than three months and is particularly dangerous in infants under twelve months of age.[432]

Even when a cold is just a cold, there is the potential for other illnesses to develop.

Croup occurs when the trachea becomes inflamed and the airway constricts. This only occurs with children under the age of eight years, but can become very serious in any child under the age of three.

Bronchitis and **pneumonia** can develop from colds as well and can be particularly detrimental in the very young and very old.

"Simple" colds aren't necessarily so simple. An infection that one person's body can fight off extremely well may be life-threatening to another individual. Just because Little Johnny has only a slight runny nose and really wants to play with the other children doesn't mean that he should. In a world where higher medical care may not be available, parents need to be parents and make hard decisions that may sadden their children. It comes with the territory.

COUGHS

Coughing isn't actually a sickness; it is a sign of any number of different conditions that affect the throat, bronchi, or lungs. A person coughs because his body is attempting to expel the phlegm and microbes in the respiratory system. For most rapid recovery, the coughing shouldn't be stopped. Rather, it's best to loosen the phlegm and mucus so that the body can expel them more easily. Even with a severe, dry cough, the body is still trying to expel mucus and microbes. However, in order to recover, the body also needs to be able to rest. Which is more important differs from one patient to the next and even for a single patient from one hour to the next.

First and foremost, the most essential treatment is to drink lots of water to loosen the mucus. Next, breathe hot water vapors. This is most easily accomplished with a pot of boiling water on a table or between the patient's feet, with a towel draped over the patient's head and pot to concentrate the vapors. Breathe deeply for 10-15 minutes, several times per day. The steam alone is sufficient, but essential oils or fresh leaves, especially peppermint or eucalyptus, may be added (but not for a person with asthma).[433]

Cough syrup may be given for all kinds of coughs, but it is most effective with a dry cough. To make your own, mix equal parts honey and lemon juice. Offer a teaspoonful every two to three hours. Alternatively, a spoonful of honey may be taken alone without any lemon juice. Do not give honey to infants under one year of age. Make a syrup with sugar instead.

Mucinex is an expectorant for loosening mucus. It does not work for a dry, non-productive cough. It works well for coughs with a lot of phlegm.

Doctors used to prescribe codeine for severe, dry coughs. One-quarter of a Tylenol-3 has enough codeine in it to calm most coughs.[434]

Type of cough, associated illness, and treatment options		
Type of cough	Illness	Conventional and alternative treatments
Dry cough with no phlegm or very little phlegm	Cold or influenza	Thyme, honey, catnip, Japanese honeysuckle, gumweed, lomatium
	Measles	Juniper, Japanese honeysuckle, calendula
	Smoker's cough	
	Worms (when passing through the lungs)	Mebendazole
Cough with a little or a lot of phlegm	Bronchitis, pneumonia	Usnea, thyme, Mucinex, plantain, gumweed
	Asthma	Caffeine, honey, Brigham tea, plantain, gumweed, oregano
	Smoker's cough, esp. in the morning	
Cough with wheezing or whooping and difficulty breathing	Asthma	Caffeine, honey, Brigham Tea, plantain, gumweed, oregano
	Whooping cough	Blackberry, red clover, gumweed, thyme
	Diphtheria	Echinacea
	Heart problems	
	Foreign object in throat	
Cough that sounds like a seal bark	Croup	Primatene Mist, cold air, steam, oregano
	Foreign object in throat	
Chronic/ persistent cough	Asthma	Primatene Mist, caffeine, honey, Brigham tea, plantain, gumweed, oregano
	Chronic bronchitis	Usnea, thyme, plantain, gumweed
	Emphysema	Plantain, gumweed
	Smoker's cough	
	Tuberculosis	Usnea, Japanese honeysuckle, juniper, peppermint
Coughing up blood	Pneumonia (yellow, green, or blood-streaked phlegm)	Usnea
	Cancer of the throat or lungs	
	Tuberculosis	Usnea, Japanese honeysuckle, juniper, peppermint
	Worms	Mebendazole

CROUP

Croup is an odd condition that stresses parents out. Typically a late fall and winter occurrence, it generally affects young children about six months to three years in age. It's seen more frequently in boys than in girls, and it's more common in odd-numbered years.[435]

Croup, laryngotracheobronchitis, is usually caused by any number of viruses, as a result of influenza, a common cold, respiratory syncytial virus, and more. The trachea swells and thus constricts the airway. As the area affected surrounds the vocal cords, laryngitis or hoarseness sometimes occurs. In more severe cases the swelling is significant and can make it difficult to breathe, but most cases are managed without incident at home.[436]

Beyond that, croup is typified by a loud, barking cough that is exacerbated by coughing, crying, anxiety, or agitation—basically anything that makes the child breathe more rapidly. That seal-like barking cough is key to diagnosis; without it, it's not croup. The illness usually begins like a regular cold but progresses to the seal bark cough, and often includes a fever, hoarse voice, and noisy or labored breathing, called stridor, due to the turbulent airflow in the larynx. A secondary infection can make the symptoms worse. The symptoms worsen at night and last anywhere from one to five days.[437]

Croup afflicts about 15% of children, and about 4% of these cases are severe enough to warrant hospitalization. Steroids are administered in more severe cases. Lacking steroids, epinephrine may also be used. However, it is not systemic epinephrine; epinephrine injections are not likely to work. The epinephrine needs to be on the vocal cords. *[438] For that a nebulizer like Primatene Mist is needed. †

Other options for reducing the swelling, irritation, and coughing for milder cases include:

- Liquid Advil. Reduce the dosages and administer more frequently without ever exceeding the total daily dosage. As Advil is an anti-inflammatory, the idea is that it will decrease inflammation of the trachea. If the child can gargle, dilute the Advil in a little water and have him gargle it thoroughly before swallowing.
- If outside temperatures are cold, wrap the child up well and take him outside to breathe the air. If it is not cold, open up the freezer and have the child breathe deeply. Alternatively, put ice cubes in a bowl, bend the child over the bowl with a towel over the child, and have him breathe deeply.
- Use a cool-mist humidifier or steam from a hot shower for ten minutes. You really want a steam room, not just some humidity by the bed.
- Have the child propped up in a sitting position.

---

* "After decades of controversy and rigorous study, corticosteroid treatment has been established as the treatment of choice for children with croup of all levels of severity. However, areas requiring further study are the most effective corticosteroid dose range and whether there is benefit from repeated doses of corticosteroid in the treatment of more severe croup. Although there is comparatively less literature on epinephrine treatment, there is sufficiently strong evidence to support its use for the temporary relief of upper airway obstruction in more severe cases of croup. On the other hand, although mist therapy was firmly entrenched in the arsenal of outpatient croup treatment for many years, it has now been shown to be ineffective and consequently is rarely used in the acute care setting."

† Some care providers believe that there isn't actually a rebound effect with epinephrine administered for croup. Rather, the epinephrine worked for a time. But because the underlying cause of the croup was not addressed, the seal cough and stridor returned when the epinephrine wore off. As we are unlikely to have access to steroids or the decadron that is often used in emergency rooms, we would have to use something like Primatene Mist. Of course, you're not actually doing this without a doctor's supervision. You're only stocking some epinephrine to have on hand just in case.

- Keep the child well hydrated.
- Comfort and cuddle the child to keep him as calm as possible.[439]

EAR INFECTIONS

One of the more horrifying thoughts entertained by a parent who prepares is the idea of having a small child in pain and not being able to help. Many of us have seen our children in pain. While some babies and toddlers escape childhood without experiencing an ear infection, they really are a common occurrence that most every family deals with at least once or twice.

Fortunately, a middle ear infection is rarely a true emergency for children or adults. However, the pain can be intense, on par even with kidney stones or labor contractions.[440] Knowing your little child is in this kind pain is torture to a parent.

Otitis media is the typical ear infection of infants and toddlers. It is most easily identified with an otoscope. An otoscope is not difficult to use, and identifying whether an ear is infected is as easy as can be. (Grayish—not infected. Red—infected.) There are so many choices and a huge range in prices. One in the $60-90 range would probably be good.

When checking for a potential ear infection, the normal ear is viewed first to prevent transferring bacteria from the infected ear. The eardrum should be a light gray color. Then the ear that is causing pain is checked. If it's infected, it will be pink or red, and the eardrum may even be bulging out. If it's not pink or red, then is there debris, a foreign object, or ear wax?[441]

Signs and symptoms. Without an otoscope, how are you going to determine whether a child has an ear infection? Symptoms include:

- Pain, which may worsen when lying down
- Difficulty sleeping
- Crying
- Irritability
- Fever

- Loss of appetite
- Holding or pulling the affected ear[442]

Otitis media infections can occur alone, but they most often develop as a result of a cold causing congestion and blockage of the nose and Eustachian tube. Bacteria get trapped and fluid and pus accumulate[443], and then your child is in pain.

Treatment. For the past half century or so, antibiotics have been the standard treatment, but before that most every doctor knew how to lance an eardrum. Current beliefs are that neither antibiotics nor lancing is necessary for most infections. It's best not to dip into the antibiotic supply if it's not necessary.[444]

However, you know your child is in extreme pain. He is not sleeping, so neither are you. Pain relief is the goal. Tylenol or Advil or both should reduce the pain. Herbal remedies and or warm compresses may reduce the pain and eliminate the infection. If they do not, and if the patient gets worse, look for a professional.

In most cases when an eardrum ruptures, whether in adults or children, antibiotics are not necessary. Do not irrigate the ruptured ear. This will force water and potential contaminants, including bacteria, past the ruptured eardrum, which may cause a worse infection.[445]

If antibiotic treatment is recommended, the most commonly used antibiotics are Keflex, Zithromax, amoxicillin, penicillin, and erythromycin. Cipro is an option in adults. Augmentin, doxycycline, and tetracycline may also be prescribed.

Physicians often prescribe the following antibiotic dosages for ear infections:

- Amoxicillin, 25-50 mg/kg per day in divided doses, 3x per day, 7-10 days for children; 500 mg, 3x per day, 5-7 days for adults[446]
- Penicillin, 80-100 mg/kg per day, in divided doses, 3x per day, for 10 days or until 2 days after the fever has passed in children[447]

- Keflex, 500 mg, 2x per day, 7-14 days[448]
- Erythromycin, 250-500 mg, 4x per day, 7-14 days[449]

Prevention. In order to reduce the incidence of ear infections, do not feed infants or toddlers while they are lying flat. No nursing to sleep, no bottles to sleep. This will also help prevent rotting teeth, which is another problem best avoided.[450]

EUSTACHIAN TUBE DYSFUNCTION

What if a child is complaining of ear pain, but there is no fever? That suggests there is no bacterial infection. This is often a Eustachian tube dysfunction, where the middle ear is blocked, like with a middle ear infection, but there is no bacteria involved. It often occurs with colds and hay fever.

Treatment. Because this is not a bacterial infection, antibiotics will do nothing. In previous generations, before antibiotic use became widespread, such an ear would often be lanced by the family physician. However, this is something most practicing physicians, with the exception of ENTs, are totally unfamiliar with. Regardless, the dysfunction usually resolves on its own, without any treatment at all.[451]

Unfortunately, the child is still in pain. While pain relief is the main purpose of treatment, treatment is also a way of ruling out other more serious issues and confirming the diagnosis. Normal doses of Tylenol or Advil should significantly lessen the pain, as will hot compresses or a heating pad. Sudafed and/or Afrin may also be used, especially if there is significant nasal congestion. If, on the other hand, the patient worsens, the problem could be meningitis, and a physician should be located.[452]

Just as with an ear infection, a Eustachian tube dysfunction may rupture the eardrum and fluid (possibly bloody mucus or pus) may leak out. Do not wash the ear out under any circumstances. Do not risk introducing bacteria into the eardrum in this situation. In most cases a ruptured eardrum will heal just fine without any other intervention or antibiotics.

FOREIGN BODY IN NOSE

It is the dreaded FBIN. Foreign body in nose. Your otherwise brilliant toddler decided TEOTWAWKI would be a great time to see if shoving peas up her nose would keep her from having to eat them.

This is not good. And because you are not a physician with the cool tools of the emergency department, the options for removing the FBIN are limited. However, if you start to panic, your child is going to stress out as well, and that will make everything worse. Just to add more pressure, statistics show that your child is only going to allow one or two attempts at most for clearing her nose. This has to be done right the first time.

The very first thing to do, as soon as you know you've got a problem, is to get the child to breathe through her mouth. Sniffling may move the object farther up the nasal passage. Depending on exactly what is up her nose and how painful it is, pain medication may be required to help calm her down. In a situation like this, many doctors turn to an anti-inflammatory like Advil and in some cases would consider a sedative as well.

Most of the time, you are going to know what is up her nose. She was playing with beads, Legos, candy, batteries, magnets, or pencil erasers. Beans, seeds, or bugs. Maybe pebbles. How you approach removing the FBIN is going to depend largely on what exactly it is. Is it hard? Soft? Round? Square? Smaller? Larger? Smooth? Rough? Metallic?

A physician has several options in a grid-down situation where there is no ER:

Positive pressure (child). The child pinches the clear side of the nose closed, takes a deep breath, and exhales forcibly through the side with the foreign body. This method is good for solid objects like beans and beads. It is difficult for small children to perform.

Positive pressure (parent, kissing technique, mouth-to-mouth). While pinching the clear side of the nose closed, a parent performs mouth-to-mouth, forcefully blowing air through the child's mouth in an effort to dislodge the object.

Positive pressure (straw). It's the same as the positive pressure parent technique above, but using a straw between the two mouths instead. Quick puffs are delivered through the straw.

Bulb syringe. This is primarily for removing round, smooth objects. Make sure you have a good seal with the nostril and suck the foreign body out. The syringe may need to be trimmed to work. Do not risk pushing the object further up the nasal passageway with a bulb syringe that is too long.

Derma-Bond or Vet-Bond (do not use super glue!). Put a little of this glue on a small stick, like a Q-tip with the cotton removed. Make contact with the foreign body and hold in place for at least 60 seconds before attempting to remove.

Saline washout. Fill a bulb syringe with 7 ml of sterile saline. Insert the bulb syringe in the opposite nostril and advance it until you form a tight seal between the nostril and the bulb syringe. Squeeze the bulb forcibly to eject the saline to the other side. The saline will hopefully carry the object out the other nostril. This method is good for friable objects like crackers.

Tweezers. May work for some objects. Don't risk pushing the object further up the nasal passage.

A bent paper clip or a wire loop held by a hemostat. Either of these can be used to rotate around the inside of the nostril between the object and the mucous membrane to dislodge and remove the foreign object.

Sometimes children do things that escape our notice, and some of the foreign bodies children choose to shove up their noses don't cause immediate discomfort or even any discomfort. Peas and raisins are nice and soft and squishy. Something like that is going to eventually start giving off a very foul odor. And there will be a runny nose, but only on one side. (Unless, of course, the objects were shoved up both nostrils. A parent's natural reaction is to panic, thinking there's some type of infection. However, there will be no fever. Careful questioning may reveal that the child did indeed shove something up her nose.

Other items you are going to want for this situation include a very good headlamp with a strong light and a small pair of pliers to hold the nostril open.

INFLUENZA

Prior to the advent of antivirals to mitigate influenza, the treatment was largely supportive, just trying to make the patient comfortable and hoping to avoid developing pneumonia. Antivirals such as Tamiflu haven't changed the scene a whole lot, because the antiviral has to be started pretty quickly and it requires a prescription.

However, there was a study published by researchers in China last year.[453] Some of the authors disclosed a loosely related financial interest, but being as the topic of this study was Aleve and its efficacy as an antiviral, it appears that their financial interest would have no real bearing on the results of the study.

The researchers studied Aleve's antiviral activity against influenza A and influenza B. It had previously been reported that Aleve had some effect against influenza A. This study found that Aleve inhibited virus replication both in the culture medium (*in vitro*) as well as in mice (*in vivo*). The researchers also found that Aleve worked better than Tamiflu in mice. Aleve was also shown to be more effective against influenza B than influenza A.

The authors conclude,

> "If Aleve is an effective anti-influenza drug for humans, it could be implemented into influenza treatment protocols more quickly than other antivirals in development."

In a nutshell, their preliminary research shows that Aleve is more effective than Tamiflu. In mice, not people. This isn't medical advice. Speak with a physician before using any medication.

PINK EYE

Conjunctivitis, commonly referred to as pink eye, is a drag in a functioning society. For kids it means no playing with friends, and for parents it means extra laundry and a trip to the doctor. What does it mean post-collapse?

First off, it's important to cover the various forms of conjunctivitis, which include:

- Allergic
- Bacterial
- Chemical
- Foreign body
- Viral[454]

The chemical and foreign body forms aren't really the focus here. If there is soap (hopefully nothing worse) or dust in the eye, flush with cool water for several minutes.

For the remaining forms, the treatment is the same regardless of the cause, *in a disaster*. If society hasn't collapsed, go to the doctor. These are *eyes* we're talking about.

Signs and symptoms

Allergic conjunctivitis is the most common form. It can be distinguished from bacterial or viral conjunctivitis in that there is usually no milky discharge, just clear, watery eyes, and both eyes are always affected. Antihistamines like Benadryl usually work well.[455]

Viral conjunctivitis, the next most common form, is passed by person to person contact very easily, particularly among children. Even when children receive antibiotic drops from the pediatrician, it's still usually a viral form that is being treated, and the antibiotics won't work! So why do doctors do this? Well, there are a few reasons. For one, they aren't too concerned about antibiotic resistance developing in this situation. For another, being sure about which form it is would require a culture, which takes time and money, and by which time the infection will most likely be resolved anyway.[456] And children can't go back to school or daycare until they've been on antibiotic drops for at least 24 hours, so there's that incentive. It's easier to just prescribe the eye drops. (Of course, if it's viral, and the child goes back to school, the virus spreads everywhere, and the doctors get more patients.)

The discharge from eyes with viral conjunctivitis is typically more watery and clear, as opposed to bacterial conjunctivitis. Viral conjunctivitis is contagious as long as the eye is pink or red. One or both eyes may be affected.

Bacterial conjunctivitis is actually pretty uncommon.[457] One or both eyes may be affected. (Bacterial conjunctivitis may also occur due to chlamydia or gonorrhea infections, which may or may not present with the usual symptoms in the genitals.) Bacterial eye drops may be hard to come by in a collapse, so it can be treated with doxycycline, 100 mg, twice per day, for 7 days.[458]

Conventional Treatment. However, that's probably not the best use of a limited valuable resource. Here's why: Both bacterial and viral forms of conjunctivitis are very likely to resolve on their own without any treatment at all. In fact, the bacterial forms usually resolve a bit more quickly than the viral forms.

Alternative Treatment. There are numerous alternative options for relieving the discomfort associated with conjunctivitis, or pink eye, and many have the benefit of being anti-viral and/or antibacterial as well. Suggested use for all of them is to apply the compress to the affected eye for ten minutes, every two hours.

- Cool compress using:
    - Wet chamomile or goldenseal tea bag[459]
    - Tea or infusion prepared from yarrow, plantain, elder, Japanese barberry, Oregon grape, *Usnea*, or Japanese honeysuckle, singly or in combination
    - A slice of cucumber
- Warm compress using:
    - Turmeric, two tablespoons in one cup boiling water and then cooled down to a comfortably warm temperature
- Eye wash using:
    - Any of the herbs listed above
    - One teaspoon baking soda in two cups cool water[460]

- One tablespoon raw, natural honey dissolved in one cup hot water and cooled[461]
- Colloidal silver[462]

PNEUMONIA

Pneumonia is an acute infection of the lungs that often develops after another respiratory illness like influenza, bronchitis, or asthma. However, it may also occur following measles, whooping cough, or any other very serious illness, especially in the very young and very old.[463] Without a laboratory for testing specimens, there is no way to definitively determine whether a patient has viral pneumonia or bacterial pneumonia. It will take an educated guess to decide whether to use the precious supply of antibiotics.*

Differentiating between viral and bacterial pneumonia. In children, pneumonia is more likely to be viral. A sick child who takes more than fifty shallow breaths per minute likely has pneumonia and must be carefully observed. If he cannot maintain fluid intake orally, it must be administered intravenously, subcutaneously, or rectally. Tylenol can be used for reducing fever.[464]

In adults, pneumonia is more likely to be bacterial but that doesn't necessarily mean antibiotics are needed.

Babies and the elderly (or anyone who seems a bit feeble) are at greater risk for unilateral pneumonia, meaning that the pneumonia is only in one lung. It can be due either to aspirated food or microbes that get trapped in one lung

---

* Dr. Joseph Alton, in his book *Alton's Antibiotics*, shares a quick guide for determining which antibiotic may be best for pneumonia based on the symptoms. *Streptococcus pneumoniae* has rusty-colored sputum. It's commonly treated with penicillin, erythromycin, or Cipro. *Legionella pneumophila* involves abdominal pain, diarrhea, and confusion (in the elderly). Zithromax or erythromycin works best. *Klebsiella pneumoniae* presents with dark bloody sputum. Fluoroquinolones may work, but IV antibiotics are usually necessary. *Mycoplasma pneumoniae* usually involves ear problems, swelling of lymph nodes, and joint pain. Zithromax or erythromycin works best. *Haemophilus influenza* starts off like a cold with a low fever but descends into the lungs within a few days and involves wheezing and difficulty breathing, as well as gray/beige sputum. Penicillin, tetracycline, Cipro, and erythromycin are options.

and cause a localized infection. Left unchecked, the fluids accumulate in the lung, preventing gas transfer—no oxygen in and no carbon dioxide out. The patient literally drowns in his own fluids. However, the infection can also enter the bloodstream, causing sepsis and death. Listening to the lungs will reveal that the affected side rattles or wheezes, while the unaffected lung is clear without any sounds. If respiration is very shallow, you may not be able to detect a difference between the two sides. The nostrils may flare with each breath. The patient may complain of one-sided chest pain, particularly when coughing or inhaling deeply. There may be no respiratory symptoms at all and the patient may simply feel weak or sick. There may be sudden chills and then a high fever. For these patients, a doctor will want to use antibiotics.[465]

The next factor a physician looks at is whether the patient "looks" well or not. In a patient that looks well, the pneumonia is more likely to be viral or the very early stages of a bacterial infection. And by "looking" well, a doctor means that the patient is physiologically stable. She can still be quite miserable, but the vital signs are normal, respiration is normal, the patient is eating and drinking and not confined to bed. These patients should continue eating and drinking and be given fever reducers and pain relievers to be kept comfortable. Antibiotics are not warranted, but the patients should be carefully observed for any changes.[466]

Signs and symptoms. Patients that do not "look" well display abnormal physiological reactions, including:

- Elevated heart rate
- Rapid breathing
- Labored breathing
- Vomiting
- Inability to take food and drink[467]

When will a doctor want to use antibiotics? They are most likely needed with:

- One-sided (unilateral) pneumonia

- A sick-looking patient, baby, or feeble adult
- When a patient has other respiratory conditions such as asthma and COPD
- In any patient that does not improve or gets worse after three to four days

Treatment. If infection develops, most doctors would prescribe Keflex, Augmentin, or erythromycin as first choices. Second-line options would be doxycycline, Cipro, or Levaquin. Treatment would be continued for two days beyond the resolution of the infection.[468]

After two to three days on antibiotics, the patient should be improving. If he is not improving by day three to four, or if he is worsening, the doctor will switch antibiotic classes. Antibiotics will usually do the job in five days in an otherwise healthy adult; it may take seven to ten days for those who are older or chronically ill. The cough may linger for weeks but is not a cause for concern.[469]

Regardless of whether the pneumonia is bacterial or viral, there are a few other measures that can be taken. The patient should take several deep breaths every hour.[470] Warming and humidifying the air will help loosen mucus secretions in the lungs. The patient can be given a balloon to blow up or he can blow bubbles through a straw into a cup of water. Both of these methods provide some back pressure when exhaling to prevent lung collapse. The vibrations from the bubbles also help loosen the mucus.[471] The patient can also yell. These measures are better than nothing but, unfortunately, not as effective as antibiotics.

In the days before antibiotics, physicians used a stethoscope to determine where the pneumonia was concentrated and then had the patient lie on the affected side to facilitate drainage. The caregiver then cupped his hand and clapped it against the chest rapidly and firmly enough to loosen the mucus, but not so hard as to cause pain or bruising.[472] This was performed several times each day, and the patients didn't like it.

RESPIRATORY SYNCYTIAL VIRUS

One of the most common viruses in the world, respiratory syncytial virus (RSV) hits just about everyone at some point in their lives. The vast majority of us experience it before the age of two years. We, or rather our parents, never even realized it. That's because it looks just like a cold. The children who have it act just like they've got a cold.[473]

Transmission. RSV is spread through the air, through droplets, and by person-to-person contact. The virus lives for several hours on hard and soft surfaces.[474]

Risk Factors. RSV is the most common cause of bronchiolitis and pneumonia in infants under one year of age. Those at greatest risk are premature infants, young children with congenital heart or lung problems, and anyone with a compromised immune system. In these people, RSV can become very serious, even life-threatening. Symptoms of a more serious course of the disease include fever, severe cough, wheezing, and rapid breathing or difficulty breathing. The skin may develop a bluish tinge due to the lack of oxygen. The child's chest muscles and skin pull inward as the child struggles to breathe. Irritability, lethargy, and poor feeding are also common.[475]

Older adults with heart and lung issues or compromised immune systems are also at risk for developing pneumonia from RSV, but the course of the disease is generally not so severe.

Signs and symptoms. The incubation period is four to six days before symptoms appear. In a normal course of the illness, the patient has a congested, runny nose, dry cough, fever, sore throat, and/or headache. A person usually sheds the virus and is contagious for about eight days. However, individuals with compromised immune systems can shed the virus for a lot longer, up to several weeks after symptoms have disappeared. That's something to keep in mind if you've got a baby who's at risk for complications.[476]

If you think you are dealing with a serious case of RSV, especially in an infant, get him to a physician as quickly as possible. If it develops into mild pneumonia, a physician will treat it as such. If it develops into moderate to severe pneumonia, she will also approach treatment as such.

STREP THROAT

Why does the mere thought of strep throat scare parents? It's a phenomenon that doctors everywhere observe, but parents can't usually articulate what they're afraid of.[477] Maybe it's because strep throat is something everyone can relate to. It really hurts, and you know your child is really in pain.

Good news. The average parent can be every bit as good at diagnosing strep throat as an experienced family doctor just by looking at a child's sore throat. The bad news is that even the best pediatricians are only right half the time. More good news is that your child has a 99.9% chance of recovering completely without any antibiotics at all.

What about rheumatic fever? (Maybe that's what parents are afraid of when their child has strep.) In the United States, less than one in one thousand cases of strep throat go on to develop into rheumatic fever. Does it make sense to use a precious supply of antibiotics on a presumed strep throat? Remember, without a lab test, one can't even be sure it's strep. It is a bacterial infection, but it's one of those infections that most people get over without antibiotics. Again, do you want to use your antibiotics that may save a life on an illness that will pass and that is nowhere near life-threatening? It's easy to be strong now and say your child will do without; it's a lot harder when your five-year-old is in great pain.[478]

Signs and symptoms. Maybe digging a little deeper can help determine whether it is strep throat. One option is to use a rapid strep test. The kits are available online and are easy to use. Unfortunately, they have a really short shelf life.

Two signs that make strep more likely are a rash on the abdomen and tiny red spots on the roof of the mouth.[479] The Centor Criteria for diagnosing strep throat can also help determine whether an individual has strep.[480]

Centor Criteria for Strep Throat		
Age	Under 3 years, strep is highly unlikely	0
	3-14 years	+1
	15-44 years	0
	45+	-1
Pus on tonsils	No 0	Yes +1
Tender, swollen neck glands	No 0	Yes +1
Fever above 100.4 F	No 0	Yes +1
Cough	No +1	Yes 0

According to the CDC, physicians shouldn't even check for strep unless at least two of the above criteria are met. Antibiotics shouldn't be prescribed until at least three criteria are met unless there is a positive strep test. If four criteria are met, strep is likely. However, even if the criteria are not met for strep throat, it does not mean that the patient doesn't have a serious illness or bacterial infection. It just means that the patient does not have strep throat. If the sore throat persists more than three days, the patient should really be evaluated for other causes for the pain. If the patient's condition worsens, there could be other serious conditions which would warrant the use of antibiotics.[481]

If you and your physician decide to go the traditional antibiotic route, here are the common dosages used for treating strep throat:

- Amoxicillin, 500 mg, 2x per day, 10 days; in children, 250 mg 2-3x per day; or 25-50 mg/kg total per day[482]
- Keflex, 250 mg, 2x per day, 7-14 days[483]
- Erythromycin, 250 mg, 4x per day, 7-14 days[484]
- Penicillin, 500 mg, 2-3x per day, 10 days[485]

17. GASTROINTESTINAL AND ABDOMINAL ISSUES

Gastrointestinal issues run the gamut from uncomfortable and benign to excruciating and fatal and everything in between. The ones we've got previous experience with generally aren't so scary, but the new ones can be absolutely terrifying. Is that intense cramping norovirus or salmonella? Can children really get ulcers? How does a family manage if there is no pharmacy? (Over-the-counter medications to treat the vast majority of gastrointestinal issues a family encounters are covered in chapter 6.) Unfortunately, there are a few other illnesses that can afflict us.

FOOD POISONING

There are over 40 million cases of food poisoning each year in the US, with about 3,000 fatalities. Most are attributed to poor personal hygiene and poor refrigeration post-preparation.[486]

While people do get sick from eating spoiled food (which is differentiated from food poisoning), the bacteria that cause food spoilage differ from those that cause food poisoning. Spoiled food usually smells and looks bad, and so people do not eat it. Food with the pathogens that cause food poisoning generally does not smell bad. It doesn't look bad. In fact, it looks *great.* That's why people ate it.

Food poisoning presents the greatest risk to the following:

- Infants and young children
- Pregnant women
- Those over the age of 60
- Immunocompromised

For the vast majority of cases, the treatment is the same:

- Rest

- Fluids to prevent dehydration
- Avoid anti-diarrheal medications
- Avoid food for a few hours to allow the stomach to settle
- When ready to resume eating, begin with bland, non-fatty foods such as crackers, toast, or rice
- Avoid caffeine, soda, alcohol, dairy, spicy, and fatty foods
- About 10% of cases, primarily among those in the risk groups listed above, will warrant antibiotic treatment.

The charts highlight some of the sources and symptoms of foodborne illnesses as well as potential treatments.

Foodborne illness sources and likely pathogens							
	Shellfish	Meat	Eggs	Milk	Produce	Water	Food handler
Norovirus	x				X	x	x
Salmonella		X	x		X		
Clostridium perfringens		Beef, poultry, gravy, pre-cooked foods					
Staphylococcus aureus		X					x
Campylobacter		X		X		x	
Shigella	x				X	x	
E. coli		X		X	X		x
Giardia intestinalis						x	x
Listeria		X			X	x	
Clostridium botulinum	x	X			X		

Foodborne illness symptoms and likely pathogens					
	Bacterial	Symptom onset after eating	Symptoms	Duration	Most common season
Norovirus		24-48	Diarrhea, vomiting, nausea, low fever, abdominal pain, headache	24-60 hours	November through April
Salmonella	X	6-96 hours	Diarrhea, fever, abdominal cramps	4-7 days	Summer
Clostridium perfringens	X	6-24 hours	Intense cramps, diarrhea. Usually no fever or vomiting.	24 hours	—
Stapylococcus aureus	X	30 minutes to 8 hours	Nausea, vomiting, stomach cramps, diarrhea	24 hours	—
Campylobacter	X	2-5 days	Diarrhea, fever, cramps, sometimes nausea or vomiting	Up to one week	Summer
Shigella	X	1-2 days	Diarrhea, often bloody; fever; cramps	5-7 days	—
E. coli	X	2-5 days	Sudden onset of cramps, abdominal pain. Diarrhea starts 24 hours later, becomes watery, then bloody	7 days	—
Giardia intestinalis		7-14 days	Watery diarrhea, gas, bloating. Fever uncommon.	4-6 weeks	Late summer
Listeria	X	3-70 days, usually about 21 days	Fever, muscle aches, nausea, diarrhea		—
Clostridium botulinum	X	6 hours to 10 days, usually 18-36 hours	Entirely inconsistent with other forms of food poisoning	May be fatal w/o treatment	—

Botulism

Clostridium botulinum is often fatal even with modern medicine. It is the most deadly type of food poisoning and is of special interest to those who can their own foods at home. Historically, the most common source of foodborne botulism has been improper canning of foods at home.[487]

Botulism stands alone in the field of pathogens linked to food poisoning. There is no diarrhea or abdominal cramps. No fever. Vomiting and nausea *may* occur with two less common forms of the disease, and only after the onset of other symptoms. There's really nothing to link it to food.

There are three types of botulism:

Wound botulism accounts for about 29% of all botulism cases. It is contracted primarily by drug abusers injecting heroin. The injection site itself does not often look infected. As it is a disease that affects people who aren't likely to survive long in a collapsed society due to their addiction, it won't be discussed any further.[488]

Infant botulism comprises the majority of botulism cases in the United States. As all parents are warned, honey is never to be given to an infant under twelve months of age. Honey has been shown to contain the *Clostridium botulinum* spores that cause botulism. The spores reproduce in the infant's intestines and release the toxin that causes botulism. However, honey is implicated in only about 20% of cases in infants. Many of the remaining 80% of cases are believed to originate from dust in the soil and air.[489] It's been observed that many infants with botulism live near construction sites.

Foodborne botulism arises from eating contaminated foods. Most of the 20-30 cases of foodborne botulism that occur in the United States each year arise from home-canned foods, especially vegetables and fish. Some occur due to a relatively unknown source—baked potatoes wrapped in foil.[490] Statistics from the CDC for 1950-1996 showed that 65% of botulism cases came from home-canned foods, while 7% were from commercially canned products. The remaining were undetermined. Of the foods that were implicated, 40% were vegetables, 13% fish, 7% marine mammals, 2% fruits and pork, 1% each of condiments, dairy, beef, and poultry; 4% other, and 30% unknown. While "unknown" seems high, keep in mind that botulism can take several days to manifest.[491] By that time, the food to blame is already long gone to the dump. Although there can be "outbreaks" of botulism because two or more people ate the same food, botulism is not transmitted by person to person contact.

Signs and symptoms. All forms of botulism have the same symptoms. As mentioned previously, there are no gastrointestinal complaints. The toxin that causes botulism affects the central nervous system. The incubation period ranges from 6 hours to 10 days, with 18-36 hours being average. In infants, the first sign of botulism is constipation, followed by lethargy, weakness, difficulty feeding, and an altered cry, progressing to paralysis where the baby becomes very floppy. (Infantile botulism was first described as "floppy baby syndrome.") With intensive hospital care, the survival rate is almost 100%.[492]

In older individuals, weakness and paralysis start from the top and work their way down. Signs and symptoms start with the droopy eyelids, blurred or double vision, difficulty chewing and swallowing, and a dry mouth. Facial paralysis sets in, followed by postural hypotension (inability to stand without the risk of passing out). This near-paralysis descends down the spinal column affecting the neck, followed by the shoulders, upper arms, forearms, and fingers. It progresses to the chest muscles, and then it hits the thighs, lower legs, and feet. Respiratory paralysis may set in anywhere along the way and the patient will need mechanical support to survive. Recovery may take months. Only a few cranial nerves may be affected, or it may be the whole body. Progression may take hours or days and appears to be dose-dependent. Paralysis occurs due to the toxin binding to the nerve endings.[493] While there is nothing that can be done to remove the toxin, the nerve endings do eventually regenerate. The paralysis eventually resolves but outpatient therapy may be required for months.[494]

Interestingly, the sensory system is completely intact and patients are entirely cognizant. Assuming they are still able to breathe (via intubation), they can respond to questions, even if only by moving fingers or toes. That is, of course, assuming the paralysis has not extended that far. Death in botulism patients is due to pharyngeal muscle paralysis and insufficient respiratory intake due to paralysis of the diaphragm and other muscles necessary for respiration.

The symptoms of botulism are very similar to those for myasthenia gravis, disease most common in women under 40 and men over 60 years. It also occurs in infants whose mothers have the condition. Myasthenia gravis is uncommon in children. Botulism also looks similar to Guillain-Barre. Both myasthenia gravis and Guillain-Barre are autoimmune diseases with rapid onset as well. However, neither occurs in an outbreak. If there are two or more cases, the diagnosis is botulism. Anything similar to botulism does not occur in outbreaks.[495]

After considering the symptoms and sources, and undoubtedly because the *Clostridium botulinum* bacteria is the culprit implicated here, some may wonder why antibiotics aren't used in treatment. It's because antibiotics are effective only against *bacteria.* Botulism is an illness that arises because the botulinum toxins produced by the bacteria have attached to the nerve endings. The bacteria simply produced the toxin. Botulism antitoxin is only available from the CDC.[496]

Let's now take a look at exactly how botulism happens. *Clostridium botulinum* bacteria are found everywhere in the soil at low levels. They don't reproduce really well there. They just kind of hang out, not really doing much with their lives. Maybe a few grow near some beans or carrots or beets and hang onto those veggies when they're harvested and taken inside. The veggies get washed and still a few bacteria might hang on and get eaten. They do nothing. No one gets sick. Their miserable little bacteria lives have been a waste.

The beans are slated for canning. They get washed pretty well. No one can *see* any dirt. They get carefully processed according to directions. The temperature reaches 250°F and stays there for at least 3 minutes.* The *Clostridium botulinum* bacteria are killed off. Their lives were also wasted. The heat under the canner is turned off, and life in that house proceeds as usual.

Next up for the canner are the beets. But something goes wrong. Nobody really remembers what. Maybe the gauge on the canner wasn't working or the gasket cracked. For some reason, the requisite temperature and pressure aren't reached. Maybe Grandma forgot when the weight started jiggling and thinks it's been 90 minutes when it has only been 30 or 60. Maybe society's been a wreck for a while and people are getting more desperate to preserve food and cut corners. Whatever the cause, the proper temperature isn't reached. Those *Clostridium botulinum* bacteria have been awakened. They are really excited. Really super happy. They indulge in wild non-stop orgies and reproduce faster than mice and rabbits ever dreamed. They're subtle about it. They don't want anyone to know, so they don't change the color of the food and they don't make a stink. If they do, then people might suspect something. They won't eat the food and won't get sick.

Properly home-canned and commercially canned foods are safe to eat straight from the can. Improperly canned stuff may kill you. However, it's hard to tell if food was improperly canned. It doesn't smell or have an off appearance. And you can't taste a difference, either. To be safe (and this comes from the CDC), all home-canned low-acid foods should be boiled for 10 minutes plus an additional minute for every 1,000 feet above sea level to neutralize the toxin.[497]

Conventional treatment. In the US today life is still pretty normal. Anyone suspected of botulism poisoning is given antitoxin and may do some time with a ventilator. Weeks or months wouldn't be unusual. Post-

* Note. This isn't the total processing time, which usually ranges from 40 to 90 minutes, depending on what is being canned. It's just the temperature that must be reached and maintained during the canning process.

collapse, there will not be any antitoxin. Ventilation will have to be done round-the-clock with a bag-valve mask. Most families won't be able to do it.

Alternative treatment. There are very limited accounts of using activated charcoal, even several hours after the suspect food was ingested.[498] The studies suggest that the botulinum toxin remains in the stomach for a while where the activated charcoal can bind to it.[499] As the progression and outcome of the disease appears to be dose-dependent, a case of botulism is not always fatal. Getting the patient to swallow copious amounts of activated charcoal before those muscles become affected may be critical to a positive outcome.

Escherichia coli

Escherichia coli was first isolated and identified over 130 years ago. There are the good *E. coli* bacteria that we are supposed to have in our intestines, and there are the bad actors that make us sick and have been implicated in a myriad of illnesses, including urinary tract infections, meningitis, pneumonia, and cholecystitis. Some strains can cause food poisoning as well.

Transmission. Most cases of this type of infection are contracted through feces-contaminated food, especially ground meats and unpasteurized milk and cheese, lettuce, spinach, sprouts, unpasteurized juice, and water. Other sources are cows, petting zoos, contaminated food handlers, and failing to wash thoroughly after helping a small child with the toilet or changing a diaper have also been implicated.

Signs and symptoms. The Centers for Disease Control and Prevention provides information on the four most common types of *E. coli* foodborne infections. Symptoms take from one to ten days to develop after exposure, but most commonly appear within three to four days. All types of *E. coli* food poisoning have the following symptoms in common:

- Severe abdominal cramping
- Profuse, watery, usually bloody diarrhea
- Other symptoms that may occur include:
- Low-grade fever (below 101°F)

- Nausea
- Vomiting
- Chills
- Headache
- Muscle aches

The illness usually concludes within five to seven days, but in some cases may last up to three weeks.

Diarrheagenic *E. coli* is often referred to as traveler's diarrhea. It makes its victims very uncomfortable but doesn't do any lasting damage.[500]

Enterotoxigenic *E. coli* (ETEC) is very similar to diarrheagenic *E. coli*, another form of traveler's diarrhea, and is not common in the US. While physicians used to prescribe antibiotics for travelers going abroad, this practice is being increasingly curtailed. In general, TMP-SMZ DS and ampicillin are usually not effective. Cipro often works, but it's not without side effects and risks. Most physicians believe that it is best to let the illness run its course.[501]

Enterohemorrhagic *E. coli* (EHEC) O104:H4 caused a large outbreak in Europe in 2011.

Shiga-toxin producing *E. coli* (STEC) O157:H7 is the most common of all the STEC strains and the one that gets all the press. The others making headlines include O26, O103, O111, and O145. The O157:H7 strain sometimes causes hemolytic uremic syndrome, which begins about 7 days after the onset of the first symptoms in 5-10% of cases. The very young and very old are at the greatest risk for complications.[502]

Conventional treatment. Treatment is largely supportive care with fluids. Most strains have developed antibiotic resistance, and the CDC suggests that antibiotic use, especially in the case of *E.coli* O157:H7, may increase the risk of hemolytic uremic syndrome. One physician recommends treatment with Zithromax or Cipro (but provides no dosing regimen for these) or doxycycline, 100 mg twice a day for the first day, and then 50-100 mg once or twice per day for 10 days.[503]

In no case should Imodium or any other anti-diarrheal medications be administered. Imodium works to keep bodily fluids *in*, but in the case of a bacterial infection, the patient needs to get the bacteria *out*.

Alternative treatment. The berberine family of herbs have been demonstrated to be effective against these *E. coli* infections.[504]

Giardia

Giardia intestinalis, also known as *Giardia lamblia* and *Giardia duodenalis*, is the most common disease-causing parasite in the world. While North America escaped getting her fair share when it comes to parasites, *Giardia* didn't pass us by. There are approximately 15,000 cases reported each year; undoubtedly many go unreported, as the protozoa don't cause any symptoms in some people. It is estimated that 20-40% of the world's population has giardiasis.

Risk factors and transmission. As the most common protozoal infection in the United States, giardiasis is more common in northern states and afflicts children under the age of 10 years and adults 35-44 years most frequently.[505] Infections are most common in late summer, when people ingest the cysts by drinking contaminated water. Yes, even those crystal clear mountain streams can harbor *Giardia*. After ingestion, the cysts are activated by stomach acid. They develop into trophozoites, attach to the intestinal walls, and make more cysts to infect other people. These new cysts then are excreted with feces. The cysts can also be passed by infected food handlers or in swimming pools and recreational waters. Even chlorinated swimming pools don't eliminate the risk as it requires about 45 minutes of exposure to chlorine before the cysts are killed.

Signs and symptoms. One to two weeks, sometimes more, after ingesting the cysts, the following symptoms begin:

- Diarrhea. It's described as quite foul, watery and greasy, yellow, and frothy--full of bubbles, but without any blood or mucus.[506]
- Burping. There is a great deal of burping, and the burps taste like sulfur.
- Gas. There is likewise a lot of gas.
- Bloating. The abdomen is rather swollen.[507]

For most individuals, the illness passes in four to six weeks.

Conventional treatment. Standard treatment is with metronidazole, 250 mg, 3x per day, 5-7 days, with food.[508]

Alternative treatment. Options not approved by the FDA include albendazole, 400 mg per day for 5 days, or mebendazole, 100 mg, 2x per day, 5 days (but not in the first trimester of pregnancy).[509] A tincture of Japanese barberry or Oregon grape may also be effective.[510]

Listeria

This form of food poisoning is not addressed in any off-grid medicine books, likely because most healthy people will recover without incident, and it will be difficult to identify without a laboratory. However, the outcome is serious for some groups of people, and knowing what foods to avoid and where *Listeria* thrives is essential to reducing your risk.

Prevention. Unlike most bacteria that cause food poisoning, *Listeria* bacteria thrive at refrigerator temperatures. Dairy products--milk, cheese, ice cream--these bacteria love it all. They especially thrive in raw, unpasteurized dairy products. Hot dogs and deli meats have also caused serious outbreaks. Avoiding these foods is the best choice for preventing a *Listeria* infection, but it is absolutely critical for pregnant women.[511] And finally, it's estimated that about 5% of the population are asymptomatic carriers of the bacteria, so careful handwashing is essential.[512]

Signs and symptoms. For most people, *Listeria* causes only mild flu-like symptoms. But for the immunocompromised and pregnant, it can cause miscarriages, meningitis, and sepsis, and as such, may be fatal.[513] The more serious symptoms of listeriosis include:

- Flu-like symptoms, including fever, headache, and achy muscles
- Stiff neck
- Joint pain
- Dizziness
- Loss of balance
- Confusion
- Convulsions[514]

Fortunately, there are only about 1500 cases of listeriosis documented in the US each year. However, of these cases, 260 will be fatal.[515] Without a functioning laboratory and because symptoms are very similar to many other illnesses, listeria will be difficult to identify. Another factor complicating diagnosis is the fact that the illness can begin the same day the offending food was eaten, or *up to seventy days later*. Gastroenteritis due to *Listeria* usually begins within a few hours to two to three days.[516] The severe, invasive form of the disease incubates anywhere from three days to three months.

The statistics for mortality from *Listeria* are as follows:

- Severe infections have an overall 15-30% mortality rate.
- Severe infections involving septicemia have a 50% mortality rate.
- Severe infections with meningitis have a 70% mortality rate. This is the most common route in the elderly and immunocompromised.
- Severe infections in newborns have an 80% mortality rate.[517]
- One-third of maternal cases result in miscarriage and stillbirth.[518]

Risk factors:

- Pregnant women are 10 times more likely to contract *Listeria* than the general population.[519]
- Hispanic and pregnant women are 24 times more likely to contract *Listeria*.[520]

- Infants of someone who had listeriosis while pregnant are susceptible.[521]
- People over the age of 65 are four times more likely to develop a listeria infection than the general population. It is due to decreased stomach acid production (stomach acid kills listeria), a weaker immune system, and/or taking medications that weaken the immune system.[522]
- Those taking stomach acid-reducing medications are at elevated risk.[523]
- Anyone with a compromised immune system is at risk.[524]

Conventional treatment. Physicians administer intravenous ampicillin and gentamicin for two to three weeks. Intravenous TMP-SMZ 3-5 mg/kg for three weeks is another option.[525]

Alternative treatment. Listeria are Gram-positive bacteria. Listeria infections may possibly be treated with juniper,[526] honey, usnea, colloidal silver, apple cider vinegar, lemon juice, oregano, and/or garlic.

Norovirus

Norovirus is the culprit for the most common type of food poisoning in the US. It is found on raw fruits and vegetables and in shellfish from tainted waters. Symptoms include nausea, diarrhea, vomiting, low fever, abdominal pain, and headache. The single largest source happens to be infected food handlers.[527]

Norovirus is a lovely little pathogen that makes the rounds every year. It is extremely contagious, so much so that it frequently closes schools. Formerly known as the Norwalk virus, it causes about 20% of acute gastroenteritis cases. It is the leading cause of foodborne illness in the world and ranks fourth in deaths due to food poisoning. This includes over 50,000 deaths of children each year, mostly in developing countries.[528] Like the common cold, norovirus comes in several genotypes that evolve over time so they can make you sick again. This virus afflicts about 20 million people in the US each year, and results in 600-800 fatalities, primarily among young children and the elderly. Fortunately, there is a lot we can do to protect ourselves.[529]

Transmission. The virus is passed in stool and vomit. If you get it, it's possible that you got someone else's bodily grossness into you somewhere along the way, probably by eating or drinking it. Primary person-to-person transmission of the virus happens that way. Probably because they didn't wash their hands after using the toilet. Perhaps because you didn't wash yours after touching whatever they touched and before touching your face or mouth, or because you didn't wash your hands well enough.[530]

Secondary person-to-person transmission occurs by sharing food, drinks, or utensils. If those were the only ways norovirus spread, thorough handwashing and not sharing food or drink would protect us. However, water can also be contaminated with norovirus, and thus contaminate everything it contacts—ice, eggs, fruits, and salads. Infected food handlers can pass it on to cooked foods. Unfortunately, norovirus also survives pretty well on doorknobs, stairway railings, and other surfaces for days to weeks.[531] That's why schools get closed down and disinfected during outbreaks. There are also some recent studies indicating that norovirus may become aerosolized during vomiting so that it can be passed by droplets in the air.

Signs and symptoms. Norovirus in the northern hemisphere is most common from November to April, with the peak season being December through February. Symptoms of a norovirus infection include nausea, vomiting, and abdominal cramps. Diarrhea is less frequent. There may be a low-grade fever. Unlike a lot of other illnesses, the moment you contract norovirus, long before exhibiting symptoms, you are contagious to others. While the symptoms usually pass in one to two days, the patient is still contagious for at least three days and perhaps up to two weeks afterward.[532]

Prevention. Careful handwashing is the best way to prevent contracting a norovirus infection. Hand sanitizers are of little efficacy because norovirus is a non-enveloped virus.[533] It's a tough bugger. Vigorous, meticulous scrubbing of the hands with soap and water and bleach and hot water for surfaces are essential.

Treatment. Treatment is primarily supportive care with fluids and rest.

And now, because this is a foodborne illness, let's bring it back to food safety. Once a person has caught norovirus, before the symptoms appear, that person is shedding norovirus and infecting people and contaminating food. It's not a problem if the food is thoroughly cooked, like in canning. But what if Grandma was exposed to norovirus on Monday morning, and then prepared some food for the freezer, to be eaten later? Grandma gets sick Tuesday evening. Everything Grandma touched, all that food, is contaminated—even if it's not eaten for months, because freezing temperatures don't affect norovirus. It has to be cooked to be killed.

Salmonella

There are just two species of *Salmonella: Salmonella enterica* and *Salmonella bongori*; the latter, found only in reptiles, won't be further discussed. *Salmonella enterica* has 6 subspecies and over 2,600 serotypes that are found in all warm-blooded animals and in the environment all over the world. The full given name of members of the *Salmonella enterica* serotypes goes like this: *Salmonella enterica* subsp. *enterica* serotype Typhimurium. So that's why you'll see what looks like all different species of *Salmonella*, when in fact, there are only two. Typhoidal serotypes cause typhoid fever and paratyphoid fever, and while they cause severe illnesses, they are not related to food poisoning.

The non-typhoidal serotypes like *Salmonella enterica* subsp. *enterica* serotype Enteritidis are more common and the source of many cases of food poisoning, up to 1.5 million each year in the US alone. While salmonellosis is definitely unpleasant, it passes within three to five days without any lasting effects for the vast majority of healthy individuals. Those most at risk for severe illness include:

- Infants (especially those who are not breast-fed[534])

- Elderly
- Immunocompromised
- Those taking proton-pump inhibitors[535]
- Organ transplant recipients

Signs and symptoms. Symptoms of salmonella food poisoning manifest 6-72 hours after consuming tainted food. Symptoms include:

- Fever
- Chills
- Diarrhea (possibly bloody)
- Stomach cramps
- Nausea
- Vomiting
- Headache[536]

Transmission. Foods most commonly infected include pork and chicken, sprouts and vegetables, and eggs, the latter accounting for 150,000 illnesses each year.[537] Other foods that may be contaminated with salmonella include nut butters, fruits, and processed foods. Not only can salmonella bacteria survive outside a host for years, they also survive boiling, freezing, and frying. An egg must be fried hard or boiled for nine minutes to kill the bacteria.[538]

Prevention. Salmonella illnesses are best prevented by frequent and thorough handwashing, especially after any contact with animals, using the toilet, or helping someone else use the toilet or change a diaper.

Conventional treatment. Antibiotic treatment is reserved for severe cases and those at greatest risk for serious complications. Rarely, salmonella may enter the bloodstream and cause sepsis. In this case, prompt treatment with antibiotics is essential. If a doctor determines that antibiotics are warranted, commonly prescribed antibiotics are Zithromax or Levaquin, each 500 mg, once per day, 7-10 days. Cipro and doxycycline may also be suggested.

Alternative treatment. While pharmaceuticals are reserved for only the most severe cases of *Salmonella* food poisoning, anyone may use colloidal silver, activated charcoal, and/or honey to bring faster relief and to conserve antibiotic supplies.

Caution: Imodium should not be administered if salmonella food poisoning is suspected. It may relieve cramping but will also likely prolong the illness. Imodium works to keep fluids in the body; the salmonella bacteria need to get out of the body for the patient to recover.[539]

Other Types of Food Poisoning

Staphylococcus aureus is the most common bacterial cause of food poisoning and, like norovirus, is passed by food handlers. *S. aureus* is commonly found all over the skin. It multiplies extremely well at temperatures around 100°F. Symptoms usually start within 30 minutes to 8 hours, and include vomiting, diarrhea, and cramps that last about 24 hours before the person starts recovering. It is most frequently found on meats, cheeses, custards, and starchy foods that stand at room temperature for hours before serving. Though this illness stems from bacteria, it is the toxin produced by the bacteria that makes people sick. As such, antibiotics are ineffective in treatment.[540]

Campylobacter infections in the US are most often due to consuming undercooked or raw poultry, although contaminated milk and water are also sometimes to blame. Symptoms manifest two to five days after consuming the tainted product and last for about a week. Diarrhea, fever, and cramps are common and are sometimes accompanied by nausea or vomiting. Antibiotic treatment is reserved for those with compromised immune systems.

Clostridium perfringens is often referred to as "cafeteria poisoning" because it occurs when food is allowed to stand for long periods, like on buffet warming tables. The foods most frequently affected are cooked meats, gravy, casseroles, and stews. These bacteria are found in soil, sewage, and human and animal waste. Symptoms begin within 8-22 hours after eating and include abdominal pain, nausea, and diarrhea. Vomiting is rare. Symptoms usually last 12-48 hours.[541]

Shigella bacteria cause shigellosis, a highly contagious illness transmitted through feces. Anyone who gets it somehow got somebody else's feces into his mouth. This is just one reason why we wash hands extremely well whenever it is called for. And because fresh produce can also be contaminated if grown in fields with human waste, it is why we also wash fresh produce very well before eating it. Diarrhea, which is often bloody, fever, and cramps begin one to two days after infection. The illness lasts five to seven days.

APPENDICITIS

Just over 1% of all hospitalizations in the US are for appendicitis. Nearly 12% of all hospitalizations for gastrointestinal problems are related to appendicitis. Those numbers aren't so concerning, but let's look at some other numbers.

Keep in mind that appendicitis can happen to anybody, but is most common in those under the age of 40. About 7% of the US population has had or will have appendicitis and the resulting appendectomy. That number is a little more disconcerting, especially when the data are inconclusive about the risk factors for developing appendicitis.

Risk factors. It is believed that the risk is lower for those who consume high fiber diets and for infants and children who are/were breast-fed. The risk is higher for those with a first-degree relative who had appendicitis.[542] The disease is 40% more common in males than females, and rates are 50% higher for whites than for non-whites. The majority of cases, 74%, occur in people between the ages of 5-34 years, with most cases occurring in 10- to 19-year-olds. To make the numbers even more interesting, the rates of appendicitis are 11% higher in summer than in winter, and there is a higher incidence of appendicitis cases in the west north central region of the US. ("[W]est north central" is exactly how the article worded it—sounds like Eastern Washington, Eastern Oregon, Idaho, Northern Nevada and Northern Utah.)[543]

Doctors have been performing appendectomies for over 100 years. It's one of the first surgeries budding surgeons ever do and supposedly pretty simple and easy to learn. For most of the last century, doctors have routinely advised appendectomies for their patients with appendicitis, but recently this habit has come under scrutiny. More and more, especially in Europe, doctors are using antibiotics in an effort to resolve uncomplicated appendicitis and prevent the need for surgery.[544]

Unfortunately, without lab equipment it's going to be difficult to determine whether any particular case of appendicitis is complicated and likely to lead to a rupture of the appendix, or whether antibiotics alone should do the job. One study showed that in cases of mild to moderate appendicitis, antibiotics were effective about 88% of the time. However, in about 24% of these patients there was a recurrence of appendicitis, with most of these recurrences occurring within one year, and surgery was undertaken.[545]

While antibiotics may not be a perfect solution for appendicitis, they may buy you some time in being able to procure supplies or until you can get to a functioning hospital.

Without a functioning medical system and without a medical professional, how are you going to determine whether a family member has appendicitis?

Signs and symptoms. Usually appendicitis begins with a vague discomfort in the area of the belly button. It then moves to the lower right section of the abdomen, about two-thirds of the way from the navel to the top of the right pelvic bone, within 12-24 hours.

Other common symptoms include:

- Nausea and vomiting
- Loss of appetite
- Fever and chills
- Abdominal swelling
- Pain that worsens when walking[546]

A patient with appendicitis will move as if he is walking on eggshells, as any movement of the legs causes movement of the abdominal muscles. (Children under the age of two years may also present with a limp.[547]) If you are suspecting appendicitis at this point, continue with this test to get a better idea of what is going on:

Press down on the lower right section of the abdomen. Someone with appendicitis should find this painful.

Now press on the same spot but on the left side of the abdomen. Does this also cause pain on the right side?

Finally, for an idea of whether the appendix has ruptured, press down again on the right side. Does it hurt even more when you release the pressure? If so, there's a greater likelihood that the appendix has ruptured.[548]

Two other diagnostic tests to conduct:

Ask the patient to hop on his right leg. If there is a significant increase in pain, appendicitis is likely.

Have the patient lie flat on a bed or a table. Ask the patient to raise the right leg. If this causes pain in the right lower quadrant, appendicitis is likely.[549]

Treatment. As soon as appendicitis is diagnosed, the patient should be restricted to small amounts of clear liquids.[550] Surgery in a medical facility is the best option for most people, but if it really is not possible:

- IV antibiotics, like cefoxitin or Rocephin, for at least 3 days followed by oral antibiotics for 8-10 days have the best outcome.
- A combination of Cipro and metronidazole *may* work and would be especially indicated for those allergic to penicillins.[551]
- Augmentin, 500 mg, 3x per day OR TMP-SMZ DS or Cipro, 500 mg, 2x per day PLUS
- Metronidazole, 500 mg, 3-4x per day.
- Both options should be continued until three to four days after symptoms have resolved.[552]

- Surgeons in third world countries commonly perform appendectomies under local anesthesia.*

Before going the surgical route, make sure you are dealing with appendicitis. Here are some quick tests for differentiating between appendicitis and other conditions that mimic appendicitis:

- Ectopic pregnancy (a woman with a missed period, positive pregnancy test, and severe pain on one side of the lower abdomen is more likely to be an ectopic pregnancy)
- Diverticulitis (symptoms are very similar, but most patients are older and have pain in the lower left side, rather than the lower right)
- Pelvic inflammatory disease (only in women, pain is on both sides of lower abdomen, there is a fever and sometimes foul vaginal discharge)
- Ovarian cysts (differentiation from appendicitis is difficult without diagnostic equipment)[553]

DIVERTICULAR DISEASE

As we age, the risk of appendicitis decreases and the chances increase for another disease with similar symptoms and similar risks for complications and death. It's called diverticular disease and encompasses diverticulosis and diverticulitis. It's kind of like appendicitis for the older generation.

Diverticulosis involves the formation of sacs or pouches in the colon. It affects about 10% of Americans over the age of 40. It causes no symptoms nor pain, so most are quite blissfully unaware they have the condition. However, between 10 and 25% of those with diverticulosis will eventually develop diverticulitis, and that *is* a problem. Still, it only affects 1 to 2.5% of all people over the age of 40. Diverticulitis is what happens when those asymptomatic diverticulosis pouches become inflamed or infected. At best, most cases of

---

* If you are going to go the surgery route, the procedure is described in detail in *Survival and Austere Medicine, 3rd Edition.* Of course, you will want to have a clean operating field, with sterile gown, gloves, and drapes, at least a local anesthetic, and scalpels, clamps, and sutures.

diverticulitis are painful, and they only require bed rest and gradual dietary changes. However, severe diverticulitis may necessitate hospitalization, intravenous antibiotics, and surgery.[554]

Signs and symptoms. The inflamed/infected diverticula can perforate or burst just like the appendix, spilling the contents into the abdominal cavity, and can be just as deadly as a ruptured appendix. The symptoms of the two diseases are very similar. Appendicitis patients generally have pain on the lower *right* side; diverticulitis usually presents with pain on the lower *left* side.[555] This pain is also very sudden and severe. Other symptoms include abdominal tenderness, fever, nausea, constipation, diarrhea, bloating, and rectal bleeding.[556]

Risk factors. The risk factors for developing diverticular disease as far as diet is concerned are high animal protein/high fat diets that are very low in fiber. Obesity, a sedentary lifestyle, age, genetics, smoking, steroids, and opiates may also contribute.

However, Metamucil is not the answer. After the body has rested and recovered from its bout with diverticulitis, *gradual* changes to the diet should be made to reduce the number of flare-ups and opportunities for recurrence. If a person has had diverticulitis once, he's at greater risk for having it again. The best diet for preventing diverticulitis includes a lot of fiber and probiotics like yogurt. In addition, exercise is very beneficial to maintaining gut flow, as is going when you've got to go rather than holding it in.[557]

Conventional treatment. Conventional therapy for diverticulitis is complete bed rest. Physicians will sometimes prescribe antibiotics, with Levaquin being the drug of choice. Cipro and metronidazole are other options. Each is taken for 10-21 days.[558] None of these is without the risk of side effects. Do not consume alcohol while taking metronidazole.[559] Side effects of Levaquin and Cipro include a risk of tendinitis and/or tendon rupture during treatment and for several months after. Tylenol may be used for pain. NSAIDs are to be avoided due to the risk of bleeding.

BEZOARS

Bezoars (*BE-zors*) are hard, compacted clumps of fiber much like hairballs in cats. While cats can cough up hairballs, people cannot cough up a bezoar. This undigested or partially digested material can build up and cause blockages anywhere along the gastrointestinal tract, but they are most commonly found in the stomach. Fortunately, many bezoars are completely asymptomatic and cause no problems at all. Unfortunately, surgical intervention is sometimes required for the others.[560]

Diagnosing a bezoar in a patient isn't going to be all that easy. It will be necessary to obtain a very thorough patient history and detailed information on the diet. Without lab equipment, it may be next to impossible to do anything more than make an educated guess.

Signs and symptoms. The symptoms of bezoars include:

- Feeling full after eating very little food
- Lack of appetite
- Nausea
- Vomiting
- Abdominal pain
- Weight loss
- Anemia[561]

Types of bezoars. There are six types of bezoars. Older adults are generally at greater risk for developing bezoars, but trichobezoars and lactobezoars are more common in children.

Phytobezoars are the most common type, making up about 40% of all bezoars. They form quickly and present with nausea, vomiting, and gastric outlet obstruction. These have been treated with good success using a 12-ounce can of Coke, regular or diet, twice per day for 6-8 weeks.[562] Other studies showed good resolution of the bezoar with just a few cans of Coke.[563]

Diospyrobezoars are a type of phytobezoar due to eating too many persimmons. These bezoars cannot be dissolved by Coke and must be surgically removed.[564]

Trichobezoars are most commonly found in adolescent girls who suck on, chew, and swallow hair and often indicate some underlying psychiatric issue, as might happen in a time of stress in a collapsed society. The condition is also called Rapunzel's syndrome. These bezoars take a considerable amount of time to develop, sometimes years. The patient usually presents with nausea and early satiety, and perhaps anorexia and weight loss. These usually require removal through endoscopy or surgery.[565] Coke does not work.

Pharmacobezoars arise due to medication that doesn't get digested. These patients are usually older and are more likely to have gastric outlet obstruction.[566]

Lactobezoars occur most frequently in infants and arise due to dehydration, prematurity and low birth weight (underdeveloped gastrointestinal tract), high calorie formula (not mixed according to directions), or the addition of thickening agents like pectin to formula. They present with problems in feeding intolerance, abdominal distension, irritability, and/or vomiting. A palpable mass may be detected in these patients.[567]

Foreign body bezoars, most often tissue paper and Styrofoam cups.

Risk factors. Bezoars most often develop in people with the following risk factors. If you don't have at least one risk factor, you're probably in the clear for this condition.

- Gastric surgery or gastric band for weight loss[568]
- Reduced stomach acid production or decreased stomach size
- Cystic fibrosis
- Delayed gastric emptying due to diabetes complications[569]
- Autoimmune disorders
- Mixed connective tissue disease

- Gastroparesis[570]
- Ulcers
- Hypothyroidism
- Not chewing food properly, due to poorly fitting dentures or missing teeth (more common among the elderly)[571]
- Excessive intake of fiber, especially in a rapid change from a modern American diet to a high fiber diet, like what may happen post-collapse[572]

Those at risk for developing bezoars should chew their food thoroughly before swallowing and should avoid following foods:

- Pumpkins
- Celery
- Persimmons
- Sunflower seed shells
- Prunes and raisins
- Leeks
- Beets

CHOLECYSTITIS

Gallstones may trigger an infection or inflammation called cholecystitis. The symptoms are pain in the right upper quadrant of the abdomen and fever, and sometimes nausea, vomiting, and jaundice. Treatment in challenging circumstances is as per other abdominal infections, to wit:

- Fluids
- Pain relievers and fever reducers
- Augmentin, intravenous (preferred)

However, intravenous Augmentin may be hard to come by. An alternative that may work would be to administer an anti-nausea drug such as Bonine or

Zofran to help the patient keep down oral antibiotics, such as Augmentin, Keflex, Cipro, or TMP-SMZ DS plus metronidazole.[573]

CHOLANGITIS

Cholangitis results from a stone lodged in the bile duct and is difficult to differentiate from cholecystitis without a functioning laboratory as the symptoms are basically the same. Cholangitis is a medical emergency. The gallbladder needs to be removed, but it is beyond the scope of care in an austere environment. A doctor may administer pain relievers, fluids, and high doses of the antibiotics, but these are unlikely to be effective.[574]

GALLSTONES

Gallstones are something 90% of people will never experience. However, because the other 10% of people do get the totally unforgettable opportunity to be in pain described as worse than childbirth, it's a good idea to learn all we can about it now.[575] Those of Scandinavian and Mexican-American descent[576] are 1.5-2 times more likely to experience gallstones, and American Indians are 80% more likely. Individuals with a first degree relative[577] with gallstones are 1.5 times more likely to experience them as well.

Gallstones are solid deposits that form in the gallbladder and block the passage of bile. Attacks are often triggered by eating a fatty meal. For most patients, the abdominal pain is constant. It may even hurt to breathe. Other symptoms include jaundice, gray or gray-white stools, nausea, and vomiting. In a grid-down situation if you're not sure the patient's pain is due to gallstones, have the patient eat some fatty foods. That will usually make the pain worse.

Signs and symptoms. The pain is generally in the upper right quadrant of the abdomen, but in some patients it occurs immediately below the breastbone in the center of the abdomen. In others, it occurs in the right shoulder or between the shoulder blades.[578] Classic onset of gallstone pain occurs over 30-

60 minutes, lasts several hours, and then slowly dissipates. While the patient is in pain, she can't get comfortable in any way and often paces the floor.[579]

Risk factors. The classic risk factors for gallstones are the four F's:

- Fat
- Female
- Fertile (has had children)
- Forty (over the age of forty)[580]

It should be noted that while most patients have the classic risk factors, gallstones can affect either sex at any age. Other risk factors include diabetes, cirrhosis of the liver, and anemia.[581] Unfortunately, the only sure treatment is surgical removal of the gallbladder.

Gallstones are extremely painful; however, they are not life-threatening (unless infection develops—that's another topic). If you're female, you may not be able to do much about some of your risk factors, but you can lose weight.

ULCERS

Technically speaking, an ulcer is an open sore where the skin or lining has been worn away gradually (in contrast to an abrasion, which happens suddenly). However, most often when we are speaking of an ulcer, we are referring to the lining of the esophagus, stomach, or duodenum that has become compromised for any number of reasons and is causing pain.

The reasons why excessive acid production compromises the intestinal mucosa lining are varied and will be covered later. The first objective is to determine whether the pain a person is complaining of is, in fact, attributable to an ulcer. It's important to make that determination quickly, because the pain can also be confused with angina and other heart issues. While there is very little that can be done for heart issues, calming down a patient's pain due to excess acid production will make a difference and prevent further pain.

Prevention. Most causes of ulcers will be reduced or eliminated with societal collapse. There will be less alcohol consumption, less smoking, and less overeating, especially of fatty foods. Advil and aspirin use, other agents that can cause ulcers, will continue until those supplies are exhausted. Some ulcers are actually caused by a bacterial infection and require antibiotic treatment. Stress levels may increase, and chronic stress will increase stomach acid production. The best prevention is to avoid alcohol, tobacco, overeating, and stress.

Signs and symptoms. Without laboratory tests and endoscopy, a diagnosis can tentatively be suggested based on the patient's symptoms. Occasional pain in the stomach is associated with heartburn, especially if the pain worsens after eating a large meal or after lying down. If it occurs more than twice a week, or other symptoms are involved, other causes should be considered.

Pain due to ulcers often is felt in the pit of the stomach, on the left or in the upper-mid abdomen and radiating toward the breastbone up to the esophagus. It's usually a chronic, dull pain, but it may become sharp at times. The pain may occur right after eating (which suggests a gastric—stomach—ulcer) or several hours later (which suggests a duodenal ulcer). It's also described as being somewhat like hunger pangs or indigestion and can be confused with angina. To differentiate ulcer pain from angina, have the patient drink some milk (the higher the fat, the better) or take an antacid. Either of these will alleviate the pain if it is due to an ulcer or acid reflux. They will do nothing for angina.[582] Frequent and lasting pain suggests an ulcer. Pain that lessens when food is eaten or when a lot of water is consumed, pain that worsens at night or after eating, or with alcohol or spicy or fatty foods also points toward an ulcer.

A severe ulcer may cause vomiting, with either fresh blood or partially digested blood. Stools with blood from an ulcer are usually black. And some ulcers are painless and the first sign is blood in the vomit and black, sticky stools. This is a medical emergency and professional care must be sought quickly. The patient may be bleeding to death.[583]

Treatment. To prevent pain and allow the ulcer to heal:

- Don't overeat. Eat small meals and healthy snacks in between meals. Focus on foods that soothe and calm.
- Avoid foods that cause pain, including:
    - Alcohol
    - Coffee and tea
    - Soda
    - Spicy foods, including pepper
    - Fatty foods
    - Chocolate
    - Milk. While milk, especially whole milk or half-and-half, calms the pain, it actually increases stomach acid production, so it should be avoided.
- Avoid Alka-Seltzer, Tums, and similar products. These also quickly calm the pain, but should only be used for occasional indigestion, not ulcers.
- If the pain is worse at night, prop the upper body with pillows for sleeping.
- Drink a lot of water, at least a pint before and after each meal and in between meals as well. Drink even if there is no pain.
- Do not eat within four hours of going to bed.
- Do not lie down after eating.[584]

There are several over-the-counter treatment options. Prilosec and Zantac are two of the most common and inexpensive, and therefore, easily stockpiled. Dosages are provided on the packages. Most packages are for a single course of treatment, usually about two weeks. However, in some cases, treatment will take longer. Also, what is sold over-the-counter is about half the prescription strength, which a physician will recommend in some cases.

Prilosec dosages physicians commonly prescribe for individuals 16+ years of age:[585]

Active duodenal ulcer—20-40 mg per day, for 4-8 weeks, either all at bedtime or in divided doses.

Duodenal ulcer with *H. pylori* infection—20 mg, 2x per day, 10 days, *plus* one of the following:

1. amoxicillin, 1000 mg, 2x per day, and Biaxin (500 mg 2x per day) OR metronidazole (400-500 mg, 3-4x per day) OR

2. metronidazole, (400-500 mg, 3-4x per day) and tetracycline (500 mg 2x per day) OR Biaxin (500 mg 2x per day).[586]

If the patient isn't substantially improved within ten days, discontinue treatment. Persistent symptoms in a middle-aged or older patient may be due to stomach cancer.

Gastric ulcer—40 mg, once per day at bedtime, for 4-8 weeks.

GERD—20 mg, 1x per day, up to 4-6 weeks. Smaller, more frequent doses help curb acid production.

Again, these are not prescriptions or recommendations. The information provided herein is a guideline for what quantities you may wish to procure for your family. There is actually a wide range in both the dosages and durations that physicians recommend. Proton-pump inhibitors and acid blockers are often recommended for preventing ulcers; however, such usage increases the patient's risk of other infections, including *Clostridium difficile* and some kinds of food poisoning.

It may be worth noting that Prilosec has been shown to be more effective than Pepcid.[587]

Alternative treatment. Honey, one tablespoon per day, has been shown to be of help.[588]

18. UROGENITAL CONCERNS

KIDNEY STONES

A kidney stone can be differentiated from a urinary tract infection in that the onset of pain from a kidney stone is very sudden, while the onset of pain from a urinary tract infection is much more gradual.[589]

There are two bits of good news when it comes to kidney stones. The first is that kidney stones are usually not due to an infection.[590] The second is that over 95% of stones pass without needing surgery.[591] The bad news is that if you've had one, there's a 50% chance you'll have another within the next 10 years.[592]

Risk factors. Men are more likely to suffer from kidney stones than women, especially between the ages of 20 and 50. Individuals with a family history of kidney stones are 2.5 times more likely to experience kidney stones themselves. And kidney stones are more common in the southeastern part of the US than the rest of the country. In general, 10% of Americans will experience at least one kidney stone in their lifetime.[593]

Signs and symptoms. While kidney stones are formed in the kidneys, they usually don't cause pain until they start moving down the ureters, the tubes that carry urine to the bladder. The pain can be absolutely excruciating due not only to the urine backing up into the kidneys, but also due to the stone (some of them look like little spiked balls) traveling through the ureter.[594] The pain is usually felt on only one side of the back and is often accompanied by abnormal urination. Tapping on the flank at the level of the lowest rib on the same side the stone is on will cause significant pain in a patient with kidney stones. Also, as the stones travel down the ureter, so does the pain.[595]

Other symptoms include:

- Blood in the urine (the stone scrapes the ureter as it travels)

- Strong urge to urinate frequently
- Inability to urinate
- Nausea and vomiting
- Sweating[596]

The pain may subside when the stone reaches the bladder and then resume as it travels from the bladder through the urethra and out. Though pain is not usually relieved by changing position, patients are often restless and prefer to move around. Some patients have found relief by passing urine lying down. Gravity allows the stone in the bladder to roll away from the opening and lets urine pass.[597] Pain may come in waves or be quite constant.

If the stone is too large and doesn't pass, it will cause pressure to build on the kidney. Without a functioning medical system, there is absolutely no possible intervention. The kidney will be permanently damaged, but the pain will eventually subside. However, if an infection develops in the blocked kidney, it may be fatal.[598]

Treatment—Dietary management

The biggest single factor contributing to kidney stones is dehydration. It's really a basic chemistry lesson: the stones form when there is not enough water to keep them dissolved. While everyone is supposed to be drinking a half-gallon of water per day, people who have had kidney stones should be drinking a bit more to prevent recurrences.[599]

Other than staying very well hydrated, what can people with a history of kidney stones do to prevent having more? Post-collapse, there probably won't be a laboratory to identify the type of stones a patient makes.

The most common type of kidney stone is the **calcium oxalate** form. They occur more often in men than in women, usually men aged 20-40 years.[600] Supplementing the diet with 400 mg of magnesium and 50 mg of vitamin B6 helps prevent the formation of this type of kidney stones.[601] Increasing the amounts of fruits, vegetables, and whole grains in the diet is critical.[602]

Struvite stones occur more in women, with chronic and frequent infections being a risk factor. Frequent catheterization also contributes to the formation of struvite stones. These account for about 10% of kidney stones. Lowering sodium consumption may reduce the formation of struvite stones.[603]

Uric acid stones are more common in men and are linked with gout. Approximately 10% of stones are this type. A diet rich in animal protein contributes to the formation of uric acid stones. Reducing the consumption of animal protein in favor of plant protein will diminish the formation of uric acid stones.[604]

Cystine stones are associated with a recessive genetic disorder and comprise about 1% of all kidney stones. The only dietary adjustment other than increasing fluid intake is that lowering the consumption of animal protein may help prevent future stone formation.[605]

If you are unsure which kind of stone you suffer from, just do everything:

- Avoid spinach, rhubarb, chocolate, parsley, and beets.[606]
- Avoid vitamin C supplements. People who consumed a gram or more per day were 40% more likely to get kidney stones.[607]
- Reduce sodium consumption.[608]
- Keep protein intake moderate, around 50 grams per day.[609]
- Get adequate vitamin D from the sun or through a supplement.[610]
- Eat lots of fruits and vegetables and whole grains.[611]
- While some doctors recommend reducing dietary calcium, recent research indicates the opposite: calcium binds the oxalate and phosphate normally found in kidney stones and helps remove them from the body before the kidneys have to.[612]

Treatment—Pain and infection management. If the patient has experienced kidney stones in the past and is sure of the diagnosis, physicians indicate that stronger pain medications are acceptable to use. Otherwise, Advil (600-800 mg, every 4-6 hours) may be alternated with Tylenol (500-1000 mg, every 4-8 hours). Tramadol, 50-100 mg every 3-6 hours, is another option.[613]

If the pain is not too intense and the patient needs help sleeping, Benadryl may be used.[614] If nausea or vomiting is a problem, Bonine may be taken, 25 mg, every 6-12 hours. Azo or Uristat are good OTC options for pain as well.

In patients with a prior history of infection or considerable bleeding, physicians may prescribe an oral antibiotic for one to three days. Either Cipro, 250-500 mg, 2x per day, Macrobid, 50-100 mg, 2x per day, or TMP-SMZ DS, 2x per day, would be acceptable.[615]

URINARY TRACT INFECTIONS

The two most common types of urinary tract infections (UTIs) are cystitis, which is a bladder infection, and pyelonephritis, which is a kidney infection. The usual offending pathogen is *Escherichia coli*, and it wends its way from outside the body up through the urethra to the bladder.[616]

Cystitis

The urethra is much shorter and straight in women, while it is two to three times as long in men and travels a winding path. The short, straight shot makes it very easy for women to develop these infections; indeed, women are about twenty times more likely than men to suffer UTIs. However, women are also much more easily treated. Men are far less likely to contract a UTI, but when they do, it is also more difficult to treat and must be approached more aggressively.[617]

Signs and symptoms of a bladder infection include the following:

- Fever
- Painful urination
- More frequent urination
- Lower abdominal pain, especially just above the pubic bone
- Cloudy urine
- Blood in the urine (but not often visible to the naked eye)
- Mental changes, most especially in the elderly[618]

Elderly individuals with a UTI generally have less specific symptoms like confusion and unsteadiness. A UTI must always be suspected in a confused elder, especially one in whom this change in mental status has been fairly rapid.[619]

A definitive diagnosis is best achieved with urinalysis strips. They've got about a two-year shelf-life unopened, and are good for 90 days after the bottle is opened. If the dipstick shows protein, blood, and leukocytes, the patient most likely has a UTI.[620]

Treatment. A conservative approach to treatment is utilized in women who appear well. For many, increasing fluid intake to wash the bacteria out will be sufficient. Alkalinizing the urine is also recommended by using either 1 teaspoon of baking soda or 1 1/2 teaspoons of cream of tartar mixed in a cup of water. Vitamin C is reported to be very helpful, as are cranberries and cranberry juice. Cranberries are not effective for kidney and severe bladder infections.[621]

Physicians often prescribe unwell women TMP-SMZ (Bactrim, Septra) for three days, and if that is ineffective, then cotrimoxazole or Augmentin for five to seven days. Men are generally prescribed a longer course of treatment, for seven to ten days. Other options include the following treatment protocols:

- Ampicillin, 500 mg, 4x day, 7 days[622]
- Keflex, 250 mg 4x day OR 500 mg 2x day, 7 days[623]
- Cipro, 250-500 mg, 2x day, 7-14 days[624]
- Doxycycline, 100 mg, 2x day for the first day, 100 mg day, 10 days[625]
- TMP-SMZ DS, 2x day, 10-14 days[626]
- Other antibiotics that are sometimes used include amoxicillin, Macrobid, Cipro, and ampicillin.[627]

Azo or Uristat is recommended for reducing the pain of urination. Both of these medications will turn the urine a reddish-brown temporarily.[628]

Prevention. The incidence of UTIs can be reduced or eliminated by practicing the following:

- Wipe front to back
- Urinate after intercourse
- Go when you need to go
- Refrain from taking bubble baths or using strong soap on the genitals[629]

Pyelonephritis

The symptoms of a kidney infection are similar to those of a bladder infection, but much more severe. There is more pain and a higher fever, which are often accompanied by nausea and vomiting. The pain may radiate from the back just below the ribs and down to the thighs. The same antibiotics are used, but for 10-14 days. Failure to treat pyelonephritis may result in sepsis and death.[630]

The following treatment protocols are routinely prescribed for pyelonephritis:

- Ampicillin, 500 mg, 4x day, 14-28 days[631]
- Keflex, 250 mg 4x day OR 500 mg 2x day, 7 days[632]
- Cipro, 250-500 mg, 2x day, 7-14 days[633]
- Doxycycline, 100 mg, 2x day for the first day; 100 mg day thereafter, 10 days total[634]
- TMP-SMZ DS, 2x day, 10-14 days[635]

SEXUALLY TRANSMITTED DISEASES

This is definitely a topic I don't want to think or write about, but because there will be some unfaithful spouses and innocent victims, it's important to address. Readers should already be pretty well aware of risk factors and methods of prevention.

Chlamydia and gonorrhea

These diseases are caused by different bacteria, but they are discussed together because they sometimes appear together and because there will be no lab work to differentiate them.

In women, STDs are difficult to diagnose. An STD must be considered in any woman with pain above the pubic bone, a low-grade fever, and offensive vaginal discharge. Women may experience slight pain when urinating.[636] If the woman is pregnant and untreated, the baby's eyes can become infected, resulting in blindness. However, many individuals will have no symptoms or only minimal symptoms. Symptoms may not develop for weeks or months. Sterility may result.

Men may experience pain or difficulty when urinating. Pus may drip from the penis and there may be painful swelling of the testicles. Weeks or months later, one or both knees, ankles, or wrists may swell painfully. Symptoms usually begin two days to three weeks after sexual contact. Untreated, sterility may result.

Women with an offensive vaginal discharge but no risk factors are more likely to have vaginal thrush or trichomoniasis. These infections are treated with a single dose of tinidazole or a five-day course of metronidazole.[637]

Treatment options physicians commonly prescribe for chlamydia include:

- Zithromax, 1 gram, single dose;
- Doxycycline, 100 mg, 2x per day, 7 days;
- Erythromycin, 500 mg, 4x per day, 7 days;
- Levaquin, 500 mg, 1x per day, 7 days.[638]

Treatment options for gonorrhea are more limited as some strains develop resistance. The commonly used antibiotics listed above are given as intramuscular injections along with cefixime. Zithromax is used in addition to those, in a one-gram single dose, and may be effective on its own.[639]

Syphilis

There are three stages to syphilis, with three opportunities for identification.

Primary syphilis presents with a painless penile ulcer, a *chancre*, which looks like a pimple, blister, or open sore that appears a few weeks after sexual contact. It's full of bacteria that are easily passed to another person. In women, this chancre generally occurs on the cervix or vaginal wall and is usually unnoticed. Both sexes may present with an enlarged lymph node in the groin. This chancre lasts a few days to a few weeks and then disappears.

Secondary syphilis appears a few months later, often as a rash all over the body that may be painless or painful. It can look like small pus-filled spots, or ring-shaped welts, like hives. It lasts a few weeks and then disappears.

Tertiary syphilis appears years later. It affects the heart and brain primarily and will eventually kill the patient if untreated.[640]

Treatment. Syphilis is best treated with intramuscular penicillin injections, again, an option unlikely to be available in a long-term collapse. The CDC suggests Zithromax in a single two-gram dose for primary and secondary syphilis. Doxycycline (100 mg, 2x day, 14 days) and tetracycline (500 mg, 4x day, 14 days) are other options, but not for pregnant women.[641]

If the infection was contracted more than one year previously, the standard treatment protocol is 1.2 million units of penicillin in each buttock, once per week, for 3 weeks. Again, that may be difficult to come by.[642] An alternative is tetracycline, 500 mg, 4x day, for 30 days. Pregnant or breastfeeding women can take erythromycin in the same dosage as tetracycline.[643]

These are the most common STDs. There are others, but they're difficult to diagnose without a laboratory and training.

19. ENVIRONMENTAL INJURIES

FROSTNIP AND FROSTBITE

Frostnip is an early warning sign for frostbite. Exposed skin becomes bright red. It's cold and feels prickly (to the patient), like pins and needles. The treatment is simple: rewarm the skin and protect from further exposure to cold.[644]

Frostbite is an entirely different matter requiring much more care. The body parts at the greatest risk of frostbite are the nose, ears, chin, toes, feet, fingers, and hands. They're smaller, with less circulation, and farther from the body core. They easily become numb, and the patient is unaware that frostbite is occurring.

Signs and symptoms of superficial frostbite include:

- Numbness
- Skin discoloration—white, red, blue-white, grayish-yellow
- Hard, waxy skin
- Joint and muscle stiffness
- Tingling of the affected areas, like pins and needles
- Swelling, blistering, and peeling of the skin after rewarming
- As the skin re-warms it will become bright red and warm to the touch, and the top tissue layers may turn black.

A deep frostbite tissue injury will be characterized by the following:

- Skin turns deep purple
- Skin is cool to the touch
- Small, bleeding blisters
- Slow swelling

In the course of weeks to months, deep structures mummify

Conventional treatment for frostbite begins as soon as the injury is observed:

- Put frostbitten hands under armpits
- Put hands and feet in warm, not hot, water
- Do not allow the patient to walk on frostbitten feet
- Offer Advil for pain and help in restoring circulation
- Remove constrictive clothing and jewelry, but keep the skin covered
- Elevate the afflicted body part to reduce swelling
- Do not break blisters
- Offer warm, non-alcoholic, non-caffeinated fluids (yes, both make a patient *feel* warmer, but due to the vasodilating effects they accelerate heat loss from the body)[645]

Do not do any of the following:

- Do not let tissues freeze again
- Do not rub or massage frostbitten tissue, even though they do it on TV
- Do not use heat lamps or fire to warm tissue
- Do not amputate, even for months, unless signs of systemic infection occur sooner[646]

It may take months to determine if the afflicted tissues are dead or alive. It's definitely a wait-and-see type of thing.

HYPOTHERMIA

When was the last time you gave a thought to how you would treat hypothermia—real hypothermia—as opposed to the kind of cold your child is after playing in the snow for an hour? It seems strange, but for some reason a lot of people worry more about dealing with the "elephants" in the jungle (gunshot wounds, pneumothorax, appendicitis, and other things that are "possible" but pretty uncommon) as opposed to the "elephant" in the room.

Hypothermia is one of those elephants in the room. If we cannot heat our homes, have no heated vehicles, or don't have adequate winter clothing and blankets, we had better be prepared to deal with hypothermia. Hypothermia will kill and will do so rapidly.

Prevention. As with absolutely everything, prevention is better than cure. The extent to which you prepare is naturally going to depend a lot on where you live. The clothing requirements are different in Minnesota than they are in Florida.

The most important item is a good hat, as up to 80% of body heat loss occurs through the head. While the ushanka, a fur hat worn by Russians, might be over the top in some areas, if it works in Siberia, it'll work here. Regardless, the dollar store knit beanies are not what is needed. At the very least get a wool cap that will cover the ears as well, not just a single layer, but one that can be folded up to provide a double layer of protection around the ears and extra coverage on the neck and forehead. If it contains angora or alpaca fiber, so much the better. Angora is eight times warmer than sheep's wool; alpaca is four times warmer. Wool absorbs water; angora and alpaca repel it.

Next, choose mittens instead of gloves. Mittens keep the fingers together so that heat is conserved. Again, skip the cheap dollar store offerings and get real animal fibers. (Knitting mittens and hats is very easy, if anyone in your group is so inclined.) Make sure to have plenty of wool socks—pure wool socks if possible.

For the rest of the clothing, wear layers of loose-fitting light-weight clothing to provide better insulation. Tightly-woven water-repellent material is ideal for protecting against the wind. Wool and silk are great for the inner layer. They hold heat much better than cotton, which should be avoided at all costs in the winter. The outer layer should ideally be both wind- and water-resistant and preferably include a hood. Finally, a scarf will not only help keep the neck warm, but placed over the nose and mouth will help warm cold air before it enters the lungs.

Teach children this simple mnemonic for preventing hypothermia--**COLD:**

C—Cover. Cover as much skin as possible.

O—Overexertion. Avoid it. Sweating accelerates the loss of heat from the body.

L—Layers. Have several layers of clothing. Thin, loose clothing can be easily added or removed to retain more heat or prevent sweating and chilling.

D—Dry. Keep dry and especially check hands and feet frequently to make sure snow hasn't gotten into mittens and boots.[647]

All of the above serve to protect the body from losing heat in the four ways that it does, whether it's by:

- Evaporation—sweat
- Radiation—any time the surrounding temperature is below the core temperature of 98.6°F (a body loses heat much more rapidly when the air temperature is 20°F than when it is 85°F)
- Conduction—direct contact with cold temperatures (falling into a pond of icy water)
- Convection—a cooler object moving against the body (wind chill. When the weather guy says the temperature is 32°F outside but the wind chill makes it feel like 5°F, the body loses heat as if it were 5°F outside)[648]

Those most at risk are the very young and elderly, diabetics, and those with low thyroid levels.

Signs and symptoms. A person experiencing mild hypothermia will:

- Have bright red, cold skin, if an infant
- Have uncontrollable shivering
- Have a body temperature of 95°F or less
- Be unable to think clearly
- Stumble when walking
- Have slow, unclear speech
- Be very tired[649]

If a person has stopped shivering but has *any* of the rest of the signs, the degree of hypothermia is much more serious. As these moderate hypothermia symptoms worsen, the person becomes apathetic and uninterested in helping himself and may fall asleep.

Bear in mind that hypothermia may not be able to be diagnosed using a thermometer. Standard glass thermometers don't register below 94°F. Battery operated thermometers may quit working altogether. If someone has these signs, assume the cause is hypothermia and treat accordingly.

Treatment. First, get the patient to a dry place protected from the wind. Remove all wet clothing and dry the body completely. Wet clothing rapidly accelerates the loss of heat from the body. Cover with dry clothing and dry blankets. Keep the hands and feet covered as well.

Do not warm the patient too quickly, as this may cause heart problems and death. The goal is a one degree increase in body temperature per hour.

Do not apply direct heat to the patient. Burning the skin will only make matters worse.

If you can get the patient to drink, offer warm non-alcoholic, non-caffeinated fluids. Alcohol does not help a person suffering from hypothermia. Do not administer it. Yes, it gives a warm feeling, but that is due to the blood vessels expanding, which results in more rapid heat loss from the body. The same goes for caffeine. It dilates the blood vessels, again resulting in rapid heat loss from the body.[650] Sweet foods like candy, sugar, honey, and ripe fruit may be offered. If those aren't available, starchy foods like potatoes, rice, and bread also work.

Use warm, dry compresses. Those little hand-warmers and toe-warmers are great. Keep some in the medical kits for just such a purpose. Do not place them directly on the skin; make sure there is at least a layer or two of clothing protecting the skin. Alternatively, heat stones in or next to a fire and wrap them in a towel or cloth. Another option is to put warm water in a water bottle. Alternatively, you can place rice in a sock and heat it in a can near the fire. All of these should be placed where they will do the greatest good, and that is in the armpits, between the thighs, the back, chest, and neck. The core of the body needs to be warmed first. Warming the extremities sends cold blood back to the core of the body, reducing the core temperature and possibly inducing death.[651]

If the patient is very young, old, or ill, it may be better to place him on a cot, cover him with blankets, and put pans with hot coals or stones under the cot. Make very sure that it is not so hot as to cause a fire or burn the patient.

Have the patient empty his bladder. It takes a lot of energy to heat urine, so it's best to get the urine out. Skin-to-skin contact is ideal for rewarming everyone, especially babies and young children.

Finally, there is the Mylar blanket. The cheap Mylar blankets will tear if you look at them crossly. A sturdier, larger blanket will cost more, but it's far less likely to tear when it's most needed. It will not reflect any more heat than a thin, cheap blanket; it just won't shred so easily. Do not place the Mylar blanket right next to the skin. Doing so has the opposite effect—it works in a conductive manner to suck heat *away* from the body. Mylar works by radiant heat—reflecting heat back to the body.[652] The shinier the blanket, the better it works. Dirty, dusty blankets will not work as well. (Think of how foil works in the oven—the shiny side is toward the food to reheat left-overs; the shiny side is out to prevent over-browning, like with pie crusts.)

If the patient is really unresponsive, you may need to take additional measures: a rectal warm water enema. For that you just need an enema bag and warm water. Lay the patient down, get something to lubricate, and up it goes.

Hypothermia can happen to anyone at any time of the year. It occurs with traumatic injuries and other blood loss. As a caregiver in an emergency situation, you and everyone around you may be working up a sweat, but if your patient has sustained an injury—and it doesn't even have to be that serious, that patient may experience some degree of hypothermia. Even if the patient doesn't want it, make sure a blanket is available for someone who has been injured and is shivering.

In the case of a traumatic injury, especially where bleeding is concerned, keeping the patient warm is critical. Cold blood does not clot very well; warm blood clots much better, and in an emergency, it can make a difference between life and death. Don't discount the need to keep patients warm at any time of the year.

HYPERTHERMIA

Heat illnesses span the spectrum ranging from heat stress, where a person is just uncomfortable, to heat exhaustion, where physiological problems are setting in, to heatstroke, which can become fatal. Knowing the risk factors and causes as well as preventative measures will help avoid problems when the temperatures rise.

Heat edema

This is temperature-induced swelling that may occur in the extremities. The treatment is to administer fluids and to elevate the limbs affected whenever possible. The swelling may persist for weeks.[653]

Heat cramps

These muscle spasms generally occur in people working hard in hot temperatures, but children may also experience these as a result of running around and playing in extreme heat. They can even develop in overdressed skiers in winter if they aren't rehydrating. The muscle spasms can be quite painful and usually only affect the arms and legs, but sometimes abdominal muscles are also involved. The patient should be directed to lie down in a cool area. Treatment consists of administering oral rehydration salts or a teaspoon of salt in a quart of water. In addition, massaging the painful muscles will help relieve the soreness. The body temperature is normal and the patient is fully conscious.[654] Both heat edema and heat cramps are considered a warning sign for the onset of heat exhaustion.

Heat exhaustion

This acute heat injury occurs due to dehydration and is usually accompanied by hyperthermia. The body can no longer dissipate the heat adequately as a result of extreme environmental conditions. The patient may be pale, weak, and nauseous, with cool, moist skin. Symptoms may include headache, dizziness, loss of appetite, and vomiting. The pupils may be dilated and the patient will have a weak, rapid pulse and rapid, shallow breathing. The mental status is normal, and the patient may have a fever of up to 103.5°F.[655] The treatment is to have the patient lie down and elevate the feet above the heart. Oral rehydration solution or saltwater, one teaspoon of salt per quart of water, should be administered hourly.[656] If the patient is unable to drink, fluids may be administered intravenously, rectally, or subcutaneously.

Heatstroke

Heatstroke sets in when the heat-regulating mechanisms in the brain fail. This is a medical emergency and treatment by a licensed provider must be sought out if at all possible. It can occur even if the patient hasn't been in the sun. It can happen with the young and old in hot temperatures in the shade, and especially in those with underlying illnesses and is often referred to as classic heatstroke. It is the disease that is triggering the body's response. Exertional heatstroke occurs in younger people exercising in the heat.[657]

Regardless of the cause, the treatment is the same. The skin is usually red, very hot, and dry (not even the armpits are moist), though not always. This is why the temperature must be taken. If the core body temperature is above 104°F, heatstroke may occur without rapid treatment. The pupils are dilated and there is generally headache, confusion, and loss of consciousness. Seizures and blood in the urine or vomit may also occur.[658]

Treatment. The treatment for all heat illnesses is to remove the patient from the hot environment to a cool and shady place. Clothing should be removed and cold, wet sheets placed on the skin with fans blowing to cool the body. Ice packs should be placed in the groin, armpits, and neck. (Instant cold packs are not effective in this situation.[659]) If the body can be immersed in cold or icy water, so much the better.[660] Intravenous fluids administered by a licensed professional would be best, but fluids given orally (if the patient is conscious), rectally, or subcutaneously are acceptable options.[661]

Unlike with hypothermia where body temperature should be restored to normal gradually, with heatstroke the body temperature must be reduced below 104°F as rapidly as possible. Note that Tylenol and Advil will not work to lower the body temperature in cases of heatstroke; those medications only lower fever due to an infection.[662]

Those at greatest risk for developing heat-related illnesses are:

- Alcoholics
- Elderly (some say anyone over the age of fifty)
- Individuals with hyperthyroidism, diabetes, Parkinson's, or dystonia
- Infants and small children
- Obese individuals
- Those taking medications such as diuretics, anticholinergics, or under the influence of drugs[663]

Risk factors may be mitigated by dressing appropriately for the weather and avoiding dehydration and physical exertion in hot temperatures.[664]

RADIATION

Potassium iodide tablets are recommended for preventing radiation sickness and future thyroid cancer in the wake of a nuclear event, whether that situation arises due to human error or faulty construction, like Chernobyl, or terrorist actions, or a natural disaster. The radiation contaminates the entire atmosphere locally and then prevailing winds carry the radiation downwind, and it is radioactive iodine that is the most common component in fallout outside the immediate area of a nuclear event. People and animals then inhale and ingest the radioactive iodine, about one-third of which will accumulate in the thyroid. This, in turn, may cause thyroid cancer years down the road. Young children are at greatest risk.*

Potassium iodide, also known as KI, when taken 30 minutes to 24 hours before exposure, saturates the thyroid with regular iodine and thus prevents it from taking up any radioactive iodine.[665] The radioactive iodine is then excreted from the body. Using potassium iodide post-exposure (like what the Russian government told their citizens to do following their recent disaster) is pointless. Keep in mind that potassium iodide can't prevent radioactive iodine from *entering* the body; it only prevents radioactive iodine from *staying* in the body, and only when it is taken *before* exposure. Also, potassium iodide does nothing to prevent radiation sickness due to radioactive strontium or radioactive cesium.

The people at the Centers for Disease Control say to only take potassium iodide when directed to do so by a physician or the government.[666] That will work just fine as long as communication channels are open. But if such is not the case, you might be on your own, and having a Geiger counter may be a good idea.[667]

Still, without a Geiger counter, and if there is no information forthcoming from the government, it's hard to know when to take the tablets. A single dose of potassium iodide has very little risk of harm, and not taking it could lead to thyroid cancer, especially in children. It's better to be safe than sorry and take the pill.[668]

That brings up a somewhat related point that is only briefly alluded to by physicians and merchants. The tablets smell horrible. I don't have personal experience taking one, but based on what they smell like while still sealed in the foil packets, I know it's going to be really bad. The smell permeates through just about everything. You definitely don't want to take them if you don't have

---

* Dr. Cynthia Koelker addresses nuclear fallout and preventing radiation poisoning and thyroid cancer quite thoroughly in her book *Armageddon Medicine*, and I'd highly recommend acquiring a copy if it is at all possible.

to. If you have got to get a child to take these tablets, you should probably have some really awesome treats to wash it down with—chocolate milk, soda, and loads of candy would probably be a good idea. Might not be a bad idea for adults, either.

The FDA recommendations for potassium iodide (KI) dosage are based on cases of thyroid cancer that developed in children exposed to radiation from the Chernobyl nuclear accident.[669]

As with every medication, there are side effects. In this case they're considered mild and clinically insignificant. Two percent of children had some gastrointestinal distress, which was attributed to the bad taste of potassium iodide One percent of children and adults developed a rash. Only two people out of 17 million had an allergic reaction, and both of those were known to have an iodine sensitivity. The risk of reaction from a single dose is very small.

Amount of KI to take by age based on predicted exposure		
	Predicted thyroid exposure (centiGrays)	Dose of potassium iodide (KI)
Birth through 1 month	≥5	16 mg
1 month through 3 years	≥5	32 mg
3 years through 18 years, but under 150 lbs	≥5	65 mg
12 years through 18 years, and over 150 lbs	≥5	130 mg
Pregnant or nursing women	≥5	130 mg
18 years through 40 years	≥10	130 mg
Over 40 years	≥500	130 mg

If there is a nuclear event, pregnant women, nursing mothers, and those with thyroid conditions are advised to take a single initial dose and then work with their physician to determine the best course of treatment.[670]

What if you don't have potassium iodide? What if your group suddenly expanded and there isn't enough for all? Remember, children are at greatest risk, so they get treated first. Thyroid cancer takes years to develop. The middle-aged and elderly will likely be just fine without any treatment.

However, there is another option if you start quickly enough. Betadine contains iodine and is absorbed through the skin and taken up by the thyroid.

When used prior to radiation exposure, it can help saturate the thyroid to prevent it from absorbing radioactive iodine. Apply Betadine to the abdomen or forearm 2-12 hours prior to radiation exposure and reapply each day in the following amounts:

- Adults—8 ml (a measuring teaspoon holds 5 ml)
- Children three years and up (but under 150 pounds) —4 ml
- Toddlers—2 ml
- Infants—1 ml

Continue for at least three days or until radiation levels drop.

Because radioactive potassium iodide can be inhaled and ingested, contaminated plants should not be used for food for at least two to three months.

Caution. Do not drink Betadine. Adverse reactions may occur in those taking diuretics and/or lithium. Do not attempt ingesting iodized salt to get enough iodine.[671] You'd have to eat over five cups of iodized salt to equal one potassium tablet.

20. SELECTED CHRONIC CONDITIONS

The advances of modern medicine have blessed all of us and kept many alive who, had they lived a century earlier, would be dead. If access to the advances of modern medicine becomes restricted, many people will die without life-sustaining drugs and equipment that keep them alive. There's no work-around for congestive heart failure. The same goes for organ transplant recipients who depend on anti-rejection medications. If you've got a chronic condition, you need to research it thoroughly and ascertain how you're going to manage without access to medications. Are there herbal options that will work for you? Will a generator keep your medical devices going?

It's impossible to cover all chronic conditions here; however, some of the most common ones can be addressed.

ASTHMA

Asthma is one of those conditions that would be best not to have in a time when there is no higher medical care. The physicians teaching off-grid medicine classes I have attended were not at all optimistic about the long-term survival odds for those with severe asthma once their maintenance medications run out. However, I also believe that when a person recognizes a threat to his own or a loved one's existence, that person will go to great lengths to find options.

Asthmatics need to stockpile their inhalers and other medications. It would be wise to do everything possible to make those supplies last as long as possible.

The first step is to get a peak flow meter, a device that assesses the patient's breathing to establish normal breathing flow and help determine necessary adjustments when attacks may be imminent. Another item is the pulse oximeter. They run under $20 on Amazon and are very simple to use. Just slip it on the finger, and you have the results in a matter of seconds. The pulse ox, as it is often called, can help you determine whether an asthma attack is cause for alarm—and help guide you in what measures to take to manage the problem. The pulse ox can reveal whether there's a real problem long before the lips turn blue.

Next, asthmatics are going to need to acquire boxes upon boxes of N95 masks. Without an unlimited supply of maintenance medications, vanity has to go out the window. Asthmatics are going to have to wear these masks whenever they're at risk for whatever triggers an attack. The N95 masks will trap particulates before they can wreak havoc in an asthmatic's lungs. They'll reduce chances for attacks.

Most asthmatics are already well aware that caffeine is a bronchodilator. In a TEOTWAWKI situation, caffeine is going to be an asthmatic's constant companion. As coffee won't last forever, is expensive, and takes space to store, it will be necessary to store a lot of caffeine pills. They're pretty inexpensive, and building up a generous supply isn't cost-prohibitive for those wishing to stockpile just in case, especially in families where asthma is a possibility. Doctors recommend giving 0.01 ml/kg for maintenance. In an attack, they recommend strong coffee as opposed to tablets. The caffeine must get into the bloodstream ASAP, and it will do so faster in a liquid such as coffee than in a tablet. (If you don't have coffee, grind up a caffeine pill really well and drink it with water.) And caffeine has several other uses as well, so even if you don't have any asthmatics in your family, the caffeine won't go to waste.[672]

Primatene Mist is something else to consider. Unfortunately, it doesn't have a great shelf life. And it will get pretty pricey trying to stock a reasonable quantity for an asthmatic. Still, it's nice to have options.

Mild asthma is the most common type of asthma. Patients usually have no symptoms but are often susceptible to chest colds. Any coughing, wheezing, or shortness of breath is generally triggered by something—upper respiratory infections, allergies, dust, vigorous exercise, even temperature changes. These people need no or only very occasional medication. The best bet is to avoid triggers and upper respiratory infections. Even though directions for antihistamines say the product shouldn't be used in asthmatic patients, allergic asthmatics may be helped with products such as Benadryl, Claritin, Zyrtec, and Allegra.[673] Sudafed may also help.

Moderate asthma patients are between the mild patients just discussed, and the severe patients that will be considered next. Most of the time, these patients can be treated the same as the mild asthma patients. But they had better behave like the severe patients, avoiding all triggers even if they believe they aren't really affected by them.[674]

Patients with severe asthma are utterly dependent on their maintenance meds. They have got to have their inhaled steroids, controller drugs, and rescue inhalers daily as well as oral steroids for flare-ups. Some even require oxygen. These people are not in a good situation. Avoiding triggers and making what medications they have stockpiled last as long as possible is critical.

All asthma patients can take charge of their own health. Be proactive. Maintain a healthy weight. Eat well and exercise regularly. For heaven's sake, don't smoke. Avoid triggers! Chronic exposure may elicit low-level responses that the patient doesn't necessarily attribute to an allergen. That means all pets, both mammals and birds, all feather pillows, wool sweaters, and rabbit fur.[675] Wear the N95 mask when seasonal allergies start. Keep the environment clean and dust-free. Get rid of the carpets.

Those who suffer from allergic asthma might consider getting tested for their allergies. Of particular interest would be the allergy-desensitization injections that may nearly cure asthma.

There are well over a dozen herbs and alternative treatments suggested for managing asthma. As asthma has many different causes, different people will benefit from various herbs and/or preparations and administration routes. If you're an asthmatic, try them out now, under a doctor's supervision, of course.

- Doctors a century ago advised breathing into a jar of honey and taking one teaspoon of honey in a glass of water three times per day.[676]
- Gumweed is *the* herb for asthmatics. It is readily found throughout the West but needs to be collected annually. It doesn't store very well except in an alcohol tincture. Take 15-40 drops of a tincture up to 5 times per day. It is also prepared as an infusion.[677]
- Essential oils of oregano, thyme, and German chamomile may be dropped into a pot of boiling water and inhaled for at least five to ten minutes.
- Infusions of Brigham tea, yarrow[678], red clover, plantain, thyme, and German chamomile are reported to provide some relief. Mullein, lobelia, purslane, and peppermint are also used.
- Magnesium levels are often deficient in individuals with severe asthma. Increasing your dietary intake of magnesium may help.[679]

Cautions: Asthmatics should not use Advil, aspirin, or Mobic.

DIABETES TYPE 1

In *One Second After*, the modern classic prepper fiction novel, the main character's teenage daughter is a type-1 diabetic. Spoiler alert, for maximum emotional impact, you know she has to die in the end. Dad was able to keep her insulin cool for a while in the toilet tank, but of course, the insulin ran out and there was no re-supply. The vast majority who read this book and those who have any understanding of type-1 diabetes assume this is true; the people with type-1 diabetes will die when our society collapses.

But do the diabetics have to die? History says *no*.

Eva Saxl and her husband found themselves in China after barely escaping from the Nazis in Czechoslovakia at the onset of World War II. Shortly thereafter she became a type-1 diabetic. Regular deliveries of insulin became increasingly unreliable; black market insulin was sometimes poor to deadly. They decided that they needed to make their own.

The exact protocol they followed to produce insulin has not been determined; however, they did make it and they saved Eva and about 400 other diabetics in Shanghai during World War II. The internet address for a 1926 journal article with the directions for producing insulin is in the endnotes.[680] If you have a diabetic in your family, print several copies.

The equipment Banting and Best used to first produce insulin in 1921 is not much different than what is found in a high school chemistry lab today. Eva Saxl and her husband were not scientists. If they could do it then, others can do it now. It will not be easy, but it is doable. The greatest challenge will be securing a constant supply of cow and pig pancreases.

With a little luck, the diabetics who prepare well won't have to go that far. Insulin-dependent folks already know that they can build up a supply of insulin; in this respect they have it much easier than others trying to build up a supply of maintenance medications. Blood glucose strips, monitors, batteries, pump supplies are all a bit harder, but still manageable, assuming that you have insurance footing the bill.

Pump supplies and the accompanying boutique insulin won't likely be an option post-collapse, so people are going to have to old-school it.

Urinalysis strips are relatively inexpensive and still available in this country, even at Walmart. It was the only method diabetics had for checking blood glucose levels at home until the 1970s. The urinalysis strips only show what the blood glucose levels *were* a few hours previous. But when things fall apart, they'll be useful.

Visual-read blood glucose strips came out in the early 1980s. They can be cut into halves or thirds to stretch the supply. I have not been able to locate a supplier in this country. Last year we purchased a few bottles of strips from Betachek in Australia.[681] They ship worldwide.

Once all the strips run out, the diabetic will have to turn to taste-testing. Yep, you read that right. Urine from a *healthy* person is sterile when fresh. It can safely be tasted. The kidneys start spilling sugar when the level tops 180 mg/dl. If the urine is sweet, the diabetic is above 180 mg/dl. If the urine is not sweet, the blood glucose level is below 180 mg/dl. If you happen to have a lot of sugar ants around, you may get them to do the work for you. Pour a little urine on the ground near them. Are they attracted to it? If so, the sugars are high. If not, the sugars are below 180 mg/dl.

Most diabetics will reuse syringes as long as possible. But they might run out as well, and unfortunately, they cannot be autoclaved due to the type of plastic and rubber. ShopMedVet.com sometimes carries glass syringes. If you happen to know an anesthesiologist, or someone who works with one, try getting some glass syringes from him. Epidural trays are one of the few places where glass syringes are still used in this country. Get the right size reusable needles for the syringe, and a means of sharpening as necessary.

While insulin does have a shelf-life, most have found that it still works long past the use-by date. One source states insulin can, in fact, be frozen to prolong its shelf life substantially. If you decide to give it a try, use some cheap stuff first.

Three stop-gap measures if you run out of insulin but know some will be available soon:

- Some doctors believe that metformin, a drug used to help type-2 diabetics maintain proper blood glucose levels, could be of use to type-1 diabetics who are deprived of insulin by being able to extend the time their supply of insulin lasts. It probably wouldn't be a long-term solution, but may be able to delay the onset of diabetic coma.[682]
- Another stop gap measure is exchange transfusion, where blood from a donor is transfused into a diabetic. It's extreme and only a stop-gap for a day or two, but if insulin re-supply is delayed but expected shortly, it works. Successful blood transfusions were performed 200 years ago, so it could be done now as well. Consider stocking up on some blood transfusion supplies.[683]

- Finally, adjusting the diet to just fats and animal proteins and green salads will greatly extend the insulin supply. This isn't a great long-term solution, because the body needs carbohydrates to function optimally, but it can work for a few weeks.

What about new cases of diabetes? How does a physician diagnose them? Well, it's a simple finger prick in the office, with a device just like what diabetics use. If you're suspecting a new case of diabetes, find someone with a blood glucose monitor or some urinalysis strips to check. The main symptoms of diabetes include frequent urination, extreme thirst, (those first two are pretty much required), hunger, and fatigue. For my husband and a good friend of ours, the onset came about two weeks after a bout of influenza, and indeed, new cases of type-1 diabetes increase four-fold after some strains of influenza pass through a community.

Keeping a diabetic alive post-collapse will be difficult, but it's going to be hard for everyone. You, and mostly the diabetics around you, will decide whether it's worth the effort.

DIABETES TYPE 2

The hard truth is most type-2 diabetics have a choice in the matter. Proper diet, exercise, and weight loss will reduce or eliminate the need for medications. There are many herbs that will help type-2 individuals control their blood sugars. They should be researched now to determine which will help. Finally, all diabetics should consider preparing for a very low carbohydrate diet to extend the insulin and medication supplies much longer.

HYPOTHYROIDISM

Hypothyroidism, or underactive thyroid, occurs when the thyroid gland does not produce adequate thyroid hormone for the body. Worldwide, insufficient iodine in the diet is the most common cause of hypothyroidism. The addition of iodine to salt is why we do not see more cases of hypothyroidism in the industrialized world. This is one reason it is absolutely critical to store iodized salt.*

The signs or symptoms of hypothyroidism most commonly observed include:

- Fatigue
- Intolerance to cold
- Dry skin
- Constipation
- Weight gain
- Hair loss

Less common symptoms include:

- Hoarseness
- Depression
- Menstrual irregularity
- Forgetfulness
- Fluid retention
- Poor growth (in children)

Extremely rudimentary biology lesson for understanding hypothyroidism:

Thyroid stimulating hormone (TSH) is produced by the pituitary gland. This is what is measured in a blood test to assess thyroid hormone—thyroxine—levels. TSH tells the thyroid to produce something called T4. T4 must be converted into T3 to be used by the body.

The missing or insufficiently produced hormone is called thyroxine. When the thyroid doesn't produce enough T4, physicians routinely prescribe a synthetic. The vast majority of hypothyroidism is treated with a synthetic replacement like levothyroxine (Synthroid), which ranks in the top five for most commonly prescribed drugs in the US. It comes in a wide variety of dosages and it is absolutely critical to have the exact right dosage for each patient.

* The best recommendations for dealing with hypothyroidism post-collapse are to get not only Dr. Koelker's book *Armageddon Medicine*, but also her hypothyroid self-study and preparation course. No one else covers hypothyroidism nearly as well as she does.

Simple enough; except when it isn't. This is because the body has to convert T4 into T3, and unfortunately, this critical process can be affected by a whole host of factors, like:

- Low-calorie diets
- Antacids
- Prescription medications (sucralfate, simethicone, antidepressants)
- Mineral deficiency (zinc, copper, selenium, calcium)
- Iron tablets
- Chronic stress
- Herbal medicine (ashwagandha, lemon balm, rosemary)
- Soybeans
- Cruciferous vegetables (broccoli, cabbage, Brussels sprouts, cauliflower)
- Pine nuts
- Walnuts
- Fiber

That's a whole lot of stuff that can affect the T3 and T4 levels. What's a person to do? The best advice is to take thyroid medications on an empty stomach, and at least 1-2 hours before or 1 hour after any medications or mineral supplements to avoid or reduce interactions.

Then there are the effects that Synthroid and its generic equivalents have on other medications, like insulin and those for type-2 diabetes. Synthroid can diminish the efficacy of diabetes medications. (Type-1 diabetes is an autoimmune disease, and hypothyroidism can be as well. The two often go hand-in-hand.) On the other hand, Synthroid potentiates warfarin, so that if the warfarin dose is not reduced, serious bleeding may occur.

Getting the right dose of Synthroid is essential; unfortunately, that is going to be very difficult to do post-collapse. It will require careful monitoring of signs from a physician. Getting the right dose is not something that occurs overnight, or even within a week or a month. While there is not so much risk if the dose is too low, there is significant risk if the dose is too high. Hyperthyroidism is no good, either.

As many of us often contemplate a time when DIY everything is going to be the norm, we wonder what was done before synthetic drugs were available. In the case of hypothyroidism, before synthetics were available, desiccated and powdered extracts from pig and cow thyroids were used. Armour Thyroid, derived from cows and pigs, is still on the market today. There are nutraceuticals—plants compounded into tablets and used as medicine—for treating hypothyroidism, but most physicians shy away from them. There are natural supplements like Thyromine. How well any of these options will work on any given patient depends on too many variables to be able to make any general statements.

If you have hypothyroidism, discuss with your doctor whether treatment is mandatory for you. For a significant number, treatment is not actually required. If it is required, stock up on your medications. Synthroid is very cheap from overseas pharmacies. If you get the tablets that are double your required dosage, you can then use a pill splitter to halve your cost.

Caution: Untreated hypothyroidism in a pregnant woman may result in birth defects in the baby.

LIFE-THREATENING ALLERGIES

Individuals with life-threatening allergies have got to have a good supply of Epi-pens. There are no known herbal options. The protocol for producing epinephrine in a laboratory is way beyond anything a couple of guys are going to be able to make in the kitchen.

Synthetic epinephrine is effective for all aspects of anaphylaxis, which is the first big reason to have it in the medical kit, because ***anyone*** can have a reaction to ***anything*** at ***any* time**. People who are allergic to nuts, bee stings, etc. already know they should be carrying an Epi-pen at all times and that all their family members should also know how to use it. In a true anaphylactic reaction, the patient's airway is being compromised or entirely shut down. In addition, the patient's blood pressure drops, the tongue and/ or back of the mouth may swell, further compromising the airway, the chest may become tight, and there may be hives and weakness or confusion. These symptoms most often appear during the first hour after the sting or eating the offending food. Epinephrine must be injected to act quickly enough to save that person's life.

Without epinephrine, you may be able to help the patient with Benadryl, oral steroids if you have them, and/or a histamine blocker like Zantac or Pepcid. Of course, your patient's best bet is to get to a functioning hospital where he can get intramuscular injections of epinephrine, as well as steroids and antihistamines in a clinical setting.

As it is a liquid, epinephrine doesn't have a great shelf life, usually about a year. Even Epi-Pens have a pretty short shelf-life, and once they hit their date, they're supposed to be discarded. However, there are a couple of little secrets to learn. First, they don't automatically lose effectiveness once they hit their use-by date. Even Epi-Pens five years out of date are about 60% effective and may have enough epinephrine in them to save a life. If you have a source for outdated Epi-Pens, get them and hang on to them. Much of the efficacy depends on how it was stored. A nice, moderate temperature is critical. Do not let it freeze under any circumstances and do not let it get hot. Always protect it from light, and always know exactly where it is in the medical kit.

The second secret concerning Epi-Pens is that they actually contain five full doses. But you can only use one dose at a time. Yes, it doesn't really make sense, and the manufacturers all know this, but they still continue to put the full five doses in, even though only one will be used. The Epi-Pen can be disassembled and reloaded so that it can be used again. Please note, this should only be done when you have no other options—no other epinephrine, no doctor, no hospital, no trained medical personnel whatsoever. There are YouTubes and other instructions online.[684] This requires strong hands and you and anyone else in the room will need safety glasses. It would also be best to do this in a small, enclosed area if possible. That spring is gonna go flying.

SECTION 4—MEDICAL RECORDS

21. MEDICAL RECORDS

The "necessary nuisance" of medical records is absolutely critical for doctors to render appropriate medical care. It will ensure the fastest and best care when time is of the essence. While they seem intrusive, the questions a doctor asks are to ensure a patient receives the best care possible with the resources at hand.

PERSONAL MEDICAL RECORDS

When disaster strikes, physicians and clinics may not be available. If things have truly deteriorated, they will not have the means to maintain your records for you. There may not be supplies to photocopy your medical records. You are going to have to maintain your own.

You may as well get started now while you have a clear mind and others around you to help you remember and document everything. Do not try doing this in a crisis.

There are dozens of templates for medical health history forms online and available for downloading. You can certainly use one of these to create your own if you don't want to trouble your doctor (or you don't have one). Unless you're a pretty sickly person, most of the answers to questions on those forms are no, right? You check hundreds of boxes indicating that you don't have that disease or condition, and neither has your father, mother, siblings, children, etc.

Future caregivers need to know what illnesses or conditions you (and your blood relatives as best you know) *have* had. Plain paper will work just fine to maintain your records. The information you need to include in your records is the same information you provide when you fill out those forms in the doctor offices.

First, especially for preparedness purposes, are the vaccines you've received and the dates they were administered.

Next, your family health history as best you know it for your blood relatives. Cancer, diabetes, heart disease, dementia, arthritis, document it. Illnesses and the age at death. Many of these conditions are genetic. If the caregiver is aware of any greater risk you may have due to your family history, then better care and suggestions can be offered.

Follow that up with your personal history. What injuries and surgeries have you had? Why? For women, provide the number of children as well as the number still living. Number of miscarriages and/or abortions. Document everything about your illnesses. The dates, medications administered, duration. List all your allergies. Very clearly somewhere, perhaps at the top of every page, note your blood type. Note things that are "normal" for you that are not normal for everyone else. For example, if you're in the 10% of the population that has one pupil more dilated than the other, that better be noted in your records or you're going to have care providers thinking that you've got brain damage.

It's a hassle, but start documenting every fall, every illness, and every injury. The more information you can provide a caregiver, the better. Without laboratories to assist in diagnosing illnesses, paper records are going to become invaluable. Things you might dismiss as insignificant may actually provide valuable clues.

The caregiver needs to know all drugs you have taken and are currently taking—every prescription and OTC medication, i.e., illegal drugs, coffee, tea, alcohol, and tobacco use. Whether you have used/abused in the past and have quit, every supplement you are taking and how much, and all herbal remedies must be documented. He's going to want to know dietary changes. Have you made a rapid transition from a diet high in processed foods to whole grains and high fiber? The more information provided, the more rapid and better the outcome.

Keep your medical records in a heavy duty Ziploc bag and take them with you to each and every visit with your doctor. And be sure to include enough blank paper for notes to be made. Make Murphy's law work for you—you know, perhaps if you have plenty of blank paper in your medical records the doctor will never need to use it.

TAKING AND GIVING A PATIENT HISTORY

When someone is sick or injured, there are a lot of questions that need to be asked and answered in order to provide the best outcome. Try not to view all these questions as an invasion of privacy or unwarranted curiosity on their part. Seemingly insignificant events can be of utmost importance. A doctor can also figure out pretty quickly if you are lying. Lies are often used to cover up stupid mistakes, right? If a guy gets super mad and punches the wall and as a result breaks a bone or two in the hand, he may not want to tell the doctor that he was so stupid, so he tells the doctor that he fell. The problem is, bones break in one way when a person punches the wall, and in an entirely different way when a person falls. The doctor already *suspects* the guy is lying based on which bones appear to be broken in his initial examination; he *knows* the guy is lying when the x-rays come in.

Unfortunately, without nifty diagnostic tests and x-rays, doctors are going to have to be a lot more discerning and ask more questions. They have to be told the truth. Doctor-patient confidentiality will still be a thing. They're going to have to know if you've been unfaithful to your spouse or if you've been abusing substances.

There are a lot of mnemonics care providers use to remember to gather all the information possible from a patient. This first one is devoted to the information that the patient or family member shares. Just as the nurse or doctor should not skimp on or skip taking a history, neither should the patient skimp on the information provided.

SAMPLE

This is the mnemonic most commonly used for taking a patient history. These are the questions a patient is going to be asked.

Symptoms and **S**igns. What is bothering you? What happened? What has changed? Is there a fever, pain, rash, or swelling? If there is diarrhea, is it totally watery or just loose? Bloody or mucous-y? How long has this been going on? What patient shares are the *symptoms*. What the caregiver sees are the *signs*.

Allergies. All allergies—seasonal, foods, medications, and insects—need to be reported. When it comes to a reaction due to a medication, was it a life-threatening allergy or simply a rash? A rash may develop due to an antibiotic, but it doesn't necessarily mean the patient has a life-threatening or potentially life-threatening allergy. There are some life-threatening conditions that can only be treated by antibiotics. If a patient has only experienced a rash in the past, that drug might still be used, though the patient will be much more carefully monitored. However, if it was anaphylaxis and it was recent (because some people outgrow penicillin allergies), then that drug can't be used, even if there are no other options. A primitive skin test where the skin is scratched and a paste or powder of the drug in question is applied to observe the patient's reaction may help determine whether to use that drug.

Medications. The mnemonic PORCCH covers the medications a person uses. All of these must be reported.

- **P**rescriptions
- **O**ver-the-counter
- **R**ecreational drugs
- **C**ontraceptives
- **C**ompliance (are drugs used as directed by the physician or the bottle?)

- **H**erbal supplements and vitamins and minerals

Past medical history. Has this happened before? Has this been developing slowly over time or is it a sudden onset? Does the patient have a medical condition predisposing him to what he has now? What illnesses have you had recently? Any bug bites in the last month or so? Last period? Was it normal? Have pregnancies been normal, without problems? Any chance she could be pregnant?

Last intake/output. The last time eating usually pertains more to whether there is a need for surgery, but it is sometimes helpful to know. Depending on the reason for seeking treatment, a doctor may definitely want to know the last time the patient urinated or defecated and whether everything was normal.

Events. What happened to lead up to this pain or complaint? When did it start? Where did it start? Where does it hurt? Has anyone near you experienced anything similar?

OPQRST

This is another mnemonic that is commonly used for helping to describe pain:

Onset. Was the onset gradual or sudden?

Provoke or palliate. Is there anything that makes the pain worse or better?

Quality. Is the pain constant, or does it come and go? Is it throbbing? Is it dull or sharp?

Radiate or refer. Does the pain move anywhere?

Severity. Rate the pain on a scale of 1 to 10.

Time. When did it start?

The answers to any of these questions may prompt the care provider to ask more questions, which may seem even more invasive. Keep in mind that the doctor is trying to provide the best care possible in what may be a very difficult situation with limited resources. Lots of medications can have drug interactions with other medications or with food. Some medications or herbs can make illnesses worse. Numerous conditions have rather nonspecific symptoms, but if someone else in your family is experiencing something similar even if it's not as bad, it can narrow things down.

Remember, the more information provided, the faster and more accurate the diagnosis and treatment, and the sooner the patient will begin to improve.

22. ASSESSING A PATIENT

Let's assume you are out in the middle of nowhere, hours away from civilization and any hopes of medical care. All is well until some child drops out of the sky right in front of you. (Yeah, that's not really likely, but it avoids having to discuss the wisdom of treating an adult who stumbles into your area, whether there are threats following him or observing you, whether he's faking and you're putting yourself in danger, etc. Also, imagining that it is your child you are treating may not work so well either for other reasons. Keeping this as someone else's child helps keep you detached and rational in your approach.)

Before rushing to the child's side, take a look around and above, just to make sure no one else is dropping out of the sky and on top of you. As you approach the child, put on your gloves and make a mental note of your initial impressions and the time. In other situations, you might also note the location and number of other patients.

ABC

There are a number of different initial mnemonics for this to help you remember everything. Some use DR ABCDE, ABCDE, or ABC. ABC is simple. Stop and fix immediate threats to life:

A—airway

B—breathing

C—circulation

Circulation. There is some debate among medical personnel about the order in which these threats are addressed, and you may disagree as well. We probably won't be working on each other. Lots will say to go in alphabetical order here: airway, breathing, and then circulation.

The American Heart Association changed the order in 2010 to CAB, because a body can survive a blocked airway and/or no respiration for three to five minutes without permanent damage. But a person can bleed out in less than 60 seconds, and there's no comeback from that. Circulation (bleeding) gets controlled first.

The next part of this is chest compressions, part of cardiopulmonary resuscitation (CPR). Except that most times when CPR is being performed it has to be continued until the patient arrives at the hospital. But what if there is no hospital, no advanced care, no diagnosis or treatment for whatever has caused the cardiac arrest? Most physicians teaching off-grid medicine agree, you don't do CPR in a grid-down situation. If the patient has a reasonable chance of getting care in a hospital, by all means perform CPR. Absent higher care, people dying due to heart attacks have underlying medical conditions that just cannot be managed without modern technology and pharmaceuticals. Those people have underlying medical conditions that are not going to be fixed without advanced care. Yes, it's hard to accept.

The few exceptions to this rule are for people who were otherwise healthy before needing resuscitation: those who have drowned, been electrocuted (lightning strike—yeah, it's possible to survive that), or choked. CPR may bring those people back without the need for additional hospital support.

Airway. If the patient is conscious, one way to judge the airway is by how much the patient can speak. Can he say a sentence, phrase, word, or nothing? Is the patient able to make any sound? The absence of any breathing sounds indicates total obstruction of the airway. Gurgling or snoring sounds suggest partial airway obstruction.

In an unconscious person, the head is tilted and the jaw thrust forward so that the tongue can't block the airway. Look, listen, and feel for air movement. Does the chest rise and fall?

In both groups of patients, vomit and foreign objects need to be scooped out of the mouth so that they cannot block the airway or be aspirated.

- Turn the patient to the side before scooping out the mouth so that gravity can help.
- Make sure to scoop carefully so that you do not further impact material into the airway.
- Semi-conscious patients may bite down on your fingers. A bite block may help prevent injury to the caregiver.
- Be prepared for the patient to unexpectedly vomit.
- In a survival situation, if necessary, you can safety pin the tongue to the lower lip to keep it out of the airway.

Oral and nasal airways are a simple way of maintaining the airway in an unconscious patient. They're really cheap on Amazon, like $6-12, and each set has a wide variety of sizes to accommodate infants to adults. It doesn't require any particular training to use them. They aren't perfect; there is no protection from aspiration of foreign objects or vomit. However, all the other methods of keeping an airway open—supraglottic airways, intubation, and a surgical airway—require skill and training.

Breathing. After the airway is open, check to see that the patient is breathing. If not, you have to do it for him. This is done either by mouth-to-mouth (or face mask) or using a bag-valve mask. Neither of these are long-term solutions. A patient requiring prolonged ventilation in a remote situation or societal collapse is unlikely to survive.

AVPU

After, and perhaps even during, taking care of the ABCs above, it's also important to assess the patient's level of consciousness (LOC). Most providers use the following AVPU scale:

- **A**lert and oriented to:
    - person, place, time, and events (AOx4)
    - person, place, and time (AOx3)
    - person and place (AOx2)
    - person (AOx1)

- **V**erbally responsive—responds to questions
- **P**ainfully responsive—responds to pain like pinching fingers or toes
- **U**nresponsive—no response to any stimulus

Care providers usually conduct the AVPU assessment while doing other things like you see on TV, asking the questions you might find annoying. "Do you remember what happened? Do you know what day it is? Do you know where you are? Do you know who I am?"

In all likelihood, you'll never be faced with any of this. Even trained physicians, other than those working in the ER or trauma departments, rarely see anyone in a life-threatening situation. But things like this are good to know.

VITAL SIGNS

Most every time you visit the doctor, a nurse checks your vital signs. When a patient is in the hospital, nurses monitor vital signs frequently, assuming there isn't a machine hooked up to do it for them. Vital signs not only provide information about the current condition of a patient, but they also provide baseline information for the doctor when the patient is feeling well so that the doctor can see more easily what is off when a patient is sick.

Normal vital signs vary by age, as well as by gender and overall health. This is one reason why maintaining accurate health records is critical for care providers; it helps physicians determine what is normal for any given patient and how to interpret any changes.

Normal vital signs, by age

	Pulse	Respiration Rate	Systolic Blood Pressure
Newborn	120-180	40-50	60-80
1-2 years	90-120	25-30	90-105
3-10 years	80-100	20-30	100-110
10+ years	<80	<20	100-120

The chart shows the normal ranges of the vital signs of pulse, respiration, and blood pressure for newborns through adults. The two other vital signs, temperature and oxygen saturation, do not vary by age. A temperature of 98.6°F is considered normal. Anything over 100.4°F is a fever, and anything below 96.8 is considered hypothermia. Any temperature over 103°F suggests a serious infection, but remember, it's not a perfect correlation.

While armpit temperature measurements were used for some time, they are not very accurate. Oral and rectal measurements are much more reliable. Be sure to have at least one thermometer of each kind. Glass thermometers are more accurate. Yeah, you've got to shake them down and it takes a few minutes to get the reading, but having an accurate reading is critical. Digital thermometers can vary quite a bit.

Another vital sign is the oxygen level in the blood. Measured with a pulse oximeter, it provides information on how well gas exchange in the lungs is proceeding. Normal is above 95%. Anything below 94% indicates a need for supplemental oxygen or significant respiratory disease.

The sicker a patient is, the more the vital signs will deviate from normal. There are several early warning score options; they are all pretty similar. They are useful for determining trends in patients, whether the patient is getting worse or better. It's a tool to use in conjunction with other observations.[685]

The NHS Early Warning Score (NEWS) comes to us from the United Kingdom. The system assigns a point value to abnormal vital signs. The point total from all signs gives an indication of how sick a patient is.[686]

NHS Early Warning Score (NEWS)							
	3	2	1	0	1	2	3
Temperature	≤95		95.1-96.8	96.9-100.4	100.5-102.2	≥102.3	
Respiration rate	<8		9-11	12-20		21-24	>25
Pulse	≤40		41-50	51-90	91-110	111-130	≥131
Oxygen saturation	≤91	92-93	94-95	≥96			≥220
Systolic blood pressure	≤90	91-100	101-110	111-219			
Consciousness level (AVPU)				A			V, P, or U

Total up the points to determine how ill the patient is using the chart below.

NEWS point scale for determining how ill a patient is	
0-4 points	The patient is not likely to be seriously ill at the moment.
5-7 points, or a single vital sign of three points	The patient may be quite ill. Monitor closely.
>7 points	The patient is seriously ill and needs immediate medical attention.

BLOOD TYPES

As far as blood types go, what is important to know here is that A and B are co-dominant and O is recessive. For the Rh factor, positive (+) is dominant to negative (-).

You need to know blood types for you, your family, and all the other members of your group. Each individual also needs to know what types of blood he can receive and to whom he can donate.

ABO blood groups for donation		
Blood type	Can receive from	Can donate to
A+	A+, A-, O+,O-	A+, AB+
A-	A-, O-	A+, A-, AB+, AB-
B+	B+, B-, O+, O	B+, AB+
B-	B-, O-	B+, B-, AB+, AB-
AB+	Everyone	AB+ only
AB-	A-, B-, AB-, O-	AB+, AB-
O+	O+, O-	A+, B+, AB+, O+
O-	O- only	Everyone

Because O- people can donate to anyone, they are called universal donors, or in more colorful language, walking blood banks. If you have one of these people in your group and only one set of body armor, this person gets it.

If you don't know your blood type, now's the time to find out. By the time most of us are adults, we've had occasion to find out for one reason or another. Children can be a different matter. You can take your child down to a hospital lab and pay around $100 for a test, or you can order one from Amazon and do it at home. The kit is called an Eldon card, and at the cheapest, purchased in the right quantities, they run about $3.00 each. Couples of child-bearing age should probably have a couple of extras on hand to test any children who may come along.

SECTION 5—SAMPLE MEDICAL KITS

Precious few of the first-aid kits commercially available are worthwhile. Search results on the first page alone of Amazon yielded kits ranging in price from $9 up to $574. The vast majority of reasonably priced kits have an overabundance of Band-Aids and little to nothing in the way of medications or supplies that would actually be useful. You're far better off to build your own kits.

The next few pages offer several examples of kits. The ones you assemble should range in size and scope depending on age, medical conditions, distance from medical care, and activities engaged in. Don't put items in your kit just because they're on the list. Only include those items you might possibly need.

These personal first-aid kits are carried by everyone in the family when away from home and when more than ten minutes from the car. Family members are taught to care for their own needs as appropriate for their ages. They also carry medications appropriate for their personal needs.

23. SMALL MEDICAL KITS

BOO-BOO KIT

The boo-boo kit container needs to be able to hold everything. Regular-size Altoids tins may work for some people, at least in the beginning. Eventually they become a bit too small for all that is wanted. Locating a good container or bag for a boo-boo kit can be a challenge, but if you know any diabetics, you may be in luck. The blood glucose meters that diabetics use are improved quite frequently and most diabetics will have at least a few. If you have a diabetic acquaintance, try hitting him up for a spare case. These really are the best cases. They're compact, somewhat water resistant, and often have pockets with zippers and Velcro or elastic bands for organizing small items.

Boo-Boo Kit					
Abrasions, Bleeding		Topical Creams		Personal Protection	
Adhesive bandages 3		Burn gel		Exam gloves, 2	
Alcohol wipes, 4		Hydrocortisone		N95 mask	
BZK wipe,		Benadryl			
Q-tips, 2				Tools	
Triple antibiotic packet		Oral Medications		Safety pins, 2	
Steri-strips, 5		Benadryl tablets, 2		Super glue	
Tincture of benzoin		Benadryl chewable, 6		Razor blade or scalpel	
Tegaderm		Imodium		Klever Kutter	
2x2 gauze, 4		Tylenol, 2		Splinter forceps	
4.5" kerlix gauze roll		Aleve, 2			
Cloth tape, 1" wide		Caffeine, 2		All quantities are "1" unless otherwise noted.	
Pressure dressing		Oral rehydration salts, 2			
Triangle bandage		Advil, 2			
Moleskin		Baby aspirin chewable, 6			

IFAK

The IFAK's (individual first-aid kit) history is based in the military. Troops have been responsible for dealing with their own minor issues forever. However, life-threatening situations also need to be managed quickly, especially when advanced medical care is far away. The IFAK evolved to include items for treating gunshot wounds and major bleeding as well.

Not everyone needs an IFAK. IFAKs are primarily for those carrying weapons, or hanging out with or near such people. Basically, anyone with a weapon carries an IFAK as well. It's just common sense. Create your own IFAKs based on your perceived needs.

IFAK					
Abrasions, Bleeding		Topical Creams		Personal Protection	
Band-Aids, 3		Burn gel		Exam gloves, 4	
Alcohol wipes, 4		Hydrocortisone		N95 mask	
BZK wipes, 2		Benadryl			
Q-tips, 2				Tools	
Triple antibiotic packet		Oral Medications		Safety pins, 2	
Steri-strips, 5		Benadryl tablets, 2		Super glue	
Tincture of benzoin		Benadryl chewable, 6		Razor blade or scalpel	
Tegaderm		Imodium		Klever Kutter	
4 2x2 gauze pads, 4		Mobic		Splinter forceps	
4.5" kerlix gauze roll		Moxifloxacin		Tourniquet	
1.5"-wide cloth tape		Caffeine, 2		Chest seals, 2	
Pressure dressing		Oral rehydration salts, 2		Quikclot or Celox gauze	
Triangle bandage		Baby aspirin chewable, 6		Sharpie marker, fine	
Moleskin				Mylar blanket	

24. LARGE MEDICAL KITS

The following kits are meant to be portable—to go on outings, camping trips, vacations, etc. They are not meant to carry all the supplies a family stores to last the duration of a crisis. Those excess supplies are stored separately in a cool, dry, dark area well protected from pests and environmental damage.

FAMILY MEDICAL KITS

In addition to everything contained in the boo-boo kit, the family medical kit contains a wide variety of supplies for addressing everyday medical conditions at home. It's generally kept at home, but it's also taken on various outings. This is not a comprehensive list of items and quantities to last through the apocalypse.

First, you'll want a place for your supplies, something that you'll be able to organize nicely. There are probably hundreds of options—tackle boxes, tool kits, and actual medical bags in all shapes, sizes, colors, and price ranges. Find something that works for your family and situation.

Family Medical Kit

Abrasions, Bleeding		Instruments		Environmental	
Band-Aids, 1 box		Pulse ox monitor		Chemical heat pads, 4	
Gauze, sterile, 2x2, 20		Glass thermometer		Hypothermia blanket	
Gauze, 8 ply, 4x4, 40		Trauma shears		ORS packets, 6	
Gauze rolls, 4.5" kerlix, 4		Nail clippers		Topical creams	
Tincture of benzoin, 1 oz		Bag valve mask		Burn gel, 4	
Sterile Q-tips, 10		Chest seals, 2		Lubricating jelly, 2	
Burn dressing, 4x8, 2		Multi-tool		Petroleum jelly	
Burn dressing, 4x4, 2		Splinter forceps		Ora-gel (dental pain)	
Non-adherent dressing, 3x4, 6		Tongue depressor		Miconazole	
		T-needle		*Lidocaine cream*	
Triangle bandage, 4		Nasopharyngeal airway		Antibiotics	
Tourniquet, SWAT-T, 2		Emesis basin		Amoxicillin, 4	
Pressure dressing, small, 4		Lighting		Zithromax, 2	
Z-gauze, 1-2		Chemical light sticks, 4		Keflex, 4	
Skin stapler and remover		Headlamp, LED		Cipro, 2	
QuikClot or Celox, 1-2		Penlight, LED		Doxycycline, 6	
Moleskin, 3 sheets		Flashlight		Moxifloxacin, 4	
Vet-bond, 1 bottle		Extra batteries		Penicillin, 4	
Steri-strips, 10		Credit card magnifier		Other tablets	
Orthopedics		Disinfectants		Diflucan, 2	
Ace bandage, 3", 2		Hand sanitizer, 2 oz		Mobic, 4	
Ace bandage, 4", 2		Betadine, 1 oz		Stool softener, 2	
Cloth tape, 1", roll		Alcohol, 70%, 2 oz		Tums, 6	
Cloth tape, 2", roll		BZK wipes, 8		Records and misc.	
Vet-wrap, 3" roll, 2		Hibiclens, 4 oz		Permethrin, 2 oz	
Athletic tape, 1.5", roll		Sterile saline vials, 2		Lighter	
SAM splint, 36", 2		Alcohol pads, 20		Antibiotic guide	
Duct tape, 2", small roll		Nano silver, 4 oz		Sharpie, fine point	
PPE		Sovereign silver, 1 bottle		Sharps container	
Nitrile gloves, 8 pairs		Irrigation syringe, 30 ml		Write in Rain notepad	
N95 masks, 6				Mechanical pencil	
CPR mask				Garbage bag, 4	
Eye shield					

ADVANCED MEDICAL KIT

Even if you do not have the training to use these items, they're still a good idea to have available for someone who can use them to help your family. You never know—there were a few doctors in Paradise, California, who escaped the fire with only their families and their lives. They still had their skills, but no medical kits to work with. In a long-term crisis, like in Venezuela, doctors are easier to locate than supplies. Or perhaps, in a telemedicine situation, a doctor can direct you in how to use these items.

In addition to everything in the family medical kit, the advanced medical kit includes the supplies and instruments that could be useful when higher medical care is hours or days away—in a blizzard or hurricane or on a backcountry trip. While trained medical personnel keep everything together in one bag, you may wish to keep the advanced kit separate so that those items aren't in your way when dealing with the everyday issues.

Advanced Medical Kit					
Personal Protection		**Instruments**		**Medications**	
N-99 mask, RZ 2.5 mask		Needle driver, smooth tips		Lidocaine 1%	
Sterile operating gloves, 4		Scissors, 1 point sharp		Lidocaine 2% with epi	
CPR shield		Scissors, Metzenbaum, curved, fine, 5.5"		Normal saline for injection, 25 ml	
Goggles					
Diagnostic equipment		Forceps, dressing		Rocephin 1 gm	
Stethoscope		Forceps, tissue, Adson 1x2		Tranexamic acid, 100 mg	
Blood pressure cuff		Forceps, Debakey, 6"		Epinephrine 1:1000, 1 ml	
Chemical light sticks, 8		Forceps, mosquito, 4		Triamcinolone, 10 ml	
Respiratory		Forceps, Kelly, straight, 2		Nubain, 10 mg/ml, 10 ml	
Chest seal, 2		Forceps, Allis 2x3		Toradol, 30 mg/ml, 10 ml	
Cricothoracotomy kit		Retractors, Simm's, 2		Valium, 5 mg/ml, 10 ml,	
Chest tube kit		Retractors, Gelpi, 5"		Augmentin, 875 mg, 60	
Peri bottle		Probe, straight		Zithromax, 500 mg, 20	
Blue towels, sterile, 4		Towel clamps, small, 3		Bactrim DS, 30	
Wound closure		Scalpel blades #11, 6		Levaquin, 750 mg, 30	
Skin stapler, 2		Scalpel blades #10, 2		Clindamycin, 300 mg, 14	
Staple remover		Scalpel blades #15, 2		Doxycycline, 100 mg, 30	
Sharps container		Scalpel blades #12, 2		Diflucan, 10	
Suture, assorted, 6		Scalpel handle		Albuterol MDI	
Suture, silk, 4-0, 4', 3		Folding zippered pouch		Envelops, dispensing, 12	
Suture needles, assortment of 6		**Records and miscellaneous**		Oxygen tank wrench and gasket	
		SOAP notes			
Syringe, glass, sterile, 2		Saran wrap, colored		Medicine cup	
Hypodermic needles, assortment of 12		Folding clipboard		Cold spray	
Iodoform gauze, ¼" packing, 1 bottle				Temporary dental filling	

Organizing All the Little Things in Medical Kits

In the process of assembling your larger medical kits, you will come to realize that there are a whole lot of tiny supplies to include. Because they are so small, they can become hard to find, especially in an emergency. A large, hanging travel cosmetic bag is ideally suited for this purpose.

The chart on the following page shows one way of organizing a bag. Keep like items together so they will be easier to locate. Some of the larger items just have to go where they fit best.

Travel cosmetic bag showing contents of various pockets, relative size, and layout

Hydrocortisone cream Burn gel Lubricating jelly Betadine ointment Petroleum jelly Triple antibiotic Benadryl cream Oral pain relief gel A&D ointment	Credit card magnifier	Band-Aids in various sizes Insect repellent wipes	Nail clippers Vet-bond

Baby aspirin Chewable baby aspirin Activated charcoal powder *Usnea* wound powder Chewable Benadryl Vicodin Benadryl Tylenol Chewable Tylenol Bonine Unisom Mobic Caffeine Advil	Penlights (store batteries separately) Rubbing alcohol Iodine tincture Dual tip Sharpie	Steri-strips, various sizes Thermometer Benzalkonium chloride wipes Sutures Tegaderm film dressings

5% lidocaine cream Sterile saline Lighter	Tincture of benzoin Hand sanitizer Matches	Liquid bandage Klever Kutter

Chest seal Duct tape Moleskin Medical tape Celox nosebleed dressing Hand cleaning towels	Light sticks Saran wrap Biofreeze 2x2 gauze Sterile q-tips 4x4 kerlix gauze Sterile non-adherent dressings

Plastic Straw Mini-Packages

Plastic straws make perfect tiny waterproof packages for a myriad of items that go in emergency bags, medical kits of all sizes, camping kits, etc.

So what exactly do we use plastic straws for? Lots and lots of things!

Pills: Generally in single doses. I make an exception for chewable baby aspirin, because if someone is having a heart attack, you want a lot of it. Right now! Some pills fit in regular straws; some require jumbos. They're perfect for boo-boo kits, IFAKs, car kits, and advanced medical kits without having to carry whole bottles around.

Medicinal powders: Powders, like activated charcoal, can be very messy; straws contain the mess better. Use jumbo straws for these.

DIY single uses of creams: Triple antibiotic and Benadryl and other creams (also toothpaste). Sure, you can buy single uses of triple antibiotic and many creams, but not all. So far I haven't been able to find single use packages of Benadryl cream. And it can get a little pricey if you're building kits for a lot of people or if you just need one or two packages of items that are only sold in large quantities. Small straws for these items.

Food: yeast, powdered eggs, Parmesan cheese, dehydrated butter, spices, salt, sugar, pepper, etc. Yes, you might get the little paper packages of these items, but they aren't waterproof and straws are.

Waterproof matches: make sure the end you are sealing doesn't have the business end of the match. Just sayin'.

Plastic Straw Mini-Packages

First, get some straws. My grocery store sells jumbo straws, but only colored ones. Amazon has clear jumbo straws, which are nice because it's easy to see what's inside. Colored straws just look fun. And if you actually remember what pills, powders, foods went into which color, you can find them faster. For example, Benadryl, that little pink magic pill, always goes in a pink straw. Aleve is a little light blue pill, so it goes in a light blue straw. You get the idea.

Then gather the rest of your supplies and items to put in the straws.

Supplies:
Straws, regular or jumbo, clear or colored
Pliers
Tea light or birthday candle
Matches
Ultra-fine tip Sharpie
Something to work on, like a plate or a pie tin
Filler items
Medications and creams
Medical powders
Food items
Strike anywhere matches
Whatever you want to have

General directions: Light candle. Crimp straw closed in pliers with just the tiniest bit of straw hanging out. Melt that end in the candle flame to seal it.
For dry items: Seal the first end, fill, put pliers on filled end, cut to size, seal.
For wet (cream) items: Cut the straw, fill by squeezing the cream in, and seal ends. Ends with liquid on them may take a few attempts to seal.
Caution: Do not do this with hand sanitizer. Alcohol is very flammable, and you can burn your fingers right off.

SECTION 6—APPENDICES

APPENDIX 1. RECOMMENDED READING

The following references are what I consider the best. However, I recognize that getting all of these is not an option for most people. The reviews provided will aid in the decision-making process when only one or two can be acquired. Information for obtaining copies of these books is provided at the end of the chapter.

ALTON'S ANTIBIOTICS AND INFECTIOUS DISEASE

Alton's Antibiotics and Infectious Disease: The Layman's Guide to Available Antibacterials in Austere Settings constitutes one aspect of Dr. Joseph Alton and Nurse Amy Alton's stated mission "to put a medically prepared person in every family." It is clearly not directed to medical professionals or microbiologists, but is written for the average layman with no medical training whatsoever. In fact, it's written at a level that a competent high school student could understand and utilize. It's a "primer on the infectious diseases most likely to rear their ugly heads" when our advanced medical care is no longer available. Some information is hypothetical, as the Altons extrapolate lessons from history and draw on the experiences of disasters in underdeveloped areas. They also devote significant attention to diseases that have been mostly eradicated in the US due to improved sanitation and hygiene, clean water, and antibiotics—all advances that will quickly disappear when society collapses.

The table of contents and the first 60+ pages can be seen on Amazon to get a brief overview of the topics they address. What I like in here that I haven't seen covered elsewhere, or covered as well, are the following topics:

- Distinguishing between viral and bacterial infections—without the benefit of laboratory tests for diagnosis—so that you don't waste antibiotics on viral infections
- How to treat childhood diseases that we currently vaccinate for
- Determining whether a person has a true allergy to a medication, or just an adverse side effect—this may be critical if you've got only one or two options to save a life
- Exact adult dosages of various antibiotics for specific diseases
- How to make liquid suspensions of antibiotics for young children
- The use of "expired" antibiotics

The Altons do not teach how to make intravenous antibiotics. The potential is too great for introducing a worse infection into the bloodstream than what needs to be treated.

What may escape the reader the first time looking at the title and reviews, is the word *available*. Lots of times we read about what we should have in a medical kit and supplies we want to have on hand, but because we are not licensed physicians, we can't get these critical items. What the Altons have done in this book, and what they have been doing for years, is determining whether fish and bird antibiotics can be safely used with people.

Of course, the ideal is to use antibiotics that are manufactured for people and that have been prescribed by your personal physician to treat a specific condition. This book, as stated at the beginning, end, and entirely throughout, is for a time when there is no higher help available now or in the foreseeable future. They have compared antibiotics that are for people with antibiotics that are sold, without prescription and without restriction, for use with birds and fish. They have found that they look the same and have the same batch numbers and dosages as pharmaceuticals for people. The Altons use them themselves.

In their book, the Altons only focus on antibiotics that are manufactured for fish and birds but that are sold in the same dosages as what are prescribed for people. Physicians may in some cases have other drugs they would prefer to use, but in an austere situation, we may not have what we would like to have and need to make do with something less. The Altons are striving to help people understand the basics of treating some of the more common conditions we'll encounter when advanced medical care is unavailable. Dr. Joe and Nurse Amy cover each available antibiotic, the exact dosages for adults, the exact conditions each is used for, and duration of treatment, as well as contraindications.

ARMAGEDDON MEDICINE

This book is exactly what the title suggests: medicine for the end of the world, or as the author writes, "How to be your own doctor when there's no other choice."

Dr. Cynthia Koelker, a board-certified family physician with thirty years' experience treating patients and their families, recognizes what is coming and the need to prepare accordingly. Her website, ArmageddonMedicine.net, features dozens if not hundreds of educational and thought-provoking articles not included in her book. Unfortunately, her website is not currently updated due to health issues, but I've emailed her and she has always responded and been quite helpful and encouraging.

Her years of communicating with patients in her family medicine practice shine through in her writing. Dr. Koelker writes in a conversational, very easy to understand style, like she is talking to concerned parents who need to be able to care for children or other loved ones when there is no one else. She assumes the reader has no medical background whatsoever.

The topic of managing respiratory infections and symptoms features significantly in *Armageddon Medicine,* with over twenty pages devoted to differentiating between cold and influenza; determining whether an infection is bacterial or viral (without laboratory work); whether to use antibiotics, which ones, and why; over-the-counter drugs to store and when to use them; how to proceed when your patient has an already compromised immune system; and much more.

Armageddon Medicine is 588 pages, 8.5 x 11 inches, in what looks like a 12-point font, double-spaced, so it's very easy on the eyes. As it is not available through Amazon or in bookstores, the table of contents is briefly reproduced here. The table of contents includes the following (there is more, but these are the highlights:

- Section 1: The Basics
- Section 2: Mental Illness
- Section 3: Acute Infection and Symptoms (quarantine, isolation; animal bites, rabies; respiratory infection; sore throat, mouth, lips; ear infection; gastrointestinal infection and symptoms; urinary and reproductive infections)
- Section 4: Skin conditions
- Section 5: Pain
- Section 6: Acute Injuries (burns, back strain, cuts and lacerations, knee and ankle injuries, insect bites and stings, concussion, fractures)
- Section 7: Selected Conditions (anemia, arthritis, asthma and COPD, blood clots and pulmonary embolism, botulism, constipation and diarrhea, diabetes, gout, headache and migraine, hearing loss, heart disease, heartburn, GERD, ulcers, hernia, high blood pressure, kidney stones, low back pain, sleep apnea, swelling, thyroid disease, vision) and women's health
- Section 8: Medication Concerns (simplifying your medications, expired medications, fish antibiotics, getting your doctor to help you

stockpile medications, essential OTC drugs to acquire, herbal medicine)

- Section 9: Special Topics (nuclear fallout, bioterrorism)
- Section 10: Becoming a Healer (taking a medical history, performing a physical exam)
- Appendices (Resources, free downloads, medical textbook recommendations, medical kit, useful OTC medications)

Merely stating that there are appendices for the medical kit and useful over-the-counter (OTC) medications is an understatement. The medical kit appendix is 12 pages long and includes not just the items that Dr. Koelker recommends for your kit, but also the quantities for a family (basic), small group (intermediate), or professional (advanced). Her suggestions will help you budget your medical dollars wisely. For instance, how many bottles of rubbing alcohol have you stored? Believe it or not, she advises just one bottle for a family, five bottles for a small group, and twenty for a professional level. She includes prescription medications and quantities of each. The OTC medicines appendix is seven pages long, and lists the common name, other names, primary use, and other possible uses. The first item in that list is Benadryl, which is primarily used for colds and allergies. It can also be used for anxiety and insomnia.

Armageddon Medicine is only available through Dr. Koelker's site, ArmageddonMedicine.net. At $89, it is a little pricey, but the information is invaluable, and there is so much that I have not seen elsewhere. This book is definitely the place to begin your medical preparation and will provide a solid foundation should you desire further education. If you're skeptical, go to her site and read the articles there. They are not duplicated in the book, but you will get an idea of the kind of information she provides. It's written with the hope that none of us will ever need it and that hospitals and doctors will always be there for us. But as the saying goes, we plan for the worst and hope for the best.

SURVIVAL AND AUSTERE MEDICINE, 3RD EDITION

This volume is written by the Remote, Austere, and Third World Medicine Discussion Board Moderators who are not named but include a family physician, veterinarian, emergency room physician, surgical physician assistant, nurse, and biomedical engineer. They've got experience with the military and NGOs in pre-hospital, remote, austere, and third-world conditions, such as one might expect to encounter in a societal collapse. Their belief and approach is that intelligent lay people with basic medical knowledge, skills, and equipment can be trained to deliver high quality medical care for 80-90% of health problems.

Are you skeptical?

The first page of the first chapter lists the twenty most common reasons patients came to see one physician, representing about 95% of his consultations:

- Sprains and minor fractures
- Colds and fever
- Minor wounds, some infected, most needing only to be cleaned, a few needing suturing
- Vomiting, diarrhea, abdominal pain, including appendicitis (which if found early may be treated with antibiotics)
- Allergic reactions and rashes
- Asthma
- Ear infections
- Urinary tract infections
- Burns
- Dental problems
- Skin infections
- Chest infections and chest pain
- Fainting
- Mental health problems

- STDs
- Early pregnancy problems

With training, references, and adequate supplies, most of these conditions are very manageable for an intelligent layperson. How many people in Venezuela right now would love to be able to care for their loved ones themselves instead of trying to find a doctor or hospital to help? In light of the social and political instability in the world, we'd better be prepared.

That's their premise—an intelligent layperson with training, skills, and knowledge (and supplies!) can manage an awful lot of common conditions, conditions which might even be life-threatening.

One of the best things about this book is that it's a free download.

I understand that many readers already have an off-grid medicine book or two. Money and shelf space for another book and a substantial one at that—it is 614 pages on 8.5x11" paper—are limited for a lot of us. Is acquiring this book really necessary?

I believe it is. That's because there isn't one book that covers everything. One reference might barely touch on an illness, while another goes into great depth, or at least as much depth as a layperson in TEOTWAWKI needs. Having a few resources is a really good idea.

One great advantage of this compilation over others dealing with medicine post-collapse is that these authors have actually practiced medicine off-grid and in remote areas, in stark contrast to others whose practice has been limited to their homes, offices, and hospitals. Much more so than other physician-authors, they have had to improvise treatments when the usual supplies were not available and/or when higher care would have to be delayed.

The extremely detailed table of contents, fifteen pages long, aids in locating the topic of concern quickly. The fact that one of the authors is a veterinarian is useful adjunct to other medical texts because there is some advice for treating pets and livestock as well. There's a chapter on medicinal herbs and various preparations. Throughout the book, the authors encourage you to ponder the ethical questions of triage—who gets treated, especially when supplies are limited. That really needs to be determined now, not when there's a crisis and it's harder to think.

There are a lot of topics addressed in here that aren't covered elsewhere:

- Pre-term delivery
- Administering capsules and tablets to an unconscious patient
- Peritonsillar abscess
- Pancreatitis
- Sugar for infected wounds
- Maggot therapy for wounds
- Malnutrition and treatment for deficiencies
- Performing an appendectomy
- Performing a Caesarean section
- Ectopic pregnancy removal
- Skin excisions and lumpectomies
- Surgical instrument acquisition and quality

THE SURVIVAL MEDICINE HANDBOOK

As noted on the cover, this book, by Dr. Joe Alton and Nurse Amy Alton, is "a guide for when medical help is NOT on the way." The second edition is significantly expanded and revised; don't cheat yourself by purchasing a first edition copy.

Like other off-grid medicine authors and teachers, the Altons firmly believe that an educated lay person with good training can successfully address 80-90 % of the medical issues they will encounter when society collapses and there is no advanced medical care available. Some of these cases may even be life-threatening, but they aren't necessarily complicated, and that's why the Altons have written this book.

The book has a few shortcomings. Approximately twenty pages at the beginning that are basically preaching to the choir. Those who are preparing for TEOTWAWKI don't really need any more encouragement to do so. The same goes for the chapter devoted to natural disasters; individuals living in earthquake country or tornado alley are likely to have already prepared for these scenarios. However, the information on treating smoke inhalation due to wildfire is valuable. There also isn't a lot of information on vector-borne diseases, which is probably the greatest weakness of this book. There's nothing about quarantine and isolation for preventing the spread of disease. That's also why having a few off-grid medicine resources is critical. If one book doesn't address your concern, another likely will.

Like most survival medicine books, there are lists of suggested items to include in your various medical kits and the recommended quantities. *The Survival Medicine Handbook* is written at a higher level than *Armageddon Medicine*, but it shouldn't be over the head of anyone with at least some college education, and at half the cost of *Armageddon Medicine*. However, it's probably not as thorough as *Survival and Austere Medicine, 3rd Edition*, which is free.

Now for the topics that *The Survival Medicine Handbook* covers well.

- Moreso than any other off-grid medicine book, this one includes alternative medicine and natural treatments, including essential oils, right in with conventional therapies; the alternative treatments aren't an afterthought relegated to the back of the book.
- An entire chapter is dedicated to growing a medicinal herb garden for making your own medicine, because pharmaceuticals will eventually run out.
- This book contains a glossary of medical terms; most do not.
- Dr. Alton is an OB-GYN, so there is a very solid chapter on birth control, pregnancy, and delivery.
- There is solid information on treating dental problems.
- This is the only volume I've seen that addresses altitude sickness and treatment.
- There's a good section on radiation.

- This reference includes more information on using an Epi-pen than I've seen elsewhere.
- There is a respectable section on administering local anesthesia and nerve blocks.

The Survival Medicine Handbook is nearly 600 pages of text on 6x9" pages, in what looks like a 10- or 11-point font. There's little room for note-taking, but there are helpful illustrations and photographs.

HERBAL ANTIBIOTICS

Stephen Harrod Buhner's *Herbal Antibiotics* is quite unlike the majority of other herbal medicine books that are more fluff than substance. Buhner clearly and logically discusses each herb, its Latin and common names, how it has been used throughout history, how it is used in other parts of the world, and how to prepare and dose it for specific illnesses. The only possible flaw is that there are no pictures of the plants. However, there's always Google Lady. Sometimes one species of plant looks quite different from another of the same genus, especially in different climates and parts of the country.

Buhner explains what's happening with the current health dilemma we face regarding increasing antibiotic resistance and takes a matter-of-fact approach to the doom and gloom of the end of the antibiotic era. A gifted writer, he goes into great detail about twenty great antibiotic herbals, including usnea, juniper, honey, the berberines, etc., that are pretty much widely available. He also includes a section on some lesser known plant-sourced antibiotics. Sprinkled throughout are brief forays into biochemistry, which can be daunting to readers without a life sciences background, but they're easily passed over. Buhner also informs us about where these plants can be found in the wild and offers recommendations for online sources. Unlike the vast majority of herbal medicine books on the market, for each herb he includes pages of references to technical journals so you can do your own research.

Buhner does go into some detail about how these herbals work in the body, but it's not entirely necessary to read all that to figure out how to treat yourself. I've read it three times, so far. It's that interesting. I understand and remember more each time, so that's a really good thing.

Buhner's intended audience was probably those who understand that antibiotic resistance is poised to create a worldwide crisis and who are looking for tools to defend themselves. However, this book is especially valuable for preparedness-minded individuals who recognize that even a substantial supply of traditional antibiotics will be exhausted in no time. And because drug companies just aren't doing the research to develop new antibiotics, and bacteria are so effective at defeating new antibiotics when they come out anyway, we need to be prepared to manage bacterial infections.

Herbal Antibiotics is definitely not a book to borrow and take notes on or make copies of a few good pages. You really want the whole thing for your own reference. It's one of precious few books that is worth every penny and every precious inch of shelf space.

HERBAL ANTIVIRALS

Stephen Harrod Buhner's *Herbal Antivirals: Natural Remedies for Emerging & Resistant Viral Infections* is another essential volume to acquire for the medical prepping library. Just like his *Herbal Antibiotics* book, in this volume Dr. Buhner clearly presents information for each of the herbs and viral diseases he discusses without any fluff. Everything is meticulously researched and documented, though much of the research does comes from outside the United States.

Buhner starts off this volume with an introduction to viruses, and though he includes the biological explanations of what viruses do, he pretty much keeps it to a level that most non-life science people with a couple of brain cells to rub together can understand. He keeps it at a conversational level and even a bit entertaining at times. He touches on polio, smallpox, and influenza—the stuff we're somewhat familiar with, and then brings out Chikungunya, a virus spread by mosquitoes that causes fever and debilitating pain, for which doctors prescribed Tylenol. The cause of death for many of Chikungunya's victims was—get this—liver failure from the Tylenol.

What's to be done? As Buhner points out, Big Pharma doesn't have a lot of antivirals at its disposal. About 30% of the pages in this volume are devoted to Buhner's top seven antiviral herbs: Chinese skullcap, elder, ginger, houttuynia, isatis, licorice, and lomatium, plus boneset and red root, which merit an honorable mention. However, he also lists the many herbal options and dosages for all the illnesses he discusses; he just doesn't go into elaborate detail on the others. You'll also learn or be reminded of how to use blackberry, raspberry, oregano, thyme, knotweed, berberine, and many other herbs in your treatment of viral diseases. He offers some advice and herbal suggestions for strengthening the immune system.

In the appendices, Buhner includes an introduction to making herbal medicine as well as a list of suppliers he recommends. Now, as people who prepare, we're probably happier being able to produce our own medicine. Fortunately, the author also includes with his discussion on each of the herbs, guidelines for growing and harvesting the herbs and sources for obtaining seeds or plants. In addition, the bibliography is over 50 pages long. If you want to find sources for further researching a specific disease or herb, it's all there.

Like *Herbal Antibiotics*, I think this volume would be better with pictures to help with plant identification. Another complaint some readers have is that very little attention is devoted to the common cold. To me, that's not a deal breaker. A cold doesn't kill, and if one strictly practices basic hygiene, common sense, and eats a healthy diet, there shouldn't be too many.

Like with his other books, Buhner's intended audience is those who want a natural, practical, and effective approach to treating viral diseases. In that respect it is also quite invaluable to preppers looking for tools to defend themselves against enemies they can't even see. Buhner provides treatment protocols for viral respiratory infections like influenza, pneumonia, SARS, RSV, and croup; viral encephalitis infections such as Japanese, West Nile, tick-borne, and dengue; and other viruses like enterovirus, varicella (shingles), herpes, and Epstein-Barr.

I'm glad I don't have to choose between getting *Herbal Antibiotics* or *Herbal Antivirals*. They are both must-haves, in my opinion. If I did have to choose, the nod would go to *Herbal Antibiotics*. *Herbal Antibiotics* covers the plants you want for treating respiratory diseases, which is probably huge for all of us. I live in a desert where we have almost nothing in the way of ticks or mosquitoes, and much of *Herbal Antivirals* deals with tick- and mosquito-borne diseases. If I did have to deal with ticks and mosquitoes, or if I were worried about shingles, I'd eat rice and beans for a month and save the money to get this book. There should be a copy in every group, if not every family.

THE HERBAL MEDIC

Let's start off by saying there is absolutely no wasted space in here. Author Sam Coffman's extensive experience as a medic in the military and in working with clients shines through in the book. He does really know whereof he speaks. He shares that information clearly and succinctly. In that respect this book is more like a manual.

Sam covers 50 herbs in 150 pages with color photographs to help identify the plants you're looking for. Unlike so very many herbal medicine books, Sam provides detailed instructions of exactly how and when to harvest and how to prepare the plants for medicine for maximum efficacy. For this reason alone, *The Herbal Medic* is an excellent book for individuals wanting to learn more about herbal medicine.

The *materia medica*, the 50 herbs covered in 150 pages, is actually the last half of the book. In the first half, there's so much more to be really impressed with, like setting up a clinic and how to build the equipment to tincture herbs efficiently and cheaply. It's something even I could (ask my husband to) build. He covers, childbirth, makeshift supplies for dealing with tear gas and pepper spray, and keeping a low profile even in a bad situation so that you can still help as many people as possible. There are also chapters on dealing with venomous snakebites and how to distill alcohol and how to make various herbal preparations—extracts, infusions, tinctures, salves, poultices, etc. Honestly, out of 344 pages, there are probably only 3-5 pages that I don't find particularly useful. This book is *solid.* Naturally, Sam focuses on herbs that are found more in his area of the country, which may not be as useful to someone in an entirely different climate, but most of the herbs covered in here grow in most parts of the country.

One thing I hate about buying herb books online is that I can't see what herbs they're covering. I really want to learn more about herbs I can actually grow and use here for my family. Honestly, if something only grows in China or India, I don't care about it at all. Because the herbs discussed in *The Herbal Medic* can't be found without buying the book, here is a list of herbs Sam discusses: Algerita, astragalus, bee balm, bilberry (blueberry, huckleberry), birch, boneset, burdock, butterbur, California poppy, chamomile, chaparral, chaste tree, comfrey, dandelion, echinacea, elder, elecampane, gotu kola, greenbriar, horsetail, juniper, licorice, lobelia, marshmallow, milk thistle, mugwort, mullein, myrrh, neem, nettles, Oregon grape, parsley, passionflower, plantain, poke, prickly ash, prickly pear, red root, rosemary, self heal, Siberian ginseng, skullcap, St. John's wort, sweet annie, usnea, white horehound, wire weed, yarrow. He also discusses the use of non-herbs like activated charcoal, honey, and bentonite.

It's a great reference, but a bit expensive.

NUCLEAR WAR SURVIVAL SKILLS

While obviously written to address a nuclear event, most of the material in here can be applied to any collapse-type situation. A significant bonus to this book is that it includes instructions on how to build a fallout meter using common household materials. At the time the book was written in 1987, the meters built by regular people using the instructions in this book were comparable to models selling for $375-1000.

The author, Cresson Kearny, graduated summa cum laude with a degree in civil engineering from Yale University nearly one hundred years ago and then later attended Oxford University and received two degrees in geology. He wrote *Nuclear War Survival Skills* while employed as a research engineer at Oak Ridge National Laboratory.

As Cresson Kearny states, the purpose and scope of this book is "for the majority of Americans who want to improve their chances of surviving a nuclear war. It brings together field-tested instructions that have enabled untrained Americans to make expedient fallout shelters, air pumps to ventilate and cool shelters, fallout meters, and other expedient life-support equipment. (*Expedient* in civil defense work refers to equipment that can be made by untrained citizens in 48 hours or less, while guided solely by field-tested, written instructions and using only widely available tools and materials.)" The author also outlines skills that individuals and groups can learn and apply to improve their chances for survival. Like many involved in preparedness, he believes that if one prepares for the worst, the worst is less likely to happen. Another interesting premise he shares is that if a nation is fully prepared to survive a nuclear attack, that nuclear attack is less likely to happen.

It's reasonably safe to suggest that this country is nowhere near prepared to withstand a nuclear attack.

Chapters in the book:

- Dangers from nuclear weapons, myths, and facts
- Psychological preparations
- Warnings and communications
- Evacuation
- Shelter—the greatest need
- Ventilation and cooling of shelters
- Protection against fires and carbon monoxide poisoning
- Water
- Food

- Fallout radiation meters
- Light
- Shelter sanitation
- Preventive medicine
- Surviving without doctors
- Expedient shelter furnishings
- Improvised clothing and protective items
- Minimum pre-crisis preparations
- Permanent family fallout shelters for dual use
- Trans-Pacific fallout
- Appendices with explicit directions for building six kinds of fallout shelters, a fallout meter, shelter-ventilating pump, and more

As the Prep School Daily blog is focused pretty strictly on the food and medicine aspects of preparedness, I don't usually get into shelter and communications at all. I definitely don't touch on anything dealing with construction of any sort. I'm just not wired that way at all, whereas my husband and one son live for that kind of stuff. What I find really interesting and relevant about this book is that the critical structures and devices are all designed to be built by regular people without any specialized training or skills. To be sure, I would not want to have to do any of these things, but if I had to, I could. If I could do it, so could most everybody else.

Now there are a lot of preparedness books out there. They promise a lot. A lot of them disappoint. There's nothing to be disappointed about regarding *Nuclear War Survival Skills* because you know what? It's free! A free download.

You do have to print it yourself, but you can also just take a look at it online and then only print the pages you want.

HOW TO OBTAIN THESE REFERENCES

Armageddon Medicine is available at ArmageddonMedicine.net.

Survival and Austere Medicine, 3rd Edition is available at https://docs.wixstatic.com/ugd/3b311a_6ef34fffc73447ce9a4d25a4d441b662.pdf

Nuclear War Survival Skills is available at http://www.oism.org/nwss/s73p904.htm

The remaining references are all available through Amazon.

APPENDIX 2.

THE MASTER MEDICAL SHOPPING LIST

This list is just a guideline; no one can predict what any given family will actually use in a year. Hopefully none of it, right? Tailor the list to your family and your budget, your known medical conditions, and your climate. When it comes to antibiotics, consider whether you can get by with less—are you willing to use herbal medicine? If so, you can probably reduce the quantities somewhat. If you are really careful people, you may not need so many Band-Aids. Maybe you just don't get headaches or colds. Those supplies could be reduced or eliminated from the list. This list only includes medications and traditional medical supplies. It does not include improvisational supplies.

Clean water and hygiene
Bath and hand soap, 25-30 bars per person
Calcium hypochlorite (68-73%), 1 pound
Chlorine bleach, 2-3 gallons
Coffee filters, 300
Hand sanitizer, 32 ounces per person

Skin preps and washes
Baby scrub brush, 1-2
Betadine, 16-oz bottle, 1
Benzalkonium chloride wipes, 40
Hibiclens, 16-oz bottle, 1
Hydrogen peroxide, 16 oz bottle, 1
Rubbing alcohol, 70%, 16-oz bottles, 4
Sterile saline vials, 15 ml, 24
Tincture of benzoin, crushable vials, 10
Tincture of iodine, 2-oz bottles, 2

Vitamins
Multi-vitamins for all, especially B9 for women of child-bearing age, B12 for anyone on stomach medications or over the age of 60, D for those lacking sun in winter

OTC MEDICATIONS
Anesthetics
Cold Spray, 1 can
Epinephrine, vial, 1
Lidocaine, HCL powder, 500 grams
Pain relieving patches, 40
Tattoo numbing cream, 5%, 1 jar

Antacids
Alka-Seltzer, 100
Prilosec, 3 courses of treatment
Tums, 300

Anthelmintics (dewormers)
Albendazole
Ivermectin

Antidiarrheal
Imodium, 100

Antifungals
Clotrimazole (Lotrimin), 1 tube
Terbinafine (Lamisil), 1 tube
Tolnaftate (Tinactin), 1 tube

Antihistamines
Benadryl, tablets and capsules, 600
Pepcid, 50
Zantac, 50
Zyrtec, 40

Antinausea
Bonine, 100
Dramamine, 50
Sea-Bands, 1-2 pairs

Children's chewables
Advil, 24
Baby aspirin, 100
Benadryl, 24
Tylenol, 24

Cold and cough relievers
Afrin, 2 bottles
Mucinex, 100
Primatene Mist, 1 bottle
Sudafed, 100
Vicks VapoRub, 1 jar

Pain relievers
Advil, Motrin, 300
Aspirin, 300
Aleve, 300
Caffeine, 90
Excedrin/Vanquish, 50
Tylenol, 300

Stool softener
Colace, 100

Topical creams
Capsaicin
Hemorrhoid
Hydrocortisone, 2 tubes
Zinc oxide

Urinary tract
Azo or Uristat, 24
Urinalysis strips, 1 bottle

PRESCRIPTION MEDICATIONS
Medications for managing your own chronic conditions

Antibiotics
Amoxicillin, 500 mg, 100
Augmentin, 500 mg, 100
Cipro, 500 mg, 100
Doxycycline, 100 mg, 100
Erythromycin, 400-500 mg, 100
Keflex, 500 mg, 100
Levaquin, 750 mg, 40
Metronidazole, 500 mg, 100
Moxifloxacin, 400 mg, 20
Penicillin, 500 mg, 100
Tetracycline, 100 mg, 100

TMP-SMZ, DS, 100
Zithromax, 250-500 mg, 30

Anti-fungals
Diflucan, 100 mg, 30

Anthelmintics
Mebendazole, 30 tablets

Pain relievers
Mobic, 30
Anything you've saved from previous surgeries or illnesses (keep these very well secured)

Topical creams
Silvadene, 1

Personal protection gear
N95 masks, 30
Nitrile gloves, 1 box per adult in the right size
Procedure (earloop, surgical) masks, 50
RZ mask, primary caregiver, 1 per family
Sterile gloves, 10 pairs

Tapes and Wraps
Ace bandages, 2", 3", 4", one of each
Cloth tape, 2-3" wide, 3 rolls
Ducklings, ½" wide rolls, 1-2
Duct tape, 2" wide roll, 1
Nexcare, 1-2 rolls
Paper tape, 2 rolls
Sterilization tape, 1 roll
Transpore, 6 rolls
Vet-wrap, 6

Dressings
Band-Aids, 300, assorted sizes
Band-Aids, 2x4", 50
Gauze, sterile, 2x2", 25
Gauze, sterile, 3x3", 25
Gauze, sterile, 4x4", 25
Gauze rolls, non-sterile, 2", 5
Gauze rolls, non-sterile, 3", 5
Gauze rolls, non-sterile, 4", 5
Q-tips, 200
Telfa, non-stick dressing, 3x4", 20
Triple antibiotic ointment, 1-oz tube, 2
Triple antibiotic ointment, 1-use packets, 20

Wound closure
Monofilament sutures, reverse cutting, sterile, half circle or 3/8", sizes 2-0, 3-0, 4-0, 4 each
Steri-Strips, assorted sizes, 50
Skin stapler and staple remover, 1
QuikClot or Celox, gauze, granules
Vet-bond, 2-3 bottles

Expendable Supplies
Activated charcoal, 1 pound
Chemical cold packs, 24
Disposable razors, 12
Enema bags and tubing, 4
Epsom salts, 2 pounds
Permethrin, 6 quarts
Pregnancy tests, several for each woman of child-bearing age
RID or Nix, 4 treatments
Scalpel blades, #10, 6
Scalpel blades, #11, 12
Scalpel blades, #12, 6
Scalpel blades, #15, 6

Reusable Supplies
SAM splints, 36", 2
Tourniquets, 2
Triangle bandages, 12

Instruments
Bandage scissors, 1
Bulb syringe, 2
Forceps/tweezers (Uncle Bill's, Tweezerman), 1
Glass dropper, 2
Glass thermometer, 2
Headlamp, 1
Klever Kutter, 4
Otoscope, 1
Penlight, 1
Pill splitter, 1
Pulse oximeter, 1
Trauma shears, 1

Minor surgery kit
Blue towels, sterile, 4
Folding zippered pouch, 1
Forceps, Allis 2x3, 1
Forceps, curved mosquito, 4
Forceps, Debakey, 6", 1
Forceps, Kelly, straight, 2
Forceps, tissue, Adson 1x2, 1
Hypodermic needles, assortment, 12
Needle driver, 1
Probe, straight, 1
Scalpel handle, #3, 1
Scissors, Metzenbaum, curved, 5.5", 1
Syringe, glass 5ml, 2
Towel clamps, small,

APPENDIX 3.

TRADE AND GENERIC NAMES FOR COMMON MEDICATIONS

It's important to know both the trade and generic names for common medications. The trade names medications always cost more and are no more effective than the generics. The trade names are used exclusively throughout this book to avoid confusion and because the trade names are always shorter.

Trade and Generic Names for Common OTC and Prescription Medications			
Trade name	Generic	Trade Name	Generic
Advil	ibuprofen	Mobic	meloxicam
Afrin	oxymetazoline hydrochloride	Motrin	ibuprofen
Aleve	naproxen sodium	Mucinex	guaifenesin
Allegra	fexofenadine	Nasalcrom	oxymetazoline hydrochloride
Anbesol	benzocaine	Orajel	benzocaine
Antivert	meclizine	Pepcid	famotidine
Augmentin	amoxicillin, clavulanic acid	Pepto-Bismol	bismuth subsalicylate
Azo	phenazopyridine	Prevacid	lansoprazole
Benadryl	diphenhydramine	Prilosec	omeprazole
Betadine	povidone-iodine	Primatene Mist	epinephrine
Biaxin	clarithromycin	Rocephin	ceftriaxone
Bonine	meclizine	Silvadene	silver sulfadiazine
Cepacol	benzocaine	Sudafed	pseudoephedrine
ChlorTrimeton	chlorpheniramine	Sudafed PE	phenylephrine
Cipro	ciprofloxacin	Tagamet	cimetidine
Claritin	loratidine	Tinactin	tolnaftate
Colace	docusate sodium	Tums	calcium carbonate
Diflucan	fluconazole	Unisom	doxylamine succinate
Dramamine	dimenhydrinate	Uristat	phenazopyridine
Excedrin	aspirin, acetaminophen, caffeine	Tylenol	acetaminophen
Hibiclens	chlorhexidine	Vagisil	benzocaine
Imodium	loperamide	Vanquish	aspirin, acetaminophen, caffeine
Keflex	cephalexin	Vicodin	acetaminophen, codeine
Lamisil	terbinafine	Zantac	ranitidine
Lanacane	benzocaine	Zithromax	azithromycin
Levaquin	levofloxacin	Zofran	ondansetron
Lotrimin	Clotrimazole	Zyrtec	cetirizine
Macrobid	Nitrofurantoin	Tums	calcium carbonate

ENDNOTES

---

[1] Miranda Hitti, "Greatest Medical Advance: Sanitation," WebMD, 19 January 2007, https://www.webmd.com/a-to-z-guides/news/20070119/greatest-medical-advancement-sanitation#1 (Accessed 6 February 2020)

[2] "Emergency Disinfection of Drinking Water," Environmental Protection Agency, https://www.epa.gov/ground-water-and-drinking-water/emergency-disinfection-drinking-water (accessed 20 February 2020); "Boil Water Advisory," Centers for Disease Control, https://www.cdc.gov/healthywater/emergency/drinking/drinking-water-advisories/boil-water-advisory.html (accessed 20 February 2020).

[3] Emergency Disinfection of Drinking Water," Environmental Protection Agency, https://www.epa.gov/ground-water-and-drinking-water/emergency-disinfection-drinking-water

[4] "Sanitary Control and Surveillance of Field Water Supplies," Departments of the Army, Navy, and Air Force, https://ia800505.us.archive.org/17/items/NAVMEDP501010SANITARYCONTROLANDSURVEILLANCEOFFIELDWATERSUPPLIES2010/NAVMED%20P-5010-10%20SANITARY%20CONTROL%20AND%20SURVEILLANCE%20OF%20FIELD%20WATER%20SUPPLIES%20%282010%29.pdf (accessed 20 February 2020).

[5] "Emergency Disinfection of Drinking Water," Environmental Protection Agency.

[6] "Sanitary Control and Surveillance of Field Water Supplies," Departments of the Army, Navy, and Air Force.

[7] https://web.archive.org/web/20070921045938/http://www.sodis.ch/files/Report_EMPA. pdf (accessed 20 February 2020).

[8] Samuel Luzi, et al, *SODIS Manual on Solar Disinfection,* EAWAG, https://www.sodis.ch/methode/anwendung/ausbildungsmaterial/dokumente_material/sodismanual_2016.pdf, p 20 (accessed 20 February 2020).

[9] "Emergency Treatment of Drinking Water at the Point of Use," World Health Organization, https://www.who.int/water_sanitation_health/emergencies/WHO_TN_05_Emergency_treatment_of_drinking_water_at_the_point_of_use.pdf (accessed 20 February 2020).

[10] Katherine Lawrie, et al., "UV Dosimetry for Solar Water Disinfection (SODIS) Carried Out in Different Plastic Bottles and Bags," https://www.profandrewmills.com/wp-content/uploads/2014/10/UV-dosimetry-for-SODIS.pdf (accessed 20 February 2020).

[11] "Solar Disinfection," Centers for Disease Control, https://www.cdc.gov/safewater/solardisinfection.html (accessed 20 February 2020).

[12] "When and How to Wash Your Hands," Centers for Disease Control, https://www.cdc.gov/handwashing/when-how-handwashing.html (accessed 22 February 2020).

[13] "Hand Hygiene in Healthcare Settings," Centers for Disease Control, https://www.cdc.gov/handhygiene/patients/index.html (accessed 22 February 2020).

[14] "When and How to Wash Your Hands," Centers for Disease Control and Prevention.

[15] "Hand Hygiene in Healthcare Settings," Centers for Disease Control and Prevention.

[16] "Towards better Hand Hygiene for Flu Prevention," American Society for Microbiology, 18 September 2019 https://www.eurekalert.org/pub_releases/2019-09/asfm-tbh091119.php (accessed 24 February 2020).

[17] Cynthia Koelker, MD, *Armageddon Medicine*, MD Books USA, 2012, 85.

[18] "Legal Authorities for Isolation and Quarantine," Centers for Disease Control and Prevention, https://www.cdc.gov/quarantine/aboutlawsregulationsquarantineisolation.html (accessed 24 February 2020).

[19] Eugenia Tognetti, "Lessons from the History of Quarantine, from Plague to Influenza A," *Emerging Infectious Diseases*, 19(2), February 2013, https://wwwnc.cdc.gov/eid/article/19/2/12-0312_article (accessed 24 February 2020).

[20] https://www.doomandbloom.net/sterilizing-instruments-in-austere-settings/ (accessed 22 February 2020). *Survival and Austere Medicine, 3rd Edition,* December 2017, 354.

[21] Ibid, 355.

[22] Ibid.

[23] William A. Rutala, Ph. D., MPH, et al., "Guidelines for Disinfection and Sterilization in Healthcare Facilities, 2008," https://www.cdc.gov/infectioncontrol/pdf/guidelines/disinfection-guidelines-H.pdf, p 40 (accessed 22 February 2020).

[24] Maira Marques Ribeiro, et al., "Efficacy and Effectiveness of Alcohol in the Disinfection of Semi-Critical Materials," *Revista Latino-Americana de Enfermagem,* July-August 2015, 23(4), https://www.ncbi.nlm.nih.gov/pmc/articles/PMC4623738/ (accessed 22 February 2020); William A. Rutala, Ph. D., MPH, et al., "Guidelines for Disinfection and Sterilization in Healthcare Facilities, 2008," https://www.cdc.gov/infectioncontrol/pdf/guidelines/disinfection-guidelines-H.pdf, p 40 (accessed 22 February 2020).

[25] "Why Is 70% Isopropyl Alcohol (IPA) a Better Disinfectant than 99% Isopropanol and What Is IPS Used For?" Production Automation Corporation, https://blog.gotopac.com/2017/05/15/why-is-70-isopropyl-alcohol-ipa-a-better-disinfectant-than-99-isopropanol-and-what-is-ipa-used-for/ (accessed 22 February 2020).

[26] https://www.chlorhexidinefacts.com/consumer-information.html (accessed 22 February 2020).

[27] *Survival and Austere Medicine, 3rd Edition*, 356.

[28] "Guideline to Dilution for Chlorine-Based Disinfecting Solutions," https://www.sahealth.sa.gov.au/wps/wcm/connect/d3396d00411006b8875bcf8f6fad9ea1/FactSheet-dilutions-sodium-hypochlorite_V2+2-phcs-ics-20140917.pdf?MOD=AJPERES (accessed 22 February 2020).

[29] *Survival and Austere Medicine, 3rd Edition;* 355; https://www.doomandbloom.net/sterilizing-instruments-in-austere-settings/ (accessed 22 February 2020).

[30] https://www.doomandbloom.net/sterilizing-instruments-in-austere-settings/ (accessed 22 February 2020); *Survival and Austere Medicine, 3rd Edition*, 357.

[31] https://www.doomandbloom.net/sterilizing-instruments-in-austere-settings/ (accessed 22 February 2020); *Survival and Austere Medicine, 3rd Edition*, 358.

[32] https://www.doomandbloom.net/sterilizing-instruments-in-austere-settings/ (accessed 22 February 2020); *Survival and Austere Medicine, 3rd Edition*, 357.

[33] https://www.instructables.com/id/Wrapping-Surgical-Tools-for-the-Autoclave/ (accessed 22 February 2020).

[34] Clare Gilbert, "The Eye Signs of Vitamin A Deficiency," *Community Eye Health Journal*, 2013, 26(84), https://www.ncbi.nlm.nih.gov/pmc/articles/PMC3936686/ (accessed 24 February 2020).

[35] Dr. Colin Tidy, "Vitamin A Deficiency," https://patient.info/doctor/Vitamin-A-Deficiency (accessed 24 February 2020).

[36] Clare Gilbert, "The Eye Signs of Vitamin A Deficiency."

[37] Dr. Colin Tidy, "Vitamin A Deficiency."

[38] "Vitamin A," National Institutes of Health, https://ods.od.nih.gov/factsheets/VitaminA-HealthProfessional/ (accessed 24 February 2020); Dr. Colin Tidy, "Vitamin A Deficiency."

[39] Georg Lietz, et al., "Single Nucleotide Polymorphisms Upstream From the β-Carotene 15,15'-monoxygenase Gene Influence Provitamin A Conversion Efficiency in Female Volunteers," *The Journal of Nutrition*, January 2012, 142(1), https://pubmed.ncbi.nlm.nih.gov/22113863-single-nucleotide-polymorphisms-upstream-from-the-carotene-1515-monoxygenase-gene-influence-provitamin-a-conversion-efficiency-in-female-volunteers/ (accessed 24 February 2020).

[40] David Werner, *Where There Is No Doctor*, Hesperian Foundation, 1992, 226.

[41] https://bestpractice.bmj.com/topics/en-us/633

[42] "Vitamin B12: What to Know," WebMD, https://www.webmd.com/diet/vitamin-b12-deficiency-symptoms-causes#2 (accessed 24 February 2020).

[43] Ibid.

[44] C. Petavy-Catala, et al., "Clinical Manifestations of the Mouth Revealing Vitamin B12 Deficiency Before the Onset of Anemia," *Annals de Dermatologie et de Venereologie,* 130 (2 pt 1), https://pubmed.ncbi.nlm.nih.gov/12671582-clinical-manifestations-of-the-mouth-revealing-vitamin-b12-deficiency-before-the-onset-of-anemia/ (accessed 24 February 2020).

[45] Jordi Graells, et al., "Glossitis with Linear Lesions: An Earl Sign of Vitamin B12 Deficiency," *Journal of the American Academy of Dermatology,*60 (3), https://pubmed.ncbi.nlm.nih.gov/19231648-glossitis-with-linear-lesions-an-early-sign-of-vitamin-b12-deficiency/, (accessed 24 February 2020).

[46] "Vitamin B12: What to Know," WebMD.

[47] Ibid.

[48] Gao-feng Yuan, et al., "Effects of Different Cooking Methods on Health-Promoting Compounds of Broccoli," *Journal of Zhejiang University Science,*August 2009, 10(8), https://www.ncbi.nlm.nih.gov/pmc/articles/PMC2722699/ (accessed 24 February 2020).

[49] Joris R. Delanghe, "Vitamin C: More Than Just a Nutritional Disorder," *Genes and Nutrition*, November 2011, 6(4), https://www.ncbi.nlm.nih.gov/pmc/articles/PMC3197848/ (accessed 24 February 2020).

[50] J. V. Hirschmann, et al., "Adult Scurvy," *Journal of the American Academy of Dermatology,* December 1999, 41(6), https://pubmed.ncbi.nlm.nih.gov/10570371-adult-scurvy/ (accessed 24 February 2020).

[51] Dr. Mary Harding, "Vitamin C Deficiency," https://patient.info/health/vitamin-c-deficiency-leaflet (accessed 24 February 2020).

[52] Ibid.

[53] John S. Adams, "Update in Vitamin D," *Journal of Clinical Endocrinology and Metabolism,* February 2010, 95(2), https://pubmed.ncbi.nlm.nih.gov/20133466-update-in-vitamin-d/ (accessed 24 February 2020).

[54] Dr. Josh Axe, "Vitamin D Deficiency Symptoms and Sources to Reverse It," 12 September 2019, https://draxe.com/nutrition/vitamin-d-deficiency-symptoms/ (accessed 24 February 2020).

[55] Betty Kovacs Harbolic, "Vitamin D Deficiency," https://www.medicinenet.com/vitamin_d_deficiency/article.htm (accessed 24 February 2020).

[56] "Vitamin D," National Institutes of Health, https://ods.od.nih.gov/factsheets/VitaminD-HealthProfessional/ (accessed 24 February 2020); Betty Kovacs Harbolic, "Vitamin D Deficiency," https://www.medicinenet.com/vitamin_d_deficiency/article.htm (accessed 24 February 2020).

[57] Betty Kovacs Harbolic, "Vitamin D Deficiency."

[58] "Vitamin D," National Institutes of Health; "Vitamin D Deficiency," https://medlineplus.gov/vitaminddeficiency.html (accessed 24 February 2020).

[59] "Vitamin D," National Institutes of Health.

[60] "Calcium Deficiency: Symptoms, Causes, and Treatments," 20 January 2017, https://www.doctorshealthpress.com/general-health-articles/calcium-deficiency-symptoms-causes-and-treatments/ (accessed 24 February 2020).

[61] Roberta H. Anding, "Nutrition Made Clear," Lecture 14, The Great Courses, TheGreatCourses.com.

[62] Jillian Levy, "Calcium Deficiency: Are Supplements the Answer," 24 September 2018, https://draxe.com/nutrition/calcium-deficiency/ (accessed 24 February 2020).

[63] Roberta H. Anding, "Nutrition Made Clear," Lecture 14.

[64] Jillian Levy, "Calcium Deficiency: Are Supplements the Answer."

[65] Ibid.

[66] Ibid.

[67] "Calcium," https://www.webmd.com/vitamins/ai/ingredientmono-781/calcium (accessed 24 February 2020).

[68] "Iodine," National Institutes of Health, https://ods.od.nih.gov/factsheets/Iodine-HealthProfessional/ (accessed 24 February 2020); Chris D. Meletis, "Iodine: Health Implications of Deficiency," *Journal of Evidence-based Complementary and Alternative Medicine,* 2001, 16(3), https://journals.sagepub.com/doi/pdf/10.1177/2156587211414424 (accessed 25 February 2020).

[69] Elizabeth N. Pearce, et al., "Sources of Dietary Iodine: Bread, Cows' Milk, and Infant Formula in the Boston Area," *Journal of Clinical Endocrinology and Metabolism,* 1 July 2004, 89(7), https://academic.oup.com/jcem/article/89/7/3421/2844466 (accessed 25 February 2020); Chris D. Meletis, "Iodine: Health Implications of Deficiency."

[70] "Being Deficient in Iodine Affects Thyroid Function," http://www.progressivehealth.com/iodine-deficiency.htm (accessed 24 February 2020).

[71] Chris D. Meletis, "Iodine: Health Implications of Deficiency."

[72] "Iodine: National Institutes of Health, https://ods.od.nih.gov/factsheets/Iodine-HealthProfessional/ (accessed 24 February 2020).

[73] Elizabeth N. Pearce, et al., "Sources of Dietary Iodine: Bread, Cows' Milk, and Infant Formula in the Boston Area"; Chris D. Meletis, "Iodine: Health Implications of Deficiency."

[74] Siamak N. Nabili, "Anemia," https://www.emedicinehealth.com/anemia/article_em.htm# anemia_causes (accessed 25 February 2020).

[75] Jerry R. Balentine, et al., "Anemia Symptoms, Causes, Diet, Diagnosis, Treatment, and Prevention," https://www.medicinenet.com/anemia/article.htm (accessed 25 February 2020).

[76] Rachael Link, "5 Natural Treatments for Anemia Symptoms," 12 July 2018, https://draxe.com/health/anemia-symptoms/ (accessed 25 February 2020).

[77] "Global Anaemia Prevalence and Number of Individuals Affected," World Health Organization, https://www.who.int/vmnis/anaemia/prevalence/summary/anaemia_data_status_t2/en/ (accessed 25 February 2020).

[78] Siamak N. Nabili, "Anemia."

[79] Ibid.

[80] Ibid.

[81] Rachael Link, "5 Natural Treatments for Anemia Symptoms," 12 July 2018, https://draxe.com/health/anemia-symptoms/ (accessed 25 February 2020).

[82] Ibid.

[83] Roberta H. Anding, "Nutrition Made Clear," Lecture 14.

[84] "Dirt Poor: Have Fruits and Vegetables Become Less Nutritious?" *Scientific American,* 27 April 2011, https://www.scientificamerican.com/article/soil-depletion-and-nutrition-loss/ (accessed 24 February 2020).

[85] Phuong-Chi T Pham, et al., "Hypomagnesemia: A Clinical Perspective," *International Journal of Nephrology and Renovascular Disease,* 2014 (7), https://www.ncbi.nlm.nih.gov/pubmed/24966690 (accessed 24 February 2020).

[86] D.L Bilbey, et al., "Muscle Cramps and Magnesium Deficiency," *Canadian Family Physician,* July 1996, https://pubmed.ncbi.nlm.nih.gov/8754704-muscle-cramps-and-magnesium-deficiency-case-reports/ (accessed 24 February 2020).

[87] Behnood Abbasi, "The Effect of Magnesium Supplementation on Primary Insomnia in Elderly," *Journal of Research in Medical Sciences,* December 2012, 17(12), https://www.ncbi.nlm.nih.gov/pubmed/23853635 (accessed 24 February 2020).

[88] S.B. Sartori, "Magnesium Deficiency Induces Anxiety and HPA Axis Dysregulation: Modulation by Therapeutic Drug Treatment," *Neuropharmacology,* January 2012, 62(1), https://www.ncbi.nlm.nih.gov/pmc/articles/PMC3198864/ (accessed 24 February 2020).

[89] M.R. Wills, "Magnesium and Potassium. Inter-Relationships in Cardiac Disorders, *Drugs*, 1986, https://pubmed.ncbi.nlm.nih.gov/3732091-magnesium-and-potassium-inter-relationships-in-cardiac-disorders/ (accessed 24 February 2020).

[90] Aneta Kowal, et al., "The Use of Magnesium in Bronchial Asthma, A New Approach to an Old Problem," *Archivum Immunologiae et Therapiae Experimentalis,* January-February 2007, 55(1), https://www.ncbi.nlm.nih.gov/pubmed/17277891 (accessed 24 February 2020).

[91] "Magnesium," National Institutes of Health, https://ods.od.nih.gov/factsheets/Magnesium-HealthProfessional/ (accessed 24 February 2020).

[92] Carolyn Dean, "Health Warning: Antacids Create and/or Magnify Magnesium Deficiency," http://www.nutritionalmagnesium.org/health-warning-antacids-create-magnesium-deficiency/ (accessed 24 February 2020).

[93] "Magnesium," National Institutes of Health; "Magnesium Deficiency Symptoms," https://www.drperlmutter.com/magnesium-deficiency-symptoms-causes-treatments/ (accessed 24 February 2020).

[94] Michael S. Stone, et al., "Potassium Intake, Bioavailability, Hypertension, and Glucose Control," *Nutrients,* 22 July 2016, 8(7), https://www.ncbi.nlm.nih.gov/pubmed/27455317 (accessed 25 February 2020).

[95] Anthony J. Viera, et al., "Potassium Disorders: Hypokalemia and Hyperkalemia," *American Family Physician*, 15 September 2015, https://www.aafp.org/afp/2015/0915/p487.html

[96] Ibid.

[97] "Zincin Diet," https://medlineplus.gov/ency/article/002416.htm (accessed 25 February 2020).

[98] Rachel Nall, "All You Need to Know about Zinc Deficiency," *Medical News Today*, 22 December 2017, https://www.medicalnewstoday.com/articles/320393#takeaway (accessed 25 February 2020).

[99] Josh Axe, "7 Signs of Zinc Deficiency and the Best Foods to Reverse It," https://draxe.com/nutrition/zinc-deficiency/ (accessed 25 February 2020).

[100] "Zinc in Diet," Medlineplus.gov, https://medlineplus.gov/ency/article/002416.htm (accessed 25 February 2020).

[101] Rachel Nall, "All You Need to Know about Zinc Deficiency."

[102] Ibid.

[103] "Zinc in Diet," Medlineplus.gov.

[104] Josh Axe, "7 Signs of Zinc Deficiency and the Best Foods to Reverse It."

[105] Rachel Nall, "All You Need to Know about Zinc Deficiency."

[106] Aileen Chen, et al., "Safe Use of Subcutaneous Diphenhydramine in the Inpatient Hospice Unit," *The American Journal of Hospice and Palliative Care,* December 2017, 34(10), https://pubmed.ncbi.nlm.nih.gov/27625354-safe-use-of-subcutaneous-diphenhydramine-in-the-inpatient-hospice-unit/?from_term=benadryl+for+injection&from_pos=1 (accessed 14 March 2020); Laura E. Pickett, "Injectable Diphenhydramine Used as Anaesthetic for Wide Local Excision with Flap," *Journal of Cutaneous Medicine and Surgery,* May-June 2017, 21(3), https://pubmed.ncbi.nlm.nih.gov/27920067-injectable-diphenhydramine-used-as-anaesthetic-for-wide-local-excision-with-flap-closure/?from_term=benadryl+for+injection&from_pos=5 (accessed 14 March 2020);

https://www.winonadailynews.com/news/connections/dr-frank-bures-benadryl-can-be-used-as-anesthetic/article_47cdb7f4-1d2f-11e1-9922-001871e3ce6c.html (accessed 14 March 2020).

[107] "Pyrogens, Still a Danger," 27 August 2014, https://www.fda.gov/inspections-compliance-enforcement-and-criminal-investigations/inspection-technical-guides/pyrogens-still-danger (accessed 26 February 2020).

[108] Ralph P, "How to Make Injectable Lidocaine HCL," 25 April 2015, https://griddownmed.blog/2015/04/25/from-modern-survival-online-make-your-own-lidocaine-topical-anesthetic/ (accessed 26 February 2020).

[109] "Lidocaine Hydrochloride," https://dailymed.nlm.nih.gov/dailymed/fda/fdaDrugXsl.cfm?setid=C7A7D3D2-7638-4570-9EB8-A5E2BEC82B5D (accessed 26 February 2020).

[110] Sanjai Sinha, "Ranitidine," 9 December 2019, https://www.drugs.com/ranitidine.html (accessed 26 February 2020).

[111] "Cetirizine," 2 December 2019, https://www.drugs.com/cetirizine-hcl.html (accessed 26 February 2020).

[112] Sanjai Sinha, "Diphenhydramine," 19 December 2018, https://www.drugs.com/diphenhydramine.html (accessed 26 February 2020).

[113] Ibid.

[114] Ibid.

[115] Ibid.

[116] Ibid.

[117] Ibid.

[118] Ibid.

[119] N.D. Yeomans, et al., "Is ranitidine therapy sufficient for healing peptic ulcers associated with non-steroidal anti-inflammatory drug use?" *International Journal of Clinical Practice*, November 2006, 60(11), https://www.ncbi.nlm.nih.gov/pmc/articles/PMC1636688/ (accessed 18 February 2020).

[120] Daniel S. Strand, et al., "25 Years of Proton Pump Inhibitors: A Comprehensive Review," *Gut and Liver*, January 2017, 11(1), https://www.ncbi.nlm.nih.gov/pmc/articles/PMC5221858/ (accessed 18 February 2020).

[121] "Ranitidine," Zantac, Other Generics Recalled After Cancer-Causing Chemical Detected," 10 January 2020, https://www.healthline.com/health-news/fda-warns-zantac-may-have-carcinogen#The-bottom-line (accessed 26 February 2020).

[122] "Omeprazole," 16 July 2018, https://www.healthline.com/health/omeprazole-oral-capsule-sprinkles#dosage (accessed 26 February 2020).

[123] "Ibuprofen Dosage," 14 August 2019, https://www.drugs.com/dosage/ibuprofen.html (accessed 26 February 2020).

[124] Sanjai Sinha, "Aspirin," 1 December 2018, https://www.drugs.com/aspirin.html (accessed 26 February 2020).

[125] Sanjai Sinha, "Aleve," 12 January 2019, https://www.drugs.com/aleve.html (accessed 26 February 2020).

[126] "Naproxen (Rx, OTC)," Medscape, https://reference.medscape.com/drug/aleve-anaprox-naproxen-343296 (accessed 26 February 2020).

[127] Sanjai Sinha, "Excedrin," 7 April 2019, https://www.drugs.com/excedrin.html (accessed 26 February 2020).

[128] Sophia Entringer, "Meloxicam," 4 January 2019, https://www.drugs.com/meloxicam.html (accessed 26 February 2020).

[129] Edward P. Krenzelok, et al., "Confusion: Acetaminophen Labeling Changes Based on NO Evidence in Adults," *Drugs in R&D*, June 2012, https://www.ncbi.nlm.nih.gov/pmc/articles/PMC3585765/ (accessed 26 February 2020).

[130] "Acetaminophen," 14 June 2019, https://www.drugs.com/dosage/acetaminophen.html (accessed 26 February 2020).

[131] Sharon Orrange, "Is It Safe to Take Tylenol (acetaminophen) with Advil or Motrin (Ibuprofen)?" 12 August 2019, https://www.goodrx.com/blog/is-it-safe-to-take-tylenol-acetaminophen-with-advil-or-motrin-ibuprofen/ (accessed 25 February 2020).

[132]https://www.fda.gov/EmergencyPreparedness/Counterterrorism/MedicalCountermeasures/MCMLegalRegulatoryandPolicyFramework/ucm411446.htm

https://www.ghdonline.org/uploads/drugs-Stability_Profiles-vencimiento.pdf

https://www.mayoclinicproceedings.org/article/S0025-6196(15)00667-9/pdf

http://www.formatex.info/microbiology4/vol3/1721-1725.pdf

[133] Stephen Buhner, *Herbal Antibiotics,* Storey Publishing, 2012, 14-17; Cynthia Koelker, *Armageddon Medicine,* 208; "List of Antibiotics," wikipedia.org, (accessed 4 March 2020).

[134] *Survival and Austere Medicine, 3rd Edition*, 210.

[135] Cynthia Koelker, *Armageddon Medicine*, 109.

[136] Ibid, 368.

[137] Joseph Alton MD, Amy Alton, ARNP, *Alton's Antibiotics*, Alton First Aid LLC, 2018, 150.

[138] Cynthia Koelker, *Armageddon Medicine,* 183.

[139] Joseph Alton, *Alton's Antibiotics*, 150.

[140] "Guidelines for the diagnosis, management, and prevention of typhoid fever 2010," Ministry of Health, Fiji Islands, https://www.health.gov.fj/wp-content/uploads/2014/05/Typhoid-Guideline_-Long-Version_-2010.pdf (accessed 5 March 2020).

[141] Cynthia Koelker, *Armageddon Medicine*, 207.

[142] Ibid, 172.

[143] Ibid, 178.

[144] Ibid, 191.

[145] "Augmentin Dosage," Drugs.com, https://www.drugs.com/dosage/augmentin.html (accessed 5 March 2020).

[146]Ibid.

[147] Paulina Salminen, et al., "Antibiotic Therapy vs Appendectomy for Treatment of Uncomplicated Acute Appendicitis: The APPAC Randomized Clinical Trial,"*JAMA,* 16 June 2015, https://pubmed.ncbi.nlm.nih.gov/26080338-antibiotic-therapy-vs-appendectomy-for-treatment-of-uncomplicated-acute-appendicitis-the-appac-randomized-clinical-trial/ (accessed 2 March 2020).

[148] Cynthia Koelker, *Armageddon Medicine*, 172.

[149] Cynthia Koelker, *Armageddon Medicine*, 489.

[150] Ibid, 489.

[151] "FDA warns about increased risk of ruptures or tears in the aorta blood vessel with fluoroquinolone antibiotics in certain patients," 21 December 2018, https://www.fda.gov/drugs/drug-safety-and-availability/fda-warns-about-increased-risk-ruptures-or-tears-aorta-blood-vessel-fluoroquinolone-antibiotics (accessed 2 March 2020).

[152] Joseph Alton, *Alton's Antibiotics*, 177.

[153] Ibid, 177.

[154] "Dandelion," https://vitagene.com/supplements/herbs/dandelion (accessed 2 March 2020).

[155] "Ciprofloxacin," https://en.wikipedia.org/wiki/Ciprofloxacin

[156] Joseph Alton, Alton's Antibiotics, 160; Dr. Cynthia Koelker, *Armageddon Medicine*, 489.

[157] Joseph Alton, Alton's Antibiotics, 160; Cynthia Koelker, *Armageddon Medicine*, 489.

[158] Cynthia Koelker, *Armageddon Medicine*, 489.

[159] Joseph Alton, *Alton's Antibiotics*, 160.

[160] Ibid.

[161] Joseph Alton, *Alton's Antibiotics*, 160; "Haiti Cholera Training Manual: A Full Course for Healthcare Providers," Ministry of Health and Population in Haiti/U.S. Centers for Disease Control and Prevention, 2011 https://www.cdc.gov/cholera/pdf/haiticholera_trainingmanual_en.pdf , 17 (accessed 5 March 2020).

[162] "Abstract: "Consensus Statement: Tularemia as a Biological Weapon: Medical and Public Health Management," Centers for Disease Control and Prevention, https://emergency.cdc.gov/agent/tularemia/facts.asp (accessed 5 March 2020).

[163] Joseph Alton, et al., *Alton's Antibiotics*, 161.

[164] Ibid, 158.

[165] Ibid, 158.

[166] Cynthia Koelker, *Armageddon Medicine*, 147.

[167] Ibid, 157.

[168] Ibid, 207.

[169] Joseph Alton, et al., *Alton's Antibiotics*, 158.

[170] Ibid.

[171] Cynthia Koelker, *Armageddon Medicine,* 172.

[172] Cynthia Koelker, *Armageddon Medicine,* 172.

[173] Ibid, 178.

[174] Ibid, 169.

[175] "Pelvic Inflammatory Disease," Centers for Disease Control and Prevention, 2015 https://www.cdc.gov/std/tg2015/pid.htm (accessed 2 March 2020).

[176] "Bacterial Vaginosis," Centers for Disease Control and Prevention, 2015 https://www.cdc.gov/std/tg2015/bv.htm (accessed 2 March 2020).

[177] G. Greenstein, "The Role of Metronidazole in the Treatment of Periodontal Diseases," *Journal of Periodontology,* January 1993, 64(1), https://pubmed.ncbi.nlm.nih.gov/8426284-the-role-of-metronidazole-in-the-treatment-of-periodontal-diseases/?from_term=metronidazole&from_page=2&from_pos=8 (accessed 14 March 2020).

[178] Timothy B. Gardner, et al., "Treatment of Giardiasis," *Clinical Microbiology Reviews,* January 2001, 14(1), https://www.ncbi.nlm.nih.gov/pmc/articles/PMC88965/ (accessed 2 March 2020).

[179] Kawthar Bouchemal, et al., "Strategies for Prevention and Treatment of Trichomonas Vaginalis Infections," *Clinical Microbiology Reviews,* July 2017, 30(3), https://www.ncbi.nlm.nih.gov/pmc/articles/PMC5475227/ (accessed 2 March 2020).

[180] Joseph Alton, et al., *Alton's Antibiotics and Infectious Disease*, 176.

[181] Ibid.

[182] *Survival and Austere Medicine, 3rd Edition*, 209.

[183] Ibid.

[184] Ibid.

[185] Joseph Alton, *The Survival Medicine Handbook*, Doom and Bloom LLC, 2013, 157.

[186] Ibid, 156.

[187] Ibid.

[188] Cynthia Koelker, *Armageddon Medicine*,157.

[189] Ibid, 147.

[190] Joseph Alton, *The Survival Medicine Handbook*, 156.

[191] Cynthia Koelker, *Armageddon Medicine*, 109.

[192] Joseph Alton, *The Survival Medicine Handbook*, 156.

[193] "Evaluation and Diagnosis of Penicillin Allergy for Healthcare Professionals," Centers for Disease Control, https://www.cdc.gov/antibiotic-use/community/for-hcp/Penicillin-Allergy.html (accessed 13 March 2020).

[194] Ibid.

[195] Ibid.

[196] Joseph Alton, *The Survival Medicine Handbook*, 127.

[197] Cynthia Koelker, *Armageddon Medicine*, 467; *Survival and Austere Medicine, 3rd Edition*, 211.

[198] Cynthia Koelker, *Armageddon Medicine*, 176; David Werner, *Where There Is No Doctor*, 356.

[199] Cynthia Koelker, *Armageddon Medicine*, 368.

[200] Ibid.

[201] Ibid.

[202] Ibid.

[203] "Tick-Borne Relapsing Fever," Centers for Disease Control and Prevention, https://www.cdc.gov/ticks/tickbornediseases/tbrf.html (accessed 5 March 2020).

[204] David Werner, *Where There Is No Doctor*, 356.

[205] Ibid.

[206] "Unsponsored BYU Laboratory Studies Conducted by Dr. Ron W. Leavitt, Professor of Microbiology at Brigham Young University," SilverMedicine.org, https://www.silvermedicine.org/byustudy.html (accessed 21 March 2020).

[207] Stephen Harrod Buhner, *Herbal Antibiotics*, 213, 215.

[208] Ibid, 132.

[209] Ibid, 226.

[210] Ibid, 235.

[211] Ibid, 215-16.

[212] "Parasites: Medications," Centers for Disease Control, https://www.cdc.gov/parasites/scabies/health_professionals/meds.html (accessed 19 March 2020).

[213] Bart J. Currie, et al., "Permethrin and Ivermectin for Scabies," *New England Journal of Medicine*, 25 February 2010, 362(8), https://pubmed.ncbi.nlm.nih.gov/20181973/ (accessed 19 March 2020).

[214] "Parasites: Medications," Centers for Disease Control.

[215] Terri L. Meinking, et al., "The Treatment of Scabies with Ivermectin," *New England Journal of Medicine*, 6 July 1995, 333(26), https://www.nejm.org/doi/full/10.1056/NEJM199507063330105 (accessed 19 March 2020).

[216] "Parasites: Treatment," Centers for Disease Control, https://www.cdc.gov/parasites/lice/head/treatment.html (accessed 19 March 2020).

[217] "Parasites--Ascariasis: Resources for Health Care Professionals," Centers for Disease Control, https://www.cdc.gov/parasites/ascariasis/health_professionals/index.html (accessed 19 March 2020).

[218] "Homemade Oral Rehydration Solutions," University of Virginia Health System, https://med.virginia.edu/ginutrition/wp-content/uploads/sites/199/2018/09/Homemade-Oral-Rehydration-Solutions-9-2018.pdf (accessed 25 February 2020).

[219] "Coronavirus Disease 2019 (COVID-19): Strategies for Optimizing the Supply of N95 Respirators: Crisis/Alternate Strategies," Centers for Disease Control, https://www.cdc.gov/coronavirus/2019-ncov/hcp/respirators-strategy/crisis-alternate-strategies.html (accessed 16 March 2020). https://www.cdc.gov/h1n1flu/guidelines_infection_control_qa.htm

[220] Amy Price, et al., "Stanford AIM Lab COVID-19 Evidence Service Report," Stanford Medicine Anesthesia Informatics and Media Lab, 22 March 2020, https://m.box.com/shared_item/https%3A%2F%2Fstanfordmedicine.box.com%2Fv%2Fcovid19-PPE-1-1 (accessed 24 March 2020).

[221] Joseph Alton, "Can N95 Masks Be Reused?" https://www.doomandbloom.net/video-can-n95-masks-be-reused/ (accessed 16 March 2020).

[222] Chris Martenson, PeakProsperity.com, https://www.youtube.com/watch?time_continue=2691&v=efaDuE-XEi4&feature=emb_title (accessed 16 March 2020).

[223] Stephen Chen, "Coronavirus can travel twice as far as official 'safe distance' and stay in air for 30 minutes, Chinese study finds," *South China Morning Post*, https://www.scmp.com/news/china/science/article/3074351/coronavirus-can-travel-twice-far-official-safe-distance-and-stay (accessed 16 March 2020).

[224] "Practical Disinfection Guidance for the Clinical Laboratory," Association of Public Health Laboratories, 28 March 2018, https://www.aphl.org/programs/preparedness/Biosafety-and-Biosecurity/Documents/Practical%20Disinfection%20Guidance%20for%20the%20Clinical%20Laborator y.pdf (accessed 22 February 2020).

[225] K. Naka, et al., "Adsorption Effect of Activated Charcoal on Enterohemorrhagic Escherichia coli," *The Journal of Veterinary Medical Science,* March 2001, 63(3), https://pubmed.ncbi.nlm.nih.gov/11307928-adsorption-effect-of-activated-charcoal-on-enterohemorrhagic-escherichia-coli/ (accessed 13 March 2020).

[226] J A Vale, et al., "How Useful is Activated Charcoal?" *BMJ*, 9 January 1993, 306(6870), https://www.ncbi.nlm.nih.gov/pmc/articles/PMC1676641/pdf/bmj00002-0006.pdf (accessed 13 March 2020).

[227] Sam Coffman, *The Herbal Medic,* The Human Path, 2013, 323-25.

[228] "Caffeine," MedlinePlus, https://medlineplus.gov/caffeine.html (accessed 14 March 2020).

[229] "Caffeine," WebMD.com, https://www.webmd.com/vitamins/ai/ingredientmono-979/caffeine (accessed 14 March 2020).

[230] Ibid.

[231] Cynthia Koelker, *Armageddon Medicine*, 118, 332.

[232] Ibid, 357.

[233] "Caffeine," WebMD.com, https://www.webmd.com/vitamins/ai/ingredientmono-979/caffeine (accessed 14 March 2020).

[234] Ibid.

[235] Ibid.

[236] "Caffeine," MedlinePlus, https://medlineplus.gov/caffeine.html (accessed 14 March 2020).

[237] Ibid.

[238] Ibid.

[239] Anna Liza C Agero, et al., "A Randomized Double-Blind Controlled Trial Comparing Extra Virgin Coconut Oil With Mineral Oil as a Moisturizer for Mild to Moderate Xerosis," *Dermatitis*, 15(3), Sep 2004, https://pubmed.ncbi.nlm.nih.gov/15724344-a-randomized-double-blind-controlled-trial-comparing-extra-virgin-coconut-oil-with-mineral-oil-as-a-moisturizer-for-mild-to-moderate-xerosis/ (accessed 5 March 2020).

[240] S Intahphuak, et al., "Anti-inflammatory, Analgesic, and Antipyretic Activities of Virgin Coconut Oil," *Pharmaceutical Biology*, February 2010, 48(2), https://www.ncbi.nlm.nih.gov/pubmed/20645831 (accessed 5 March 2020).

[241] Pallavi Srivastava, "Burn wound healing property of *Cocos nucifera*: An appraisal," *Indian Journal of Pharmacology*, August 2008, 40(4), https://www.ncbi.nlm.nih.gov/pmc/articles/PMC2792613/ (accessed 5 March 2020).

[242] K. G. Nevin, et al., "Effect of Topical Application of Virgin Coconut Oil on Skin Components and Antioxidant Status During Dermal Wound Healing in Young Rats," *Skin Pharmacology and Physiology*, 2010, 23(6), https://www.ncbi.nlm.nih.gov/pubmed/20523108 (accessed 5 March 2020).

[243] D.O. Ogbolu, et al., "In Vitro Antimicrobial Properties of Coconut Oil on Candida Species in Ibadan, Nigeria," *Journal of Medicinal Food*, June 2007, 10(2), https://www.ncbi.nlm.nih.gov/pubmed/17651080 (accessed 5 March 2020).

[244] "Perineal Massage In Pregnancy," *Journal of Midwifery and Women's Health,* Jan-Feb 2005, Vol 50(1),

http://www.midwife.org/ACNM/files/ccLibraryFiles/Filename/000000000656/Perineal%20Massage%20in%20Pregnancy.pdf (accessed 5 March 2020).

[245] Ian F. Burgess, et al., "Clinical Trial Showing Superiority of a Coconut and Anise Spray Over Permethrin 0.43% Lotion for Head Louse Infestation, ISRCTN96469780," *European Journal of Pediatrics*, January 2010, 169(1), https://www.ncbi.nlm.nih.gov/pubmed/19343362 (accessed 5 March 2020).

[246] Kirsty Martin, et al., "Ketogenic Diet and Other Dietary Treatments for Epilepsy," *The Cochrane Database of Systematic Reviews,* 9 February 2016, https://www.ncbi.nlm.nih.gov/pubmed/26859528 (accessed 5 March 2020).

[247] Mark A. Reger, et al., "Effects of Beta-Hydroxybutyrate on Cognition in Memory-Impaired Adults," *Neurobiology of Aging*, March 2004, 25(3) https://www.ncbi.nlm.nih.gov/pubmed/15123336 (5 March 2020).

[248] V. Van Wimelbeke, et al, "Influence of medium-chain and long-chain triacylglycerols on the control of food intake in men," *American Journal of Clinical Nutrition*, August 1998, 68(2), https://academic.oup.com/ajcn/article/68/2/226/4648722 (accessed 5 March 2020); Monica L. Assuncao, et al., "Effects of Dietary Coconut Oil on the Biochemical and Anthropometric Profiles of Women Presenting Abdominal Obesity," *Lipids*, July 2009, 44(7), https://www.ncbi.nlm.nih.gov/pubmed/19437058 (accessed 5 March 2020).

[249] Dear R. Focht III, et al., "The Efficacy of Duct Tape vs Cryotherapy in the Treatment of Verruca Vulgaris (the Common Wart)," *JAMA Pediatrics*, October 2002, https://jamanetwork.com/journals/jamapediatrics/fullarticle/203979 (accessed 5 March 2020); Rachel Nall, "What to Know About Duct Tape Wart Removal," Medical News Today, 12 July 2019, https://www.medicalnewstoday.com/articles/325734#does-it-work (accessed 14 March 2020).

[250] Joseph Alton, *The Survival Medicine Handbook*, 245.

[251] Joseph Alton, *The Survival Medicine Handbook*, 321-22; Zoriah Aziz, et al., "The Effects of Honey Compared to Silver Sulfadiazine for the Treatment of Burns: A Systematic Review of Randomized Controlled Trials," *Burns*, February 2017, 43(1), https://pubmed.ncbi.nlm.nih.gov/27576926-the-effects-of-honey-compared-to-silver-sulfadiazine-for-the-treatment-of-burns-a-systematic-review-of-randomized-controlled-trials/?from_term=honey+burns&from_pos=1 (accessed 6 March 2020).

[252] "Honey Works Better than Cough Medicine," LiveScience, 3 December 2007, https://www.livescience.com/7446-honey-works-cough-medicine.html (accessed 14 March 2020).

[253] G. Gethin, et al., "Bacteriological Changes in Sloughy Venous Leg Ulcers Treated With Manuka Honey or Hydrogel: An RCT," *Journal of Wound Care*, June 2008, 17(6), https://pubmed.ncbi.nlm.nih.gov/18666717-bacteriological-changes-in-sloughy-venous-leg-ulcers-treated-with-manuka-honey-or-hydrogel-an-rct/ (accessed 14 March 2020); Elizabeth A van der Weyden, "Treatment of a Venous Leg Ulcer with Honey Alginate Dressing," *British Journal of Community Nursing,* June 2005, https://pubmed.ncbi.nlm.nih.gov/15944502-treatment-of-a-venous-leg-ulcer-with-a-honey-alginate-dressing/ (accessed 14 March 2020).

[254] Iain S. Whitaker, et al., "Larval therapy from antiquity to the present day: mechanisms of action, clinical applications and future potential," *Postgraduate Medical Journal*, June 2007, 83(980), https://www.ncbi.nlm.nih.gov/pmc/articles/PMC2600045/ (accessed 7 March 2020).

[255] "Wound Series Part 2: Approaches to Treating Chronic Wounds," CEUfast, https://ceufast.com/course/wound-series-part-2-approaches-to-treating-chronic-wounds (accessed 7 March 2020).

[256] "Medical Maggots™ (maggot therapy, maggot debridement therapy, MDT, biotherapy, biosurgery, biodebridement, larval therapy)," http://www.monarchlabs.com/mdt (accessed 7 March 2020).

[257] R. A Sherman, "Maggot Therapy Takes Us Back to the Future of Wound Care: New and Improved Maggot Therapy for the 21st Century," *Journal of Diabetes Science and Technology*, March 2009, 3(2), https://www.ncbi.nlm.nih.gov/pmc/articles/PMC2771513/ (accessed 7 March 2020).

[258] Iain S. Whitaker, "Larval therapy from antiquity to the present day: mechanisms of action, clinical applications and future potential."

[259] Gary Greenburg, "What If the Placebo Effect Isn't a Trick?" The New York Times Magazine, 7 November 2018, https://www.nytimes.com/2018/11/07/magazine/placebo-effect-medicine.html (accessed 6 March 2020); Brian Resnick, "The Weird Power of the Placebo Effect Explained," Pocket, https://getpocket.com/explore/item/the-weird-power-of-the-placebo-effect-explained (accessed 6 March 2020).

[260] M. Murandu, et al., "Use of Granulated Sugar Therapy in the Management of Sloughy or Necrotic Wounds: A Pilot Study," *Journal of Wound Therapy*, May 2011, 20(5), https://pubmed.ncbi.nlm.nih.gov/21647066 (accessed 6 March 2020).

[261] R. A. Knutson, "Sugar for Wound Care: What Is Sugardyne?" *The People's Pharmacy*, https://www.peoplespharmacy.com/articles/sugar-for-wound-care (accessed 6 March 2020).

[262] Ibid.

[263] Ibid.

[264] R. A. Knutson, et al., "Use of Sugar and Povidone-Iodine to Enhance Wound Healing: Five Year's Experience," *Southern Medical Journal*, November 1981, 74(11), https://pubmed.ncbi.nlm.nih.gov/7302631 (accessed 6 March 2020).

[265] R. A. Knutson, "Sugar for Wound Care: What Is Sugardyne?"

[266] Zawn Villines, "Why Do We Use Pulse Oximetry?" Medical News Today, 20 July 2017, https://www.medicalnewstoday.com/articles/318489#Limitations-of-pulse-oximetry (accessed 14 March 2020).

[267] Vishakha Sonawane, "ER Visits 2016: Top Ten Reasons for Going to Emergency Department," *Medical Daily*, 12 October 2016, https://www.medicaldaily.com/er-visits-2016-top-10-reasons-going-emergency-department-400875 (accessed 6 March 2020); "Ten Common ER Visits," Beamont Emergency Center, 21 July 2015, https://beaumontemergencycenter.com/ten-common-er-visits/ (accessed 6 March 2020); Marianne Spoon, "10 Most Common Reasons for an ER Visit," How Stuff Works, https://health.howstuffworks.com/medicine/10-common-reasons-for-er-visit1.htm (accessed 6 March 2020).

[268] *Survival and Austere Medicine, 3rd Edition*, 24-25.

[269] Ibid, 25.

[270] Ibid, 122.

[271] Joseph Alton, *The Survival Medicine Handbook*, 317.

[272] Cynthia Koelker, *Armageddon Medicine*, 267.

[273] Ibid, 267-68.

[274] Ibid, 268-69.

[275] R. Maenthaisong, et al., "The Efficacy of Aloe Vera Used for Burn Wound Healing: A Systematic Review," *Burns*, September 2007, 33(6), https://pubmed.ncbi.nlm.nih.gov/17499928 (accessed 6 March 2020).

[276] Joseph Alton, *The Survival Medicine Handbook*, 320.

[277] Ibid, 319-20.

[278] Ferdaous Ghrab Ben Djemaa, et al., "Antioxidant and Wound Healing Activity of Lavandula Aspic L Ointment," *Journal of Tissue Viability*, November 2016, 25(4) https://pubmed.ncbi.nlm.nih.gov/27769632 (accessed 6 March 2020); Joseph Alton, *The Survival Medicine Handbook*, 320.

[279] Joseph Alton, *The Survival Medicine Handbook*, 320.

[280] Ibid, 319.

[281] Joseph Alton, *The Survival Medicine Handbook*, 321; Zoriah Aziz, et al., "The Effects of Honey Compared to Silver Sulfadiazine for the Treatment of Burns: A Systematic Review of Randomized Controlled Trials," *Burns*, February 2017, 43(1), https://pubmed.ncbi.nlm.nih.gov/27576926-the-effects-of-honey-compared-to-silver-sulfadiazine-for-the-treatment-of-burns-a-systematic-review-of-randomized-controlled-trials/?from_term=honey+burns&from_pos=1 (accessed 6 March 2020).

[282] Peter Oldani, "How to Treat Different Types of Burns," Inside First Aid, 13 April 2019, https://insidefirstaid.com/burns/how-to-treat-different-types-of-burns (accessed 6 March 2020).

[283] Cynthia Koelker, *Armageddon Medicine*, 264.

[284] *Survival and Austere Medicine, 3rd Edition*, 123.

[285] Joseph Alton, *The Survival Medicine Handbook*, 321.

[286] *Survival and Austere Medicine, 3rd Edition*, 123; Cynthia Koelker, *Armageddon Medicine*, 266.

[287] "Tetanus," https://en.wikipedia.org/wiki/Tetanus (accessed 6 March 2020).

[288] David Werner, *Where There Is No Doctor*, 184.

[289] Joseph Alton, *The Survival Medicine Handbook*, 196.

[290] David Werner, *Where There Is No Doctor*, 183.

[291] NM Apte, et al., "Short Report: The Spatula Test: A Simple Bedside Test to Diagnose Tetanus," *American Journal of Tropical Medicine and Hygiene*, October 1995, 53 (4), https://pubmed.ncbi.nlm.nih.gov/7485691 *(accessed 6 March 2020).*

[292] David Werner, *Where There Is No Doctor*, 183.

[293] Ibid, 184.

[294] Joseph Alton, *The Survival Medicine Handbook*, 197.

[295] Cynthia Koelker *Armageddon Medicine*, 111.

[296] David Werner, *Where There Is No Doctor*, 183.

[297] "Tetanus," Mayo Clinic, https://www.mayoclinic.org/diseases-conditions/tetanus/diagnosis-treatment/drc-20351631 (accessed 6 March 2020).

[298] Cynthia Koelker, *Armageddon Medicine*, 112.

[299] David Werner, *Where There Is No Doctor*, 183.

[300] Jillian Levy, "Shingles Symptoms, Risk Factors, and Causes," DrAxe.com, 15 February 2016, https://draxe.com/health/shingles-symptoms/ (accessed 6 March 2020).

[301] Cynthia Koelker, *Armageddon Medicine*, 215.

[302] Stephanie Watson, "New Shingles Vaccine: What You Need to Know," WebMD, 13 November 2019, https://www.webmd.com/skin-problems-and-treatments/shingles/news/20191113/new-shingles-vaccine_what-you-need-to-know (accessed 6 March 2020).

[303] "Shingles: Signs & Symptoms," Centers for Disease Control, https://www.cdc.gov/shingles/about/symptoms.html (accessed 6 March 2020).

[304] "Shingles: Complications of Shingles," Centers for Disease Control, https://www.cdc.gov/shingles/about/complications.html

[305] Cynthia Koelker, *Armageddon Medicine*, 215.

[306] Ibid, 214.

[307] "Shingles: Treating Shingles," Centers for Disease Control, https://www.cdc.gov/shingles/about/treatment.html (accessed 6 March 2020).

[308] Sam Coffman, *The Herbal Medic*, 110; Charles Kane, *Medicinal Plants of the Western Mountain States*, Lincoln Town Press, 2017, 284.

[309] Stephen Harrod Buhner, *Herbal Antivirals*, Storey Publishing, 2013, 117-18.

[310] Ibid.

[311] Joseph Alton, *The Survival Medicine Handbook*, 340.

[312] Ibid.

[313]"Tick Bites/Prevention," Centers for Disease Control, https://www.cdc.gov/ticks/tickbornediseases/tick-bites-prevention.html (accessed 7 March 2020).

[314] Joseph Alton, *The Survival Medicine Handbook*, 117.
[315] "Body Lice: Biology," Centers for Disease Control, https://www.cdc.gov/parasites/lice/body/biology.html (accessed 7 March 2020).
[316] Joseph Alton, *The Survival Medicine Handbook*, 121.
[317] "Body Lice: Prevention and Treatment," Centers for Disease Control, https://www.cdc.gov/parasites/lice/body/prevent.html (accessed 7 March 2020).
[318] Ibid.
[319] Ibid.
[320] Ibid.
[321] "Zika Virus: Prevent Mosquito Bites," Centers for Disease Control, https://www.cdc.gov/zika/prevention/prevent-mosquito-bites.html (accessed 7 March 2020).
[322] Ibid.
[323] Ibid.
[324] Ibid.
[325] Ibid.
[326] "Tick Bites/Prevention," Centers for Disease Control.
[327] Joseph Alton, *The Survival Medicine Handbook*, 123.
[328] "Tick Bites/Prevention," Centers for Disease Control.
[329] Ibid.
[330] Ibid.
[331] "Geographic Distribution of Ticks That Bite Humans," Centers for Disease Control, https://www.cdc.gov/ticks/geographic_distribution.html (accessed 6 March 2020).
[332] "Tick Bite Prophylaxis," Centers for Disease Control, https://www.cdc.gov/ticks/tickbornediseases/tick-bite-prophylaxis.html (accessed 7 March 2020).
[333] "Tick-Borne Diseases," Centers for Disease Control, https://www.cdc.gov/ticks/tickbornediseases/rmsf.html (accessed 7 March 2020).
[334] Ibid.
[335] "Lyme Disease," Centers for Disease Control, https://www.cdc.gov/ticks/tickbornediseases/lyme.html (accessed 7 March 2020).
[336] "Rocky Mountain Spotted Fever," Centers for Disease Control, https://www.cdc.gov/ticks/tickbornediseases/rmsf.html (accessed 7 March 2020).
[337] Ibid.
[338] "Ricketssiosis" Centers for Disease Control, https://www.cdc.gov/ticks/tickbornediseases/rickettsiosis.html (accessed 7 March 2020).
[339] "Ehrlichiosis," Centers for Disease Control, https://www.cdc.gov/ticks/tickbornediseases/ehrlichiosis.html (accessed 7 March 2020).
[340] "Anaplasmosis," Centers for Disease Control, https://www.cdc.gov/ticks/tickbornediseases/anaplasmosis.html (accessed 7 March 2020).
[341] "Tick-Borne Relapsing Fever," Centers for Disease Control, https://www.cdc.gov/ticks/tickbornediseases/tbrf.html (accessed 7 March 2020).
[342] "Colorado Tick Fever," Centers for Disease Control, https://www.cdc.gov/ticks/tickbornediseases/ctf.html (accessed 7 March 2020).
[343] "Heartland and Bourbon Virus Diseases," Centers for Disease Control, https://www.cdc.gov/ticks/tickbornediseases/heartland-virus.html (accessed 7 March 2020).
[344] "Insects and Scorpions: Bees, Wasps, and Hornets," Centers for Disease Control, https://www.cdc.gov/niosh/topics/insects/beeswasphornets.html (accessed 7 March 2020).
[345] Cynthia Koelker, *Armageddon Medicine*, 300.
[346] Ibid.
[347] Ibid.

[348] Joseph Alton, *The Survival Medicine Handbook*, 322.
[349] Ibid.
[350] Cynthia Koelker, *Armageddon Medicine*, 302.
[351] Joseph Alton, *The Survival Medicine Handbook*, 333.
[352] "Venomous Spiders," Centers for Disease Control, https://www.cdc.gov/niosh/topics/spiders/symptoms.html (Accessed 7 March 2020).
[353] Joseph Alton, *The Survival Medicine Handbook*, 334.
[354] Josh Axe, "Top 10 Activated Charcoal Uses, Plus Potential Side Effects," DrAxe, 5 July 2019, https://draxe.com/nutrition/activated-charcoal-uses/ (accessed 7 March 2020).
[355] William K Hayes, "Snakebite Severity and Treatment," Loma Linda University School of Medicine, https://medicine.llu.edu/research/department-earth-and-biological-sciences/biology/research/william-k-hayes-phd-ms/snakebite (accessed 9 March 2020).
[356] Joseph Alton, *The Survival Medicine Handbook*, 327.
[357] Ibid.
[358] Sam Coffman, *The Herbal Medic*, 82.
[359] William K Hayes, "Snakebite Severity and Treatment."
[360] David Werner, *Where There Is No Doctor*, 104.
[361] Eric Weiss, A Comprehensive Guide to Wilderness and Travel Medicine, 129-30.
[362] Ibid, 131-32.
[363] *Survival and Austere Medicine, 3rd Edition*, 196-97.
[364] Joseph Alton, *The Survival Medicine Handbook*, 330.
[365] "Venomous Snakes: Symptoms and First Aid," Centers for Disease Control, https://www.cdc.gov/niosh/topics/snakes/symptoms.html (accessed 9 March 2020).
[366] "Venomous Snakes: Symptoms and First Aid."
[367] Eric Weiss, *A Comprehensive Guide to Wilderness and Travel Medicine,* 130; William K Hayes, "Snakebite Severity and Treatment," Loma Linda University School of Medicine, https://medicine.llu.edu/research/department-earth-and-biological-sciences/biology/research/william-k-hayes-phd-ms/snakebite (accessed 9 March 2020).
[368] Sam Coffman, *The Herbal Medic*, 86-87.
[369] Ibid, 88.
[370] Ibid, 90.
[371] Patrick Jones, *The HomeGrown Herbalist*, 2014.
[372] Robert Ellis, et al., "Dog and Cat Bites," American Family Physician, 2014, 90(4), 239 https://www.aafp.org/afp/2014/0815/p239.pdf (accessed 9 March 2020); H. Dele Davies, "When Your Best Friend Bites," *Canadian Journal of Infectious Diseases,* September-October 2000, 11(5), https://www.ncbi.nlm.nih.gov/pmc/articles/PMC2094772/ (accessed 9 March 2020).
[373] Cynthia Koelker, *Armageddon Medicine*, 107.
[374] Ibid, 109.
[375] Robert Ellis, et al., "Dog and Cat Bites."
[376] Cynthia Koelker, *Armageddon Medicine*, 106-07.
[377] Ibid, 108-09.
[378] "Morbidity and Mortality Weekly Report," Centers for Disease Control, 7 May 2008, 2.
[379] Cynthia Koelker, *Armageddon Medicine*, 110.
[380] Joseph Alton, *The Survival Medicine Handbook*, 325; Cynthia Koelker, *Armageddon Medicine*, 111.
[381] *Survival and Austere Medicine, 3rd Edition*, 255.
[382] David Werner, *Where There Is No Doctor*, 181.
[383] Cynthia Koelker, *Armageddon Medicine*, 111.

[384] J. A. Armstrong, "Inactivation of Viruses by Benzalkonium Chloride," *Applied Microbiology*, March 1964; 12(2) https://www.ncbi.nlm.nih.gov/pmc/articles/PMC1058082/ (accessed 9 March 2020).

[385] *Survival and Austere Medicine, 3rd Edition*, 255.

[386] David Werner, *Where There Is No Doctor*, 181.

[387] Cynthia Koelker, *Armageddon Medicine*, 175.

[388] "Haiti Cholera Training Manual: A Full Course for Healthcare Providers," Centers for Disease Control, p 10, https://www.cdc.gov/cholera/pdf/haiticholera_trainingmanual_en.pdf (accessed 7 March 2020).

[389] Ibid.

[390] Cynthia Koelker, *Armageddon Medicine*, 176.

[391] Stephen Buhner, *Herbal Antibiotics*, 162.

[392] Cynthia Koelker, *Armageddon Medicine*, 490.

[393] Ibid, 489.

[394] Ibid, 489.

[395] Joseph Alton, *Alton's Antibiotics*, 160, 164, 178.

[396] "Plague: Resources for Clinicians," Centers for Disease Control, https://www.cdc.gov/plague/healthcare/clinicians.html (accessed 9 March 2020).

[397] Joel B. Pollack, "Dr Drew: Los Angeles Faces Imminent Outbreak of Pneumonic Plague," Breitbart, 19 July 2019, https://www.breitbart.com/health/2019/07/19/dr-drew-pinsky-bubonic-plague-outbreak-imminent-in-los-angeles/ (accessed 9 March 2020); A. J. Viseltear, "The Pneumonic Plague Epidemic of 1924 in Los Angeles," *Yale Journal of Biology and Medicine*, March 1974, 47(1), https://www.ncbi.nlm.nih.gov/pmc/articles/PMC2595158/ (accessed 9 March 2020).

[398] "Plant Uses: California," Arboretum, University of California—Santa Cruz, https://arboretum.ucsc.edu/pdfs/ethnobotany-webversion.pdf (accessed 14 March 2020).

[399] "Tularemia: Bioterrorism Agent Profiles for Health Care Workers," Arizona Department of Health Services, https://azdhs.gov/documents/preparedness/emergency-preparedness/zebra-manual/zm-s4-tularemia.pdf (accessed 9 March 2020).

[400] Ibid.

[401] Carrie Byington, et al., "Tularemia with Vesicular Skin Lesions May Be Mistaken for Infection with Herpes Viruses," *Clinical Infectious Diseases*, 1 July 2008, https://academic.oup.com/cid/article/47/1/e4/378987 (accessed 9 March 2008).

[402] "Tularemia Post-Exposure Prophylaxis," Oklahoma State Department of Health, https://www.ok.gov/health2/documents/Tularemia.pdf (accessed 9 March 2020).

[403] Robert Herriman, "Outbreaks and Bioterrorism: Tularemia Planned Use in Turkey's Water," *Outbreak news Today*, 21 January 2016, https://outbreaknewstoday.com/isis-and-bioterrorism-tularemia-planned-use-in-turkeys-water-67823/ (accessed 9 March 2020).

[404] Larry Bush, et al., "Tularemia," *Merck Manual Professional Version,* https://www.merckmanuals.com/professional/infectious-diseases/gram-negative-bacilli/tularemia (accessed 9 March 2020); "Tularemia Post-Exposure Prophylaxis," Oklahoma State Department of Health, https://www.ok.gov/health2/documents/Tularemia.pdf (accessed 9 March 2020).

[405] "Typhoid Fever and Paratyphoid Fever: Questions and Answers," Centers for Disease Control, https://www.cdc.gov/typhoid-fever/sources.html (accessed 10 March 2020).

[406] Ibid.

[407] "Typhoid Fever," Wikipedia, https://en.wikipedia.org/wiki/Typhoid_fever (accessed 10 March 2020).

[408] "Typhoid Fever and Paratyphoid Fever: Information for Healthcare Professionals," Centers for Disease Control, https://www.cdc.gov/typhoid-fever/health-professional.html (accessed 10 March 2020).

[409] David Werner, *Where There Is No Doctor*, 189.

[410] Ibid.

[411] Ibid.

[412] "Typhoid Fever," Wikipedia.

[413] "Typhus: Information for Healthcare Providers," Centers for Disease Control, https://www.cdc.gov/typhus/healthcare-providers/index.html (accessed 10 March 2020).

[414] Ibid.

[415] Charles Patrick Davis, et al., "Typhus," MedicineNet, https://www.medicinenet.com/typhus/article.htm#what_is_the_history_of_typhus (accessed 10 March 2020).

[416] "Typhus: Information for Healthcare Providers," Centers for Disease Control.

[417] Ibid.

[418] "Yellow Fever," Wikipedia.org, https://en.wikipedia.org/wiki/Yellow_fever (accessed 10 March 2020).

[419] Ibid.

[420] "Yellow Fever: Symptoms, Diagnosis, and Treatment," Centers for Disease Control, https://www.cdc.gov/yellowfever/symptoms/index.html (accessed 10 March 2020).

[421] Ibid.

[422] "Yellow Fever: Transmission of Yellow Fever Virus," Centers for Disease Control, https://www.cdc.gov/yellowfever/transmission/index.html (accessed 10 March 2020).

[423] Stephen Harrod Buhner, *Herbal Antivirals*, 160, 172, 218-19.

[424] "Chikungunya Virus: Symptoms, Diagnosis, and Treatment," Centers for Disease Control, https://www.cdc.gov/chikungunya/symptoms/index.html (accessed 10 March 2020).

[425] "Dengue: Symptoms and Treatment," Centers for Disease Control, https://www.cdc.gov/dengue/symptoms/index.html (accessed 10 March 2020).

[426] "West Nile Virus: Symptoms, Diagnosis, and Treatment," Centers for Disease Control, https://www.cdc.gov/westnile/symptoms/index.html (accessed 10 March 2020).

[427] "Zika Virus: Potential Range in US," Centers for Disease Control, https://www.cdc.gov/zika/vector/range.html (accessed 10 March 2020).

[428] Cynthia Koelker, *Armageddon Medicine*, 97.

[429] Ibid, 142.

[430] Ibid.

[431] David Werner, *Where There Is No Doctor*, 313.

[432] Ibid.

[433] David Werner, *Where There Is No Doctor*, 168.

[434] Cynthia Koelker, *Armageddon Medicine*, 119.

[435] Candice L Bjornson, et al., "Croup in Children," CMAJ, 15 October 2013, 185(15), https://www.ncbi.nlm.nih.gov/pmc/articles/PMC3796596/ (accessed 10 March 2020).

[436] Ibid.

[437] Ibid.

[438] Ibid.

[439] "Croup: Diagnosis and Treatment," Mayo Clinic, https://www.mayoclinic.org/diseases-conditions/croup/diagnosis-treatment/drc-20350354 (accessed 10 March 2020).

[440] Cynthia Koelker, *Armageddon Medicine*, 156-57.

[441] Joseph Alton, *The Survival Medicine Handbook*, 440.

[442] Ibid, 437-38.

[443] Cynthia Koelker, *Armageddon Medicine*, 156.

[444] Ibid.

[445] Ibid, 158.

[446] Joseph Alton, *Alton's Antibiotics*, 151.

[447] Ibid, 156.

[448] Ibid, 158.
[449] Ibid, 173.
[450] Joseph Alton, *The Survival Medicine Handbook*, 437.
[451] Cynthia Koelker, *Armageddon Medicine*, 156.
[452] Ibid, 157.
[453] Weinan Zheng, et al, "Naproxen Exhibits Broad Anti-influenza Virus Activity in Mice by Impeding Viral Nucleoprotein Nuclear Export," Cell Reports, Vol 27 Issue 6, 7 May 2019, https://www.sciencedirect.com/science/article/pii/S2211124719305261?via%3Dihub (accessed 18 February 2020).
[454] Joseph Alton, *The Survival Medicine Handbook*, 429.
[455] Ibid.
[456] Amir A. Azari, et al., "Conjunctivitis: A Systematic Review of Diagnosis and Treatment," *JAMA*, 23 October 2013, 310(16), https://www.ncbi.nlm.nih.gov/pmc/articles/PMC4049531/ (accessed 10 March 2020).
[457] *Survival and Austere Medicine, 3rd Edition*, 182.
[458] Joseph Alton, *The Survival Medicine Handbook*, 430.
[459] Ibid.
[460] Ibid.
[461] Ibid.
[462] "Colloidal Silver," National Center for Complementary and Integrative Health, https://nccih.nih.gov/health/colloidalsilver (accessed 10 March 2020).
[463] David Werner, *Where There Is No Doctor*, 171.
[464] Ibid.
[465] Cynthia Koelker, *Armageddon Medicine*, 121.
[466] Cynthia Koelker, *Armageddon Medicine*, 122; *Survival and Austere Medicine, 3rd Edition*, 116.
[467] *Survival and Austere Medicine, 3rd Edition*, 116.
[468] Ibid.
[469] Cynthia Koelker, *Armageddon Medicine*, 123.
[470] *Survival and Austere Medicine, 3rd Edition*, 116.
[471] Ibid, 117.
[472] Ibid, 116.
[473] "Respiratory Syncytial Virus," Mayo Clinic, https://www.mayoclinic.org/diseases-conditions/respiratory-syncytial-virus/symptoms-causes/syc-20353098 (accessed 11 March 2020).
[474] "Respiratory Syncytial Virus (RSV) Infection," Centers for Disease Control, https://www.cdc.gov/rsv/about/transmission.html (accessed 11 March 2020).
[475] "Respiratory Syncytial Virus," Mayo Clinic, https://www.mayoclinic.org/diseases-conditions/respiratory-syncytial-virus/symptoms-causes/syc-20353098 (accessed 11 March 2020); "Respiratory Syncytial Virus (RSV) Infection," Centers for Disease Control, https://www.cdc.gov/rsv/about/symptoms.html (accessed 11 March 2020).
[476] Ibid.
[477] Cynthia Koelker, *Armageddon Medicine*, 142.
[478] Ibid, 145.
[479] Ibid, 143.
[480] "Centor Score for Strep Pharyngitis," https://www.mdcalc.com/centor-score-modified-mcisaac-strep-pharyngitis#next-steps (accessed 11 March 2020).
[481] "Strep Throat: All You Need to Know," Centers for Disease Control, https://www.cdc.gov/groupastrep/diseases-public/strep-throat.html (accessed 11 March 2020).
[482] Joseph Alton, *Alton's Antibiotics*, 151.
[483] Ibid, 158.

[484] Ibid, 173.
[485] Ibid, 156.
[486] "Food Poisoning Treatment: What to Expect," WebMD, https://www.webmd.com/food-recipes/food-poisoning/understanding-food-poisoning-treatment#1 (accessed 14 March 2020).
[487] "Clostridium Botulinum," USDA Food Safety Information, https://www.fsis.usda.gov/wps/wcm/connect/a70a5447-9490-4855-af0d-e617ea6b5e46/Clostridium_botulinum.pdf?MOD=AJPERES (accessed 11 March 2020).
[488] Jeremy Sobel, "Botulism," *Clinical Infectious Diseases*, 41(8), https://academic.oup.com/cid/article/41/8/1167/379325 (accessed 11 March 2020).
[489] "Botulism: Prevention," Centers for Disease Control, https://www.cdc.gov/botulism/prevention.html (accessed 11 March 2020).
[490] F J Angulo, et al., "A Large Outbreak of Botulism: The Hazardous Baked Potato," *Journal of Infectious Disease*, July 1998, 178(1), https://pubmed.ncbi.nlm.nih.gov/9652437-a-large-outbreak-of-botulism-the-hazardous-baked-potato/ (accessed 11 March 2020).
[491] Larry Bush, et al., "Botulism," MSD Manual: Consumer Version.
[492] "Clostridium Botulinum: Bacterial Diseases Monograph 858," World Health Organization, https://www.who.int/csr/delibepidemics/clostridiumbotulism.pdf (accessed 11 March 2020); "Clostridium Botulinum," USDA Food Safety Information, https://www.fsis.usda.gov/wps/wcm/connect/a70a5447-9490-4855-af0d-e617ea6b5e46/Clostridium_botulinum.pdf?MOD=AJPERES (accessed 11 March 2020).
[493] Cynthia Koelker, *Armageddon Medicine*, 341.
[494] "Clostridium Botulinum: Bacterial Diseases Monograph 858"; "Clostridium Botulinum," USDA Food Safety Information, https://www.fsis.usda.gov/wps/wcm/connect/a70a5447-9490-4855-af0d-e617ea6b5e46/Clostridium_botulinum.pdf?MOD=AJPERES (accessed 11 March 2020).
[495] Larry Bush, et al., "Botulism," MSD Manual: Consumer Version, https://www.msdmanuals.com/home/infections/bacterial-infections-anaerobic-bacteria/botulism (accessed 11 March 2020).
[496] Cynthia Koelker, *Armageddon Medicine*, 342.
[497] "Botulism: Prevention," Centers for Disease Control, https://www.cdc.gov/botulism/prevention.html (accessed 11 March 2020).
[498] S J Pandian, et al., "Therapeutic Management of Botulism in Dairy Cattle," *Veterinary World*, November 2015, 8(11), https://www.ncbi.nlm.nih.gov/pmc/articles/PMC4774742/ (accessed 11 March 2020).
[499] Hernan Gomez, et al., "Adsorption of Botulinum Toxin to Activated Charcoal With a Mouse Bioassay," *Annals of Emergency Medicine,* 25(6), June 1995, https://www.sciencedirect.com/science/article/abs/pii/S0196064495702148 (accessed 11 March 2020); Christie Sun, et al., "Botulism," California Poison Control System, 1 August 2017, https://calpoison.org/news/botulism (accessed 11 March 2020); Larry Bush, et al., "Botulism," MSD Manual: Consumer Version, https://www.msdmanuals.com/home/infections/bacterial-infections-anaerobic-bacteria/botulism (accessed 11 March 2020).
[500] "Diarrheagenic *E. coli,"* Centers for Disease Control and Prevention, https://www.cdc.gov/ecoli/diarrheagenic-ecoli.html (accessed 3 March 2020).
[501] "Enterotoxigenic *E. coli*," Centers for Disease Control and Prevention, https://www.cdc.gov/ecoli/etec.html (accessed 3 March 2020).
[502] "Questions and Answers," Centers for Disease Control and Prevention, https://www.cdc.gov/ecoli/general/index.html#what_shiga (accessed 3 March 2020).
[503] Joseph Alton, et al., *Alton's Antibiotics*, 51, 160.
[504] Stephen Buhner, *Herbal Antibiotics*, 177-78.

[505] Julia E. Painter, et al., "Giardiasis Surveillance--U.S. 2011-2012," Surveillance Summaries, Centers for Disease Control and Prevention, 1 May 2015 https://www.cdc.gov/mmwr/preview/mmwrhtml/ss6403a2.htm (accessed 3 March 2020).

[506] David Werner, *Where There Is No Doctor*, 145.

[507] Ibid.

[508] Joseph Alton, *Alton's Antibiotics*, 176; Cynthia Koelker, *Armageddon Medicine*, 173.

[509] Jeffrey D. Kiser, et al., "What's the Most Effective Treatment for Giardiasis?" *The Journal of Family Practice*, April 2008, 57(4) https://www.mdedge.com/familymedicine/article/63098/infectious-diseases/whats-most-effective-treatment-giardiasis (accessed 23 March 2020); Roberto Canute, "Effectiveness and Tolerability of 3-Day Mebendazole Treatment of *Giardia duodenalis* Infection in Adults and Children: Two Prospective, Open-Label Phase IV Trials," *Current Therapeutic Research, Clinical and Experimental,* 30 November 2018, 89, https://pubmed.ncbi.nlm.nih.gov/30792825/ (accessed 23 March 2020).

[510] Stephen Buhner, *Herbal Antibiotics*, 164.

[511] "Listeria: Prevention," Centers for Disease Control, https://www.cdc.gov/listeria/prevention.html (accessed 14 March 2020).

[512] Almudena Hernandez-Milian, et al., "What Is New in Listeriosis?" *Biomed Research International*, 14 April 2014, https://www.ncbi.nlm.nih.gov/pmc/articles/PMC4005144/ (accessed 14 March 2020).

[513] "Listeria," Centers for Disease Control, https://www.cdc.gov/listeria/risk-groups/pregnant-women.html (accessed 14 March 2020).

[514] "Listeria: Questions and Answers," Centers for Disease Control, https://www.cdc.gov/listeria/faq.html (accessed 14 March 2020).

[515] "Listeria," Centers for Disease Control.

[516] "Listeria: Questions and Answers," Centers for Disease Control.

[517] Ronald F. Lamont, et al., "Listeriosis in Human Pregnancy: A Systematic Review," *Journal of Perinatal Medicine,* May 2011, 39(3), https://www.ncbi.nlm.nih.gov/pmc/articles/PMC3593057/ (accessed 14 March 2020).

[518] "Get the Facts about Listeria!" US Food and Drug Administration, https://www.fda.gov/animal-veterinary/animal-health-literacy/get-facts-about-listeria (accessed 14 March 2020).

[519] "Listeria," Centers for Disease Control, https://www.cdc.gov/listeria/risk-groups/pregnant-women.html (accessed 14 March 2020).

[520] Ibid.

[521] Ibid.

[522] "Listeria," Centers for Disease Control, https://www.cdc.gov/listeria/risk-groups/elderly.html (accessed 14 March 2020).

[523] Ibid.

[524] "Listeria," Centers for Disease Control, https://www.cdc.gov/listeria/risk-groups/weakened-immunity.html (accessed 14 March 2020).

[525] Ronald F. Lamont, et al., "Listeriosis in Human Pregnancy: A Systematic Review."

[526] Natalia Filipowicz, et al., "Antibacterial and Antifungal Activity of Juniper Berry Oil and Its Selected Components,"*Phytotherapy Research*, March 2003, 17(3), https://onlinelibrary.wiley.com/doi/abs/10.1002/ptr.1110 (accessed 14 March 2020).

[527] "FAQ: Norwalk and Noroviruses," Department of Microbiology, Mt Sinai Hospital, https://eportal.mountsinai.ca/Microbiology/faq/norwalkfaq.shtml#six (11 March 2020).

[528] "Norovirus: Global Trends," Centers for Disease Control, https://www.cdc.gov/norovirus/trends-outbreaks/worldwide.html?CDC_AA_refVal=https%3A%2F%2Fwww.cdc.gov%2Fnorovirus%2Fworldwide.html (accessed 14 March 2020).

[529] Charles Patrick Davis, "Norovirus Infection," Medicine Net, https://www.medicinenet.com/norovirus_infection/article.htm (accessed 11 March 2020).

[530] "FAQ: Norwalk and Noroviruses," Department of Microbiology, Mt Sinai Hospital.

[531] "FAQ: Norwalk and Noroviruses," Department of Microbiology, Mt Sinai Hospital.

[532] "Norovirus: Burden of Norovirus Illness in the US," Centers for Disease Control, https://www.cdc.gov/norovirus/trends-outbreaks/burden-US.html (accessed 11 March 2020).

[533] Lauren Vogel, et al., "Hand Sanitizers May Increase Norovirus Risk," *CMAJ*, 6 September 2011, 183(12), https://www.ncbi.nlm.nih.gov/pmc/articles/PMC3168661/ (accessed 11 March 2020).

[534] T F Jones, et al., "A case-control study of the epidemiology of sporadic *Salmonella* infection in infantsexternal icon," *Pediatrics*, 2006, 118(6), https://pediatrics.aappublications.org/content/118/6/2380.short?sso=1&sso_redirect_count=1&nfstatus=401&nftoken=00000000-0000-0000-0000-000000000000&nfstatusdescription=ERROR%3a+No+local+token (accessed 11 March 2020).

[535] C. Bavashi, et al., "Systematic review: the use of proton pump inhibitors and increased susceptibility to enteric infection," *Alimentary Pharmacology and Therapeutics*, December 2011, 34(11-12), https://onlinelibrary.wiley.com/doi/full/10.1111/j.1365-2036.2011.04874.x (accessed 11 March 2020).

[536] Ann Abraham, et al., *Bad Bug Book*, p 10, https://www.fda.gov/media/83271/download (accessed 11 March 2020).

[537] Stephen Harrod Buhner, *Herbal Antibiotics*, 67.

[538] Ibid, 28.

[539] "Salmonella Infection," The Mayo Clinic, https://www.mayoclinic.org/diseases-conditions/salmonella/diagnosis-treatment/drc-20355335 (accessed 11 March 2020).

[540] "Staphylococcal (Staph) Food Poisoning," Centers for Disease Control, https://www.cdc.gov/foodsafety/diseases/staphylococcal.html (accessed 14 March 2020).

[541] "*Clostridium perfringens*," Centers for Disease Control, https://www.cdc.gov/foodsafety/diseases/clostridium-perfringens.html (accessed 14 March 2020).

[542] Kiran Panesar, et al., "Antibiotic Therapy for Appendicitis in Children," *US Pharmacist*, 2013, 38(12), https://www.uspharmacist.com/article/antibiotic (accessed 12 March 2020).

[543] Kiran Panesar, et al., "Antibiotic Therapy for Appendicitis in Children," *US Pharmacist*, 2013, 38(12), https://www.uspharmacist.com/article/antibiotic-therapy-for-appendicitis-in-children (accessed 12 March 2020); O Soreide, "Appendicitis--a study of incidence, death rates and consumption of hospital resources," *Postgraduate Medical Journal*, May 1984, 60(703), https://www.ncbi.nlm.nih.gov/pmc/articles/PMC2417863/ (accessed 12 March 2020); DG Addiss, et al., "The Epidemiology of Appendicitis and Appendectomy in the United States," *American Journal of Epidemiology*, November 1990, 132(5), https://pubmed.ncbi.nlm.nih.gov/2239906-the-epidemiology-of-appendicitis-and-appendectomy-in-the-united-states/ (accessed 12 March 2020).

[544] Paulina Salminen, et al., "Five-Year Follow-up of Antibiotic Therapy for Uncomplicated Acute Appendicitis in the APPAC Randomized Clinical Trial," *JAMA*, 25 September 2018, 320(12), https://www.ncbi.nlm.nih.gov/pmc/articles/PMC6233612/ (accessed 12 March 2020).

[545] "Antibiotic Therapy for Acute Appendicitis in Adults. Fewer Immediate Complications Than With Surgery, but More Subsequent Failures," *Prescrire International,* June 2014, 23(150), https://pubmed.ncbi.nlm.nih.gov/25121154-antibiotic-therapy-for-acute-appendicitis-in-adults-fewer-immediate-complications-than-with-surgery-but-more-subsequent-failures/ (accessed 12 March 2020).

[546] Joseph Alton, *The Survival Medicine Handbook*, 174; *Survival and Austere Medicine, 3rd Edition*, 165.

[547] Kiran Panesar, et al., "Antibiotic Therapy for Appendicitis in Children."

[548] Joseph Alton, *The Survival Medicine Handbook*, 174

[549] *Survival and Austere Medicine, 3rd Edition*, 165.

[550] Joseph Alton, *The Survival Medicine Handbook*, 173-78.

[551] *Survival and Austere Medicine, 3rd Edition*, 165.

[552] Cynthia Koelker, *Armageddon Medicine*, 172, 177.

[553] Joseph Alton, *The Survival Medicine Handbook*, 176-178; Survival and Austere Medicine, 3rd Edition, 165.

[554] "Diverticulitis," Mayo Clinic, https://www.mayoclinic.org/diseases-conditions/diverticulitis/symptoms-causes/syc-20371758 (accessed 12 March 2020).

[555] Joseph Alton, *The Survival Medicine Handbook*, 177.

[556] *Survival and Austere Medicine, 3rd Edition*, 168.

[557] "Diverticulitis," Mayo Clinic.

[558] Cynthia Koelker, *Armageddon Medicine*, 172.

[559] Gary Hoffman, "Levaquin and Metronidazole for Diverticulitis," 28 November 2018, https://howtoadult.com/levaquin-and-metronidazole-for-diverticulitis-8673713.html (accessed 12 March 2020).

[560] Michael F. Picco, "Bezoars: How Do They Happen?" https://www.mayoclinic.org/diseases-conditions/gastroparesis/expert-answers/bezoars/faq-20058050 (accessed 12 March 2020).

[561] Ibid.

[562] Masaya Iwamuro, et al., "Review of the Diagnosis and Management of Gastrointestinal Bezoars," *World Journal of Gastrointestinal Endoscopy,* April 2015, 7(4), https://www.ncbi.nlm.nih.gov/pmc/articles/PMC4400622/ (accessed 24 February 2020).

[563] S. D. Ladas, et al., "Systematic Review: Coca-Cola Can Effectively Dissolve Gastric Phytobezoars as a First-Line Treatment," *Alimentary Pharmacology and Therapeutics*, January 2013, 37(2), https://pubmed.ncbi.nlm.nih.gov/23252775-systematic-review-coca-cola-can-effectively-dissolve-gastric-phytobezoars-as-a-first-line-treatment/ (accessed 12 March 2020).

[564] Nasrin Razavianzadeh, et al., "Small Bowel Obstruction Attributable to Phytobezoar," *Oxford Medical Case Reports,* 2016(12), https://pubmed.ncbi.nlm.nih.gov/28031856-small-bowel-obstruction-attributable-to-phytobezoar/ (accessed 24 February 2020); Pei Yuan-Wang, et al., "Bezoar Induced Small Bowel Obstruction: Clinical Characteristics and Diagnostic Value of Multi-Slice Spiral Computed Tomography," *World Journal of Gastroenterology*, 7 September 2015, 21(33), https://pubmed.ncbi.nlm.nih.gov/26361425-bezoar-induced-small-bowel-obstruction-clinical-characteristics-and-diagnostic-value-of-multi-slice-spiral-computed-tomography/ (accessed 12 March 2020).

[565] Michael F. Picco, "Bezoars: How Do They Happen?"

[566] Ibid.

[567] Katharine Eng, et al., "Gastrointestinal Bezoars: History and Current Treatment Paradigms," *Gastroenterology and Hepatology,* November 2012, 8(11), https://www.ncbi.nlm.nih.gov/pmc/articles/PMC3966178/ accessed 12 March 2020).

[568] Pei Yuan-Wang, et al., "Bezoar Induced Small Bowel Obstruction: Clinical Characteristics and Diagnostic Value of Multi-Slice Spiral Computed Tomography," *World Journal of Gastroenterology*, 7 September 2015, 21(33), https://pubmed.ncbi.nlm.nih.gov/26361425-bezoar-induced-small-bowel-obstruction-clinical-characteristics-and-diagnostic-value-of-multi-slice-spiral-computed-tomography/ (accessed 12 March 2020).

[569] Ibid.

[570] Katharine Eng, et al., "Gastrointestinal Bezoars: History and Current Treatment Paradigms."

[571] Pei Yuan-Wang, et al., "Bezoar Induced Small Bowel Obstruction: Clinical Characteristics and Diagnostic Value of Multi-Slice Spiral Computed Tomography."

[572] Michael F. Picco, "Bezoars: How Do They Happen?"; Sara Abou Azar, et al., "Small Bowel Obstruction Secondary to a Metamucil Bezoar Case Report and Review of the Literature," *Case Reports in Surgery,* 2017, https://pubmed.ncbi.nlm.nih.gov/29085697-small-bowel-obstruction-secondary-to-a-metamucil-bezoar-case-report-and-review-of-the-literature/ (accessed 12 March 2020).

[573] Cynthia Koelker, *Armageddon Medicine,* 178.

[574] *Survival and Austere Medicine, 3rd Edition*, 167.

[575] Ibid, 166.

[576] Jay W Marks, MD, "Gallstones: Pain, Symptoms, Causes, Diet, Treatment," https://www.medicinenet.com/gallstones/article.htm#what_causes_gallstones_who_gets_them (accessed 12 March 2020).

[577] Ibid.

[578] "Gallstones," Mayo Clinic, https://www.mayoclinic.org/diseases-conditions/gallstones/symptoms-causes/syc-20354214 (accessed 12 March 2020).

[579] *Survival and Austere Medicine, 3rd Edition*, 166.

[580] *Survival and Austere Medicine, 3rd Edition*, 166; Joseph Alton, *The Survival Medicine Handbook*, 400-01.

[581] Joseph Alton, *The Survival Medicine Handbook*, 401.

[582] Joseph Alton, *The Survival Medicine Handbook*, 386.

[583] David Werner, *Where There Is No Doctor*, 128.

[584] Ibid, 129.

[585] G. Massimo Claar, et al., "Omeprazole 20 or 40 mg Daily for Healing Gastroduodenal Ulcer in Patients Receiving Non-Steroidal Anti-Inflammatory Agents," *Alimentary Pharmacology and Therapeutics*, August 1993, 7(4), https://pubmed.ncbi.nlm.nih.gov/9663727-omeprazole-20-or-40-mg-daily-for-healing-gastroduodenal-ulcers-in-patients-receiving-non-steroidal-anti-inflammatory-drugs/ (accessed 2 March 2020).

[586] G. Treiber, et al., "Amoxicillin/Metronidazole/Omeprazole/Clarithromycin: A New, Short, Quadruple Therapy for *Helicobacter pylori* Eradication," *Helicobacter*, March 1998, 3(1) https://pubmed.ncbi.nlm.nih.gov/9546119-amoxicillinmetronidazoleomeprazoleclarithromycin-a-new-short-quadruple-therapy-for-helicobacter-pylori-eradication /?from_term=omeprazole+amoxicillin+helicobacter+pylori+metronidazole&from_page=2&from_pos=9 (accessed 2 March 2020).

[587] S. C. Misra, et al., "Omeprazole Versus Famotidine in the Healing and Relapse of Duodenal Ulcer," *Alimentary Pharmacology and Therapeutics*, May 1998, 12(5), https://pubmed.ncbi.nlm.nih.gov/8218758-omeprazole-versus-famotidine-in-the-healing-and-relapse-of-duodenal-ulcer/?from_term=omeprazole+duodenal+ulcer&from_pos=9 (accessed 2 March 2020).

[588] *Survival and Austere Medicine, 3rd Edition*, 166.

[589] Cynthia Koelker, *Armageddon Medicine*, 374.

[590] Joseph Alton, *The Survival Medicine Handbook*, 397.

[591] Cynthia Koelker, *Armageddon Medicine*, 374.

[592] Haewook Han, et al., "Nutritional Management of Kidney Stones (Nephrolithiasis)," *Clinical Nutrition Research*, July 2015, 4(3), https://www.ncbi.nlm.nih.gov/pmc/articles/PMC4525130/ (accessed 13 March 2020).

[593] Ibid.

[594] Cynthia Koelker, *Armageddon Medicine*, 374.

[595] Joseph Alton, *The Survival Medicine Handbook*, 398.

[596] Cynthia Koelker, *Armageddon Medicine*, 374.

[597] David Werner, *Where There Is No Doctor*, 235.

[598] *Survival and Austere Medicine, 3rd Edition*, 142.

[599] Cynthia Koelker, *Armageddon Medicine*, 375; David Werner, *Where There Is No Doctor*, 235.

[600] Joseph Alton, *The Survival Medicine Handbook*, 397.

[601] Mark Finger, MD, *Renal & Urology News,* 21 November 2011, https://www.renalandurologynews.com/home/departments/commentary/kidney-stone-prevention-fact-versus-fiction/ (accessed 21 February 2020); Alan R. Gaby, MD, "Magnesium and Vitamin B6 for Kidney Stone Prevention," /n-magnesium-kidney-stones (accessed 21 February 2020).

[602] Haewook Han, et al., "Nutritional Management of Kidney Stones (Nephrolithiasis)," *Clinical Nutrition Research*, July 2015, 4(3), https://www.ncbi.nlm.nih.gov/pmc/articles/PMC4525130/ (accessed 13 March 2020).

[603] Ibid.

[604] Ibid.

[605] Ibid.

[606] Ibid.; Joseph Alton, *The Survival Medicine Handbook*, 398.

[607] Haewook Han, et al., "Nutritional Management of Kidney Stones (Nephrolithiasis)," *Clinical Nutrition Research*, July 2015, 4(3), https://www.ncbi.nlm.nih.gov/pmc/articles/PMC4525130/ (accessed 13 March 2020).

[608] Ibid.

[609] Ibid.

[610] Ibid.

[611] Ibid.

[612] Mark Finger, MD, *Renal & Urology News,* 21 November 2011, https://www.renalandurologynews.com/home/departments/commentary/kidney-stone-prevention-fact-versus-fiction/ (accessed 21 February 2020); Haewook Han, et al., "Nutritional Management of Kidney Stones (Nephrolithiasis)," *Clinical Nutrition Research*, July 2015, 4(3), https://www.ncbi.nlm.nih.gov/pmc/articles/PMC4525130/ (accessed 13 March 2020).

[613] Cynthia Koelker, *Armageddon Medicine*, 375.

[614] Ibid.

[615] Ibid.

[616] *Survival and Austere Medicine, 3rd Edition*, 140.

[617] "Urinary Tract Infection," Mayo Clinic, https://www.mayoclinic.org/diseases-conditions/urinary-tract-infection/symptoms-causes/syc-20353447 (accessed 13 March 2020); *Survival and Austere Medicine, 3rd Edition*, 141.

[618] Ibid.

[619] *Survival and Austere Medicine*, 3rd Edition, 141.

[620] Ibid.

[621] Ibid.

[622] Joseph Alton, *Alton's Antibiotics*, 154.

[623] Ibid., 158.

[624] Ibid., 177.

[625] Ibid., 161.

[626] Ibid., 166.

[627] *Survival and Austere Medicine, 3rd Edition*, 142.

[628] Joseph Alton, *The Survival Medicine Handbook*, 180

[629] "Urinary Tract Infection," Mayo Clinic, https://www.mayoclinic.org/diseases-conditions/urinary-tract-infection/symptoms-causes/syc-20353447 (accessed 13 March 2020); Cynthia Koelker, *Armageddon Medicine*, 87; Joseph Alton, *The Survival Medicine Handbook*, 180.

[630] *Survival and Austere Medicine, 3rd Edition*, 141.

[631] Joseph Alton, *Alton's Antibiotics*, 154.

[632] Ibid., 158.

[633] Ibid., 177.

[634] Ibid., 161.

[635] Ibid., 166.
[636] *Survival and Austere Medicine, 3rd Edition*, 140.
[637] Ibid.
[638] "Chlamydia Infections," Centers for Disease Control, https://www.cdc.gov/std/tg2015/chlamydia.htm (accessed 21 February 2020).
[639] "Gonorrhea Infections," Centers for Disease Control, https://www.cdc.gov/std/tg2015/gonorrhea.htm (accessed 21 February 2020); *Survival and Austere Medicine, 3rd Edition*, 139.
[640] *Survival and Austere Medicine, 3rd Edition*, 139.
[641] "Syphilis," Centers for Disease Control, (accessed 21 February 2020).
[642] "Gonorrhea Infections," Centers for Disease Control.
[643] *Where There Is No Doctor*, p 238.
[644] "Frostbite," Mayo Clinic, https://www.mayoclinic.org/diseases-conditions/frostbite/symptoms-causes/syc-20372656 (accessed 13 March 2020).
[645] Ibid.
[646] *Survival and Austere Medicine, 3rd Edition*, 192.
[647] "Hypothermia," Mayo Clinic, https://www.mayoclinic.org/diseases-conditions/hypothermia/symptoms-causes/syc-20352682 (accessed 21 February 2020).
[648] Ibid.
[649] Ibid.
[650] Ibid
[651] Ibid.
[652] https://insidefirstaid.com/first-aid-kit/how-to-use-a-mylar-blanket-to-stop-hypothermiaError! Bookmark not defined. (accessed 21 February 2020).
[653] Andrew L Miners, et al., "The Diagnosis and Emergency Care of Heat-Related Illness and Sunburn in Athletes: A Retrospective Case Series," *The Journal of the Canadian Chiropractic Association*, June 2010, 54(2), https://www.ncbi.nlm.nih.gov/pmc/articles/PMC2875908/ (accessed 13 March 2020).
[654] Ibid.
[655] Ibid.
[656] David Werner, *Where There Is No Doctor*, 81.
[657] Andrew L Miners, et al., "The Diagnosis and Emergency Care of Heat-Related Illness and Sunburn in Athletes: A Retrospective Case Series."
[658]Joseph Alton, *The Survival Medicine Handbook*, 204-05.
[659] Samson Phan, et al., "Chemical Cold Packs May Provide Insufficient Enthalpy Change for Treatment of Hyperthermia," *Wilderness Emergency Medicine Journal*, 2013, 24, https://www.wemjournal.org/article/S1080-6032(12)00305-5/pdf (accessed 13 March 2020).
[660] Andrew L Miners, et al., "The Diagnosis and Emergency Care of Heat-Related Illness and Sunburn in Athletes: A Retrospective Case Series."
[661] Joseph Alton, *The Survival Medicine Handbook*, 206.
[662] Ibid.
[663] Andrew L Miners, et al., "The Diagnosis and Emergency Care of Heat-Related Illness and Sunburn in Athletes: A Retrospective Case Series"; *Survival and Austere Medicine, 3rd Edition*, 193.
[664] Joseph Alton, *The Survival Medicine Handbook*, 207.
[665] "Potassium Iodide," Centers for Disease Control, https://www.cdc.gov/nceh/radiation/emergencies/ki.htm?CDC_AA_refVal=https%3A%2F%2Femergency.cdc.gov%2Fradiation%2Fki.asp (accessed 21 February 2020).
[666] Ibid.

[667] Cresson Kearney, *Nuclear War Survival Skills*, http://www.oism.org/nwss/s73p904.htm (accessed 21 February 2020). This free download has instructions for constructing a Geiger counter.

[668] Cynthia Koelker, *Armageddon Medicine*, 473.

[669] "Guidance: Potassium Iodide as a Thyroid Blocking Agent in Radiation Emergencies," Food and Drug Administration, https://www.fda.gov/media/72510/download (accessed 21 February 2020).

[670] "Potassium Iodide, Centers for Disease Control.

[671] Ibid.

[672] Cynthia Koelker, *Armageddon Medicine*, 332; *Survival and Austere Medicine, 3rd Edition*, 126.

[673] Cynthia Koelker, *Armageddon Medicine,* 331.

[674] Ibid, 333.

[675] Ibid.

[676] Joseph Alton, *The Survival Medicine Handbook*, 245.

[677] Maria Spitari, et al., "Compilation of a Herbal Medicine Formulary for Herbal Substances in Malta and Its Usefulness Amongst Healthcare Professionals," *Journal of Young Pharmacists,* 7 March 2013, 5(1), https://www.ncbi.nlm.nih.gov/pmc/articles/PMC3758078/ (accessed 10 March 2020).

[678] Arif-ullah Khan, et al., "Blood Pressure Lowering, Cardiovascular Inhibitory and Bronchodilatory Actions of *Achillea Millefolium*," *Phytotherapy Research*, April 2011, https://pubmed.ncbi.nlm.nih.gov/20857434-blood-pressure-lowering-cardiovascular-inhibitory-and-bronchodilatory-actions-of-achillea-millefolium/ (accessed 8 February 2020).

[679] Aneta Kowal, et al., "The Use of Magnesium in Bronchial Asthma: A New Approach to an Old Problem," *Archivum Immunologiae et Therapiae Experimentalis*, January-February 2007, https://www.ncbi.nlm.nih.gov/pubmed/17277891 (accessed 8 February 2020).

[680] N.R. Blatherwick, et al, "Studies on Insulin," https://www.jbc.org/content/72/1/57.full.pdf (accessed 8 February 2020).

[681] betachek.com (visual read glucose strips)

[682] Joseph Alton, *The Survival Medicine Handbook*, 372-373; Cynthia Koelker, *Armageddon Medicine*, 345.

[683] Cynthia Koelker, *Armageddon Medicine*, 345.

[684] https://www.youtube.com/watch?v=luultUD0eK0 (accessed 8 February 2020).

[685] *Survival and Austere Medicine, 3rd Edition*, 70.

[686] Gary B. Smith, "National Early Warning Score (NEWS)," MD+Calc, https://www.mdcalc.com/national-early-warning-score-news (accessed 14 March 2020).

INDEX

2-undecanone, 240
abrasions, 140, 198, 203, 210
abscesses, 197, 203
acetaminophen, 98, 99, 100, 172, 175, 204, 249, 252, 291, 298, 336, 350, 386, 400
acid, 63, 64, 66, 78, 87, 88, 92, 93, 107, 114, 115, 116, 172, 175, 201, 229, 250, 310, 327, 384
acid reflux, 87
acne, 57
activated carbon, 172
activated charcoal, 36, 37, 97, 98, 172, 173, 250, 251, 253, 254, 258, 311, 320, 386, 387, 402
acyclovir, 228
ADHD, 78, 92
adrenal glands, 79, 96
adrenalin, 96
Advanced Medical Kit, 384
Advil, 89, 97, 98, 100, 229, 292, 357
Aedes aegypti, 279
African-Americans, 75
Afrin, 95, 283, 284, 292, 411
airway, 95, 175, 288, 363, 371, 372, 373, 382
Alabama, 34
albendazole, 133, 314
alcohol, 40, 41, 46, 64, 65, 73, 78, 83, 86, 92, 116, 124, 138, 146, 151, 152, 156, 157, 158, 172, 235, 237, 240, 241, 257, 305, 325, 330, 331, 332, 346, 357, 366, 379, 380, 382, 386, 393, 402
alcoholic, 343, 346
alcoholics, 57, 79, 350
alcoholism, 59, 67, 76, 81
Aleve, 98, 100, 229, 295, 379, 388
Alka-Seltzer, 78, 87, 332
Allegra, 356
allergies, 42, 54, 87, 89, 90, 93, 99, 126, 142, 180, 182, 201, 203, 356, 363, 366, 368, 393
allopurinol, 117
almonds, 61, 71, 78
aloe vera, 158, 216, 217, 220, 251
alpaca, 344
altered mental status, 244, 245
altitude, 27, 217, 397
aluminum foil, 47, 48, 154
Alzheimer's, 178
amebiasis, 74
amenorrhea, 71
amoebic dysentery, 124
amoxicillin, 106, 108, 110, 111, 113, 114, 115, 116, 117, 123, 126, 202, 204, 245, 260, 275, 276, 291, 303, 333, 338, 382
ampicillin, 106, 113, 126, 225, 275, 312, 316, 338
amputation, 223, 246
anaerobic, 107, 114, 224
anaerobic bacteria, 224
anaphylaxis, 88, 89, 91, 93, 96, 203, 250, 363, 368
anaplasmosis, 246
Anbesol, 83
anemia, 60, 62, 64, 65, 66, 74, 75, 76, 326, 330, 392
anesthesia, 24, 324, 398
anesthetic, 82, 85, 89, 90, 91, 163, 164, 175, 190, 249, 324
angina, 74, 330, 331
angora, 344
animal, 38, 57, 58, 60, 66, 81, 151, 224, 259, 260, 262, 320, 325, 344, 360, 392
animal feed, 38
animal waste, 38, 320
anorexia, 67, 245, 327
antacids, 72, 78, 87, 130, 331, 362
anthrax, 102, 113, 121, 126, 273
antibiotics, 18, 23, 24, 36, 42, 72, 78, 79, 87, 102, 105, 106, 107, 108, 109, 111, 112, 114, 117, 120, 121, 122, 125, 127, 128, 129, 130, 132, 176, 185, 189, 190, 202, 204, 205, 219, 225, 226, 233, 244, 245, 246, 250, 256, 258, 260, 261, 264, 265, 266, 267, 268, 271, 275, 280, 291, 292, 296, 298, 299, 300, 302, 303, 305, 309, 312, 319, 320, 322, 323, 325, 329, 331, 337, 338, 339, 340, 368, 379, 380, 386, 387, 390, 391, 392, 394, 398, 399

anti-coagulants, 82, 97, 100, 117, 280
anti-fungal, 131, 177
antihistamines, 88, 89, 204, 235, 249, 356, 364
Antivert, 94
antivirals, 228, 229, 295, 400
anxiety, 81, 88, 89, 90, 94, 176, 288, 393
apathy, 54
appendectomy, 45, 321, 396
appendicitis, 203, 321, 322, 323, 324, 343, 394
apple cider vinegar, 316
apricots, 62, 80
ariboflavinosis, 60
Arizona, 34, 245, 246
Arkansas, 34, 245
Armageddon Medicine, 93, 134, 351, 361, 363, 392, 397, 405
Armour Thyroid, 363
Artemisia annua, 270
Artemisia tridentata, 270
arthritis, 98, 99, 137, 201, 245, 366, 392
artificial nails, 39
ashwagandha, 362
asparagus, 60
aspirin, 16, 87, 93, 97, 98, 102, 172, 175, 229, 251, 280, 282, 331, 357, 379, 386, 387
asthma, 96, 97, 99, 175, 176, 182, 203, 204, 286, 287, 298, 300, 354, 355, 356, 357, 392, 394, 437
athlete's foot, 177
Augmentin, 110, 111, 112, 115, 116, 204, 219, 269, 291, 300, 323, 328, 338, 384, 411
autoclave, 48, 50, 166
autoimmune disorders, 327
AVPU, 373
azithromycin, 107, 111, 112, 123
Azo, 338
baby brush, 198
bacitracin, 106, 219
backache, 98
bacteria, 31, 32, 33, 35, 36, 45, 46, 63, 87, 90, 105, 106, 107, 108, 113, 114, 116, 120, 121, 124, 125, 128, 130, 142, 144, 151, 155, 156, 157, 159, 161, 172, 173, 174, 183, 190, 221, 224, 225, 226, 244, 259, 260, 261, 262, 265, 266, 272, 273, 276, 290, 291, 292,304, 309, 310, 319, 320, 321, 338, 340, 341, 399
Bacterial vaginosis, 123
Bacteroides, 260
Bactine, 151
Bactrim, 338, 384
bag-valve mask, 373
baked potatoes, 73, 307
baking soda, 154, 174, 175, 216, 220, 235, 250, 251, 297, 338
bandana, 32, 33, 171
bats, 262
batteries, 194, 196, 358, 382, 386
bay leaves, 232
bedbugs, 42, 43, 230, 231, 242
bee stings, 201, 248, 250, 363
beef, 57, 60, 63, 69, 81, 160, 305, 307
beeswax, 240
beet greens, 60, 61, 80
Benadryl, 83, 88, 89, 90, 92, 93, 95, 204, 232, 237, 249, 253, 296, 337, 356, 364, 379, 380, 386, 387, 388, 393
Ben-Gay, 236
benzathine, 125
benzocaine, 83
benzylpenicillin, 125
berberine, 130, 266, 313, 398, 400
beriberi, 59
beta blockers, 72
beta carotene, 57, 58
Betadine, 35, 46, 152, 153, 243, 353, 382, 386
bezoars, 326, 327, 433
bidens, 130
biotin, 63
bites, 16, 89, 90, 91, 110, 113, 115, 120, 123, 126, 137, 151, 173, 174, 177, 191, 203, 224, 225, 230, 231, 233, 236, 239, 241, 242, 243, 244, 247, 251, 252, 253, 254, 255, 256, 257, 258, 259, 260, 261, 271, 272, 281, 369, 392, 402
Bitot's spots, 57
black cohosh, 232
black tea, 76
black widow, 250, 251, 253
bladder infections, 99, 121, 338
bleach, 26, 27, 28, 29, 46, 154, 318
bleeding, 23, 66, 67, 74, 75, 76, 79, 80, 85, 96, 100, 117, 118, 149, 150, 151, 166, 168, 171, 191, 255, 281, 325, 331, 337, 342, 347, 362, 372, 380
bleeding gums, 66, 67
blisters, 165, 179, 218, 219, 227, 228, 229, 255, 342, 343
bloating, 98, 173, 306, 314, 325
blood glucose strips, 358
blood pressure, 70, 72, 77, 78, 79, 96, 97, 175, 176, 192, 225, 252, 280, 364, 374, 375, 392
blood sugar, 80, 176
blunt tip syringe, 259
body lice, 231, 237, 238, 277
body temperature, 52, 95, 156, 345, 346, 348, 349, 350
boiling, 26
bone fractures, 54, 69
boo-boo kits, 139, 151, 158, 380, 387
borax, 238
botulinum, 309
botulism, 273, 306, 307, 308, 309, 310, 311, 392
bread, 55, 58, 59, 64, 72, 74, 346
Brigham tea, 287, 357
broccoli, 61, 64, 67, 71, 362
bronchiolitis, 301
bronchitis, 111, 113, 121, 129, 275, 285, 287, 298

bronchodilator, 79, 95, 175, 355
brown recluse, 191, 250, 251, 253
brucellosis, 129
bruising, 66, 67, 255, 300
Brussels sprouts, 60, 61, 64, 362
bubonic plague, 266
buckwheat, 55
bug bites, 83
bulb syringe, 259
burns, 23, 55, 91, 115, 120, 139, 140, 153, 158, 177, 182, 185, 190, 203, 216, 217, 218, 219, 220, 221, 222, 223, 224, 392, 394
burping, 314
bursitis, 98
butter, 55, 57, 63, 69, 190, 197, 387
butterfly bandage, 164
cabbage, 67, 362
caffeine, 98, 175, 176, 287, 305, 346, 355
calamine lotion, 229, 235
calcium, 26, 29, 30, 31, 62, 70, 71, 72, 76, 130, 175, 335, 336, 362
calcium carbonate, 71, 86
calcium hypochlorite, 26, 28, 29, 30, 31
California, 34, 268, 276, 383, 402
Campylobacter, 35, 305, 306, 320
capsaicin, 229
carbapenem, 107
carbohydrates, 51, 52, 55, 360
carbon monoxide, 105, 193, 403
cardboard, 180, 244
cardiopulmonary resuscitation, 22, 372
carrots, 58, 309
cashews, 78
CAT, 169
cat bites, 260
cataracts, 54
catheters, 47, 48
catnip, 240, 241, 287
cauliflower, 362
C-collar, 167
cefixime, 340
cefoxitin, 323
celiac disease, 57, 64, 65, 69, 70, 76, 81
cellulitis, 90, 115, 122, 123, 124, 126
Celox, 149, 150, 380, 382
Centers for Disease Control, 35, 38, 227, 244, 248, 303, 341, 351
central nervous system, 51, 125, 175, 252, 255, 281, 308
Cepacol, 83
cephalosporins, 106, 121
cereals, 58, 60, 62, 64, 69
cerebral edema, 245
chamomile, 297, 402
cheese, 57, 61, 387
chest compressions, 372
chest pain, 269
chicken, 18, 44, 55, 81, 319
chickenpox, 177, 227, 228
Chikungunya, 280, 282
chills, 228, 246, 247, 253, 279, 299, 312, 319, 322
chitosan, 150
chlamydia, 113, 120, 129, 297, 340
chloramphenicol, 275
chlorhexidine, 46, 152, 155
chlorine, 27, 28, 29, 30, 31, 47
chlorine dioxide, 31
chocolate, 76, 78, 80, 229, 332, 336, 352
cholangitis, 329
cholecystitis, 311, 328, 329
cholera, 35, 41, 87, 110, 112, 120, 129, 130, 264, 265, 266,
cholesterol, 70
chronic kidney disease, 70, 174
chronic prostatitis, 116, 120
chronic stress, 331, 362
Cipro, 87, 107, 109, 110, 111, 112, 114, 117, 118, 119, 127, 129, 132, 219, 265, 267, 273, 275, 276, 291, 298, 300, 312, 319, 323, 325, 329, 337, 338, 382
circumcision, 140
cirrhosis, 57, 330
citronella, 240, 241, 242
Civil War, 184, 274
clamps, 48, 197, 324, 384
clarithromycin, 107, 111, 113, 123, 132, 333
Claritin, 356
clindamycin, 107, 110, 111, 127, 384
Clostridium, 87, 88, 128, 224, 225, 305, 306, 307, 309, 310
Clostridium difficile, 87, 88, 123, 128, 333
Clostridium perfringens, 305, 306, 320
Clostridium tetani, 224
clove, 133, 240
Coban, 165
cocoa, 78
coconut oil, 174, 177, 178, 179, 238, 240
cod liver oil, 57, 69
codeine, 95, 99, 286
coffee, 26, 27, 32, 33, 37, 76, 95, 175, 176, 217, 287, 332, 355
coffee filter, 26, 27, 32, 33, 37
Coke, 326, 327
cola drinks, 176
cold sores, 178
Cold Spray, 83
colds, 68, 87, 94, 98, 151, 283, 292, 356, 393, 394
colitis, 123
colloidal silver, 298, 316, 320
Colorado tick fever, 247
communicable diseases, 42, 264, 278
complete proteins, 54
confusion, 30, 59, 70, 74, 252, 255, 298, 315, 338, 349, 364

conjunctivitis, 63, 272, 282, 295, 296, 297
constipation, 71, 94, 140, 173, 274, 275, 308, 325, 361, 392
convulsions, 59, 315
copper, 362
copperheads, 256
coral snakes, 254, 256
corn, 62
corn syrup, 51, 101, 183
cornea, 229, 272
coronavirus, 42, 146, 192
corticosteroids, 78
cotrimoxazole, 338
cotton, 21, 49, 62, 139, 166, 220, 244, 344
cotton balls, 244
cottonmouth, 256
cough, 42, 95, 99, 175, 182, 273, 274, 285, 286, 287, 288, 289, 298, 300, 301, 326
coughing, 38, 95, 96, 175, 267, 285, 288, 289, 299, 356
COVID-19, 16, 18, 38, 41, 146, 283, 284
Coxsackie, 156
coyotes, 262
CPR, 23, 372, 384
cramps, 80, 97, 98, 138, 252, 253, 306, 307, 317, 319, 320, 321, 348
cranberries, 338
credit card magnifier, 195, 382, 386
creosote bush, 229
Crohn's disease, 57, 64, 65, 67, 69, 76, 78, 79, 81
crotamiton, 234
croup, 96, 285, 287, 288, 289, 400
crush injury, 224
Cryptolepis, 270
Cryptosporidium, 31, 32, 35
cuts, 91, 164, 199, 202, 277, 392
cyanocobalamin, 65, 76
cystic fibrosis, 57, 69, 327
cystitis, 114, 116, 122, 337
dairy products, 54, 56, 65, 70, 71, 314
Dakin's solution, 154, 155, 175
dandelions, 58
dandruff, 236
decadron, 289
DEET, 242, 271
dehydration, 32, 141, 176, 218, 222, 265, 282, 305, 327, 335, 348, 350
deli meats, 314
dengue fever, 42, 280, 282, 401
dental abscess, 114
dental infections, 111, 124, 125
depression, 66, 68, 70, 73, 81, 188, 361
Derma-Bond, 163
Dermacentor andersoni, 247
dermatitis, 42, 62, 63, 88, 90, 191
diabetes, 59, 79, 80, 81, 280, 327, 330, 357, 360, 362, 366, 392
diabetic coma, 359
diabetic neuropathy, 98
dialysis, 59, 67
diarrhea, 19, 32, 53, 59, 62, 79, 80, 81, 87, 93, 94, 112, 114, 116, 118, 126, 141, 203, 205, 246, 265, 266, 273, 274, 275, 281, 298, 306, 307, 311, 312, 314, 316, 317, 319, 320, 321, 325, 368, 392, 394
diatomaceous earth, 235, 236
diazepam, 226
difficulty swallowing, 90, 127, 263
Diflucan, 131, 204, 384
digestion, 52
digoxin, 72
diphenhydramine, 89, 90, 91, 92, 393
diphtheria, 24, 41, 126, 264
disinfecting, 45, 151, 155, 156
disinfection, thermal, 45
dislocations, 203
distillation, 36, 37
distilled water, 27, 46
diuretics, 59, 72, 79, 153, 175, 350, 353
diverticular disease, 324, 325
diverticulitis, 112, 115, 123, 324, 325
diverticulosis, 324
dizziness, 74, 94, 114, 127, 176, 315, 349
dogs, 90, 224, 236, 261, 262, 273, 276
doxycycline, 87, 102, 107, 108, 109, 110, 111, 112, 118, 119, 120, 121, 123, 127, 129, 202, 219, 226, 244, 245, 250, 260, 265, 267, 268, 273, 278, 291, 297, 300, 313, 319, 340, 341, 382, 384
Dramamine, 94
droopy eyelids, 59, 308
drowsiness, 88, 91
drug abusers, 79, 307
drug overdoses, 172
dry skin, 57, 361
duct tape, 163, 165, 179, 180, 181
duodenal bypasses, 57
duodenal ulcer, 331, 333
duodenum, 330
dust, 33, 143, 171, 184, 201, 296, 307, 356
E. coli, 116, 129, 130, 172, 266, 305, 306, 311, 312, 313
ear infection, 15, 23, 109, 111, 113, 115, 122, 126, 129, 177, 192, 202, 203, 290, 292, 392, 394
early warning score, 375
Ebola, 41
echinacea, 254, 258, 271, 402
Echinacea angustifolia, 254, 258, 275
Echinacea purpurea, 254
eczema, 90, 177
edema, 59, 245, 348
eggs, 55, 56, 57, 60, 61, 65, 66, 73, 132, 178, 230, 232, 233, 235, 237, 238, 317, 319, 387
eggshells, 71
Ehrlichiosis, 246

elder, 280, 297, 338, 400, 402
elderly, 23, 54, 65, 78, 160, 169, 234, 281, 283, 298, 317, 319, 328, 337, 345, 350, 352
Eldon card, 377
encephalitis, 228, 275, 281, 400
enema bag, 101, 140, 141, 347
Enterobacter, 120
Enterobacteria, 116
enterovirus, 35, 401
Environmental Protection Agency, 30, 239
epididymitis, 118, 120
epilepsy, 178
epinephrine, 84, 85, 88, 89, 93, 96, 249, 289, 363, 364
Epi-pen, 89, 201, 248, 249, 363, 398
erythromycin, 107, 110, 111, 112, 127, 132, 219, 246, 260, 265, 291, 292, 300, 303, 340, 341
Escherichia coli, 118, 120, 130, 172, 311, 337
esophagus, 93, 330, 331
essential oil, 130, 174, 178, 216, 231, 236, 238, 242, 251, 254
estrogen, 71, 72
eucalyptus, 231, 240, 286
Eustachian tube dysfunction, 292
Excedrin, 98
fainting, 203, 252, 255, 394
famciclovir, 228
fat, 51, 52, 53, 56, 57, 58, 67, 70, 71, 178, 221, 325, 330
fatigue, 53, 54, 62, 64, 66, 67, 68, 73, 74, 75, 80, 174, 247, 360, 361
fat-soluble vitamins, 52
fetus, 61, 193
fever, 41, 87, 88, 95, 97, 98, 99, 113, 114, 120, 121, 125, 126, 129, 156, 171, 203, 219, 225, 228, 237, 243, 245, 246, 247, 253, 263, 268, 269, 272, 273, 274, 275, 278, 279, 280, 281, 282, 288, 290, 291, 292, 298, 299, 301, 302, 306, 307, 311, 315, 316, 317, 318, 319, 320, 321, 322, 324, 325, 328, 337, 339, 340, 349, 350, 368, 374, 394, 399
fiber, 51, 55, 164, 325, 326, 328, 344, 362, 367
figs, 130
fingernails, 39, 63, 67
fish, 54, 56, 57, 60, 66, 69, 76, 80, 81, 114, 119, 307, 390, 391, 392
Flagyl, 122
flaky skin, 54
flatulence, 173
fleas, 42, 231, 242, 276
floppy baby syndrome, 308
Florida, 34, 202, 280, 282, 344
fluid retention, 361
flukes, 133
fluoroquinolone, 72, 87
flypaper, 181
folate, 63, 64, 76, 107
folic acid, 64
food poisoning, 203, 304, 306, 307, 311, 314, 316, 318, 319, 320, 333
food storage, 55, 69
forceps, 48, 198, 379, 380, 382, 384
foreign body bezoar, 327
forgetfulness, 361
formula, 218, 259, 327
foxes, 262
Francisella tularensis, 272
frostbite, 157, 180, 191, 342, 343
frostnip, 342
fruits, 51, 55, 66, 67, 80, 307, 316, 317, 319, 336
fungi, 45, 151, 155
gallbladder, 115, 123, 329, 330
gallstones, 328, 329, 330
garbage, 38, 186
garlic, 133, 316
gas, 144, 173, 299, 306, 314, 375, 401
gastric bypass, 65, 70, 76, 78
gastroenteritis, 87, 203, 315, 316
gastroparesis, 328
gauze, 21, 49, 138, 139, 140, 149, 150, 166, 170, 174, 179, 183, 185, 201, 220, 251, 379, 380, 382, 384
gentamicin, 273, 316
Georgia, 34
GERD, 88, 92, 93, 176, 392
German chamomile, 357
gestation, 56
Giardia, 31, 32, 35, 112, 305, 306, 313
Giardia duodenalis, 313
Giardia intestinalis, 305, 306, 313
Giardia lamblia, 313
giardiasis, 57, 124, 313
ginger, 62, 130, 280, 400
glossitis, 65
gloves, 31, 44, 86, 141, 142, 148, 167, 181, 207, 224, 262, 267, 324, 344, 371, 379, 380, 384
Glycyrrhiza, 130
goiter, 35, 73, 152
goldenseal, 266, 297
gonorrhea, 113, 120, 129, 297, 340
gout, 98, 175, 392
Gram-negative, 106, 113, 114, 121, 125, 190, 224
Gram-positive, 106, 113, 114, 117, 121, 190, 316
grapefruit seed extract, 37
Great Lakes, 248
Group A strep, 125
guaifenesin, 95, 287
Guillain-Barre, 309
gumweed, 287, 357
gunshot wounds, 343, 380
H2-receptor antagonists, 65
Haemophilus influenzae, 116
hair loss, 63, 74, 361
hand sanitizer, 40, 41, 158, 317, 388

handwashing, 39, 40, 41, 158, 205, 274, 314, 317, 319
hares, 271, 272, 273
Hawaii, 271, 276, 280
head lice, 237
headache, 53, 62, 87, 98, 99, 114, 116, 175, 176, 202, 244, 245, 246, 247, 253, 263, 274, 278, 279, 280, 281, 282, 301, 306, 312, 315, 316, 349, 392
headlamp, 137, 195
heart attack, 22, 97, 99, 387
heart failure, 74, 87, 99, 354
heart palpitations, 64, 66, 80
heart rhythms, 70, 176
heartburn, 86, 87, 88, 93, 97, 98, 174, 331, 392
Heartland virus infection, 247
heat exhaustion, 138, 348
heat stress, 348
heatstroke, 138, 348, 349, 350
helichrysum, 249
Helicobacter pylori, 76, 88, 92, 113, 123, 129
hemoglobin, 75
hemolytic uremic syndrome, 312
hemorrhoids, 178
hemostatic agents, 149
hemostats, 197
hemp, 55
hepatitis, 35, 41
hepatitis A, 35
Herbal Antibiotics, 270, 398, 399, 400
Hibiclens, 46
Hispanics, 67, 75
hives, 88, 90, 126, 127, 233, 341, 364
hoarseness, 269, 288, 361
honey, 51, 101, 182, 183, 184, 190, 219, 221, 222, 286, 287, 298, 307, 316, 320, 333, 346, 357, 398, 402, 422
hookworms, 74
hot dogs, 314
HTH, 29, 30
hunger, 53, 178, 360
hydrocodone, 204
hydrocortisone, 204, 232
hydrogen peroxide, 155, 156, 238
hypertension, 80, 92
hyperthermia, 138, 348
hyperthyroidism, 363
hypocalcemia, 70
hypogonadism, 81
hypoparathyroidism, 70
hypothermia, 141, 150, 181, 218, 222, 343, 344, 345, 346, 347, 350, 375, 382
hypothyroidism, 73, 76, 328, 360, 361, 362, 363
ibuprofen, 89, 97, 99, 216, 219, 249, 252, 289, 291, 331, 336, 343, 350, 379, 386
ice, 137, 138, 157, 251, 257, 289, 314, 317
ice packs, 137, 138, 157
IFAK, 380
Imodium, 266, 313, 379, 380
impetigo, 115, 122, 233
impotence, 81
indigestion, 87
infantile botulism, 308
infants, 25, 36, 54, 57, 59, 64, 69, 74, 76, 94, 116, 157, 176, 192, 202, 281, 286, 290, 292, 301, 304, 307, 308, 309, 318, 327, 350, 373
infectious mononucleosis, 284
infertility, 57
inflammation, 60, 87, 97, 162, 175, 232, 243, 245, 253, 289, 328
inflammatory bowel disease, 76
influenza, 40, 41, 98, 146, 203, 243, 266, 267, 273, 283, 284, 287, 288, 295, 298, 360, 392, 399, 400
influenza A, 40, 41, 295
ingrown toenail, 83, 197
inhalers, 204, 354, 356
inoculum, 148, 149
insect bites, 392
insect repellent, 178, 271, 386
insomnia, 77, 99, 176
instruments, 45, 46, 47, 48, 49, 50, 86, 154, 157, 197, 198, 226
insulin, 46, 79, 80, 200, 357, 358, 359, 360, 362
iodine, 26, 29, 35, 37, 46, 72, 73, 74, 150, 151, 152, 153, 155, 190, 191, 262, 350, 351, 352, 353, 360, 386
iodized salt, 73, 74, 152, 353, 361
IQ, 73, 74
IR3535, 240
iron, 46, 57, 74, 75, 76, 80, 130, 154, 170, 217, 362
irritability, 59, 66, 74, 81, 225, 290, 327
isolation, 41, 42, 44, 392, 397
isopropyl alcohol, 155
itching, 85, 90, 91, 127, 132, 232, 233, 234, 235, 237, 253
itchy eyes, 42
ivermectin, 133, 134, 234, 235
Ixodes cookei, 248
Ixodes scapularis, 248
Japanese barberry, 130, 266, 270, 297, 314
Japanese honeysuckle, 236, 270, 287, 297
jaundice, 75, 253, 279, 328, 329
joint infections, 123, 126
joint pain, 54, 67, 80, 244, 280, 281, 282, 298, 315
juice, 33, 67, 69, 101, 173, 286, 316, 338
juniper, 67, 231, 232, 270, 287, 316, 398, 402
Kansas, 247
kaolin, 150
Katadyn Micropur MP1, 31
Keflex, 78, 106, 108, 110, 121, 122, 202, 219, 260, 291, 292, 300, 303, 329, 382
ketones, 51
ketosis, 51
kidney failure, 98, 246

kidney infections, 114
kidney stones, 23, 53, 80, 97, 98, 175, 203, 290, 334, 335, 336, 392
kidneys, 61, 79, 100, 334, 336, 359
Klever Kutter, 199, 379, 380, 386
knitting, 344
Kool-Aid, 36
kwashiorkor, 54
lacerations, 140, 197, 202, 203, 211, 224, 259, 392
lactation, 56
lactic acidosis, 59
lactobezoars, 326
Lanacane, 83
Larrea tridentata, 229
latex, 44, 142, 180
lavender, 178, 216, 220, 231, 238, 240, 241, 249, 251, 254
laxatives, 79
leg cramps, 77
legumes, 60, 61
lemon balm, 229, 362
lemongrass, 240
lethargy, 81, 301, 308
Levaquin, 87, 107, 111, 112, 117, 123, 219, 268, 300, 319, 325, 340
levothyroxine, 361
lice, 42, 132, 178, 231, 236, 237, 238, 242, 244, 276
licorice, 130, 270, 280, 400, 402
lidocaine, 83, 85, 86, 89, 90, 91, 96, 159, 216, 219, 229, 249, 386
light, 33, 34, 37, 61, 81, 137, 154, 155, 193, 194, 195, 196, 216, 225, 237, 240, 248, 263, 278, 290, 344, 364, 382, 384, 388, 395
light sticks, 137, 195, 382, 384
lightheadedness, 74
lincosamides, 107
lindane, 234
liniment, 157
Listeria, 305, 306, 314, 315, 316
listeriosis, 315, 316
liver, 53, 57, 60, 61, 63, 69, 81, 97, 99, 100, 275, 279, 330, 400
lobelia, 357, 402
lockjaw, 225
Lomatium, 270
Lonicera japonica, 236
loperamide, 87, 204, 320
loss of balance, 315
Louisiana, 34, 202
low blood pressure, 53, 127, 176, 193, 223
low-calorie diets, 362
lye, 62, 172
Lyme disease, 114, 243, 245, 246
lymphadenopathy, 272, 273
Lysol, 236
Maalox, 78
macrolides, 107
macronutrients, 51
maggot therapy, 184, 185, 396
magnesium, 71, 76, 77, 78, 79, 130, 335, 357
magnesium chelate, 78
magnesium chloride, 79
magnesium citrate, 78
magnesium oil, 79
mal de caribou, 52
malaise, 59
malaria, 19, 42, 75, 202, 279
Malathion, 231
malnutrition, 70, 133, 396
manuka, 183
mask, 18, 28, 36, 44, 141, 142, 143, 144, 145, 146, 147, 148, 149, 171, 181, 267, 270, 311, 355, 356, 373, 379, 380, 382, 384
mastitis, 113, 122
maternal death, 56
measles, 24, 41, 56, 264, 287, 298
meat, 54, 56, 61, 63, 72, 76, 80, 81, 160
mebendazole, 134, 314
meclizine, 94, 328, 337, 386
medical history, 200, 201, 203, 369, 393
medical instruments, 45, 47, 152, 154, 196
Medihoney, 183, 221
memory loss, 66, 70
meningitis, 123, 124, 125, 225, 245, 281, 292, 311, 315
mental illness, 67
Metamucil, 325
methadone, 92
metronidazole, 107, 118, 122, 127, 129, 132, 133, 225, 226, 323, 325, 329, 333, 340
Micropur, 31, 32
migraine, 98, 100, 201, 392
milk, 18, 54, 55, 61, 67, 69, 70, 73, 80, 81, 92, 101, 114, 130, 221, 281, 314, 320, 331, 332, 352, 402
Milk of Magnesia, 78
minocycline, 87, 102, 107, 127, 268
mint, 220, 232
miscarriage, 58, 100, 123, 203, 315
Mississippi, 34, 277
Missouri, 26, 245, 247
mittens, 344, 345
Mobic, 99, 100, 357, 380, 382, 386
monitors, 358
mononucleosis, 42
morphine, 172, 187, 204
mosquito, 44, 181, 197, 202, 231, 239, 240, 241, 251, 279, 280, 281, 384, 399, 401
motion sickness, 90, 94
Motrin, 97
moxifloxacin, 107, 108, 110, 111, 268, 380, 382
MRSA, 41, 120, 183, 189, 250
mucus, 95, 285, 286, 292, 300
mullein, 357
multi-tool, 32

muscle, 53, 54, 68, 69, 70, 74, 80, 97, 98, 137, 160, 174, 225, 244, 245, 247, 248, 252, 253, 255, 279, 280, 281, 282, 306, 308, 342, 348
muscle aches, 98, 306, 312
muscle contractions, 70
mushrooms, 61, 62, 69
myasthenia gravis, 309
Mylar blanket, 347, 380
N100, 147
N95, 18, 44, 142, 143, 144, 145, 149, 355, 379, 380
nail brush, 39
nail clippers, 32
nail polish, 193
naproxen sodium, 388
Nasalcrom, 95
nausea, 51, 59, 62, 90, 93, 94, 123, 124, 126, 127, 245, 246, 252, 253, 255, 273, 281, 306, 307, 312, 316, 317, 320, 321, 322, 325, 326, 327, 328, 329, 335, 337, 339
needle driver, 48, 197
needle holder, 197
needles, 45, 47, 160, 163, 164, 166, 203, 342, 384
neem oil, 236, 238
Neisseria, 124
neural tube defects, 64
neuropathic
    neuropathy, 98
New Mexico, 34
niacin, 61
night blindness, 56, 57
night sweats, 269
nitrofurantoin, 337
nits, 237, 238
Nix, 238
nixtamalization, 62
Norco, 100, 132
norovirus, 35, 304, 305, 306, 316, 317, 318, 320
nosebleeds, 177, 274
NSAIDs, 79, 93, 100, 325
numbness, 59, 66, 70, 80, 127, 281, 342
nutraceuticals, 363
nuts, 78, 80, 81, 229, 362, 363
nylon, 161, 163
oatmeal, 81, 216, 229, 235
obsessive-compulsive, 81
ofloxacin, 117, 123
oil of lemon eucalyptus, 240
Oklahoma, 34, 245, 247
olive oil, 156, 179, 236, 240
omeprazole, 92, 93, 123, 132, 204, 332
ondansetron, 132
One Second After, 357
opiates, 325
opioid, 229
opium, 172
opossums, 262, 276
OPQRST, 369
Orajel, 83
oral contraceptives, 73, 117
oregano, 178, 287, 316, 357, 400
Oregon grape, 130, 266, 270, 297, 314, 402
organic poisons, 172
osteoarthritis, 97, 98
osteomyelitis, 122
osteoporosis, 70, 93
otoscope, 192, 196, 202, 290
oven, 47, 48, 347
oxygen, 75, 155, 169, 192, 224, 299, 301, 356
oxygen saturation, 374
oyster, 81, 130
P100, 144, 145
pain, 22, 23, 59, 68, 69, 85, 89, 90, 93, 94, 97, 98, 99, 100, 132, 133, 157, 160, 162, 163, 168, 174, 188, 190, 201, 202, 203, 204, 216, 218, 219, 220, 223, 228, 229, 244, 247, 248, 249, 251, 252, 253, 255, 258, 267, 272, 273, 274, 279, 280, 281, 282, 290, 291, 292, 299, 300, 302, 303, 306, 316, 321, 322, 323, 324, 325, 326, 328, 329, 334, 335, 336, 337, 338, 339, 340, 343, 368, 369, 374, 382, 386, 392, 394, 399
pain relievers, 97
painful tongue, 60
palpitations, 74
pancake syrup, 101
pancreatic disease, 81
pancreatitis, 70, 396
pandemic, 18, 146
pandemic influenza, 41
panic attacks, 81
pantothenic acid, 63
paradoxical effect, 92
paralysis, 256, 281, 308
parchment, 48
Parkinson's, 90, 97, 188
Parkland formula, 222
Pasteurella multocida, 260, 261
patent ductus arteriosus, 97
pathogens, 27, 33, 35, 142, 143, 304, 307
peak flow meter, 355
peanuts, 63, 78
pelvic fractures, 23
pelvic inflammatory disease, 120, 129, 324
penicillin, 18, 78, 106, 109, 110, 111, 113, 114, 117, 124, 125, 126, 127, 128, 225, 226, 250, 260, 291, 303, 341, 368, 382
penlights, 196, 386
Pepcid, 65, 78, 92, 249, 333, 364
peppermint, 174, 178, 231, 240, 241, 242, 249, 270, 286, 287, 357
peppers, 58, 62, 67
Pepto-Bismol, 94
Percocet, 132
peritonitis, 123

permethrin, 186, 231, 234, 235, 237, 238, 242, 244, 271
persimmons, 327, 328
petrolatum-gauze dressings, 140
petroleum, 172, 189, 235
pets, 38, 242, 261, 273, 395
pharmacobezoar, 327
phenobarbital, 226
phlegm, 285, 286, 287
phytobezoar, 327, 433
Picaridin, 240
piles, 178
pink eye, 295, 297
pinworms, 132
piperine, 270
piperonyl butoxide, 238
placebo, 44, 188
plague, 41, 119, 266, 267, 268, 273
plantain, 164, 250, 258, 287, 297, 357, 402
plumeria, 133
pneumonia, 19, 41, 81, 88, 93, 111, 113, 115, 120, 121, 123, 124, 192, 203, 228, 266, 267, 268, 273, 275, 283, 284, 287, 295, 298, 299, 300, 301, 302, 311, 400
pneumonic plague, 267
pneumothorax, 343
poison ivy, 90, 91, 174, 191
poison oak, 90, 91, 174, 191
poison sumac, 90, 91, 174, 191
polio, 156, 264, 399
polymyxin B, 106
pomegranate, 130, 275
poor appetite, 81
pork, 60, 62, 81, 307, 319
post-herpetic neuralgia, 228
postpartum infections, 123
potassium, 76, 79, 80, 152, 351, 352, 353
potassium iodide, 152, 350, 351, 352, 353
potato, 251
poultice, 250, 251, 253, 254, 258, 259
Powassan viral disease, 248
prednisone, 98, 249, 250
pregnancy, 56, 61, 73, 74, 76, 80, 86, 88, 97, 114, 121, 202, 203, 281, 324, 395, 396, 397
pregnant women, 23, 56, 64, 76, 99, 100, 114, 131, 153, 234, 235, 281, 282, 304, 341, 352
premature baby, 97
pressure canner, 47, 48, 50, 196
pressure dressing, 170
Prilosec, 65, 78, 93, 332, 333
Primatene Mist, 96, 287, 289, 355
prostate, 92
protecting the vital organs, 52
protein, 51, 52, 53, 54, 55, 70, 107, 223, 252, 325, 336, 338
protein poisoning, 52
protein starvation, 52
proton-pump inhibitors, 65, 77, 93, 265, 319, 333
protozoa, 33, 35, 36, 37, 151, 152
psoriatic arthritis, 98
pubic lice, 237, 238
pulmonary edema, 245
pulse, 192, 274, 275, 349, 355, 374, 375
pulse oximeter, 192, 355, 375
pumpkin seeds, 81, 133
purification tablets, 29
purslane, 357
pyelonephritis, 116, 122, 337, 339
pyrethroid, 231
pyrethrum, 238
pyroxidine, 63
quarantine, 41, 42, 43, 267, 268, 392, 397
QuikClot, 149, 150, 380
quinoa, 55
quinolone, 107
rabbit starvation, 52
rabbits, 52, 55, 262, 271, 272, 273, 310
raccoons, 262
radiation, 33, 35, 68, 73, 105, 181, 345, 350, 351, 352, 353, 397, 404
ragweed, 238
raisins, 130, 328
rapid breathing, 278, 299, 301
Rapunzel's syndrome, 327
rash, 42, 60, 63, 90, 91, 97, 98, 117, 126, 127, 130, 177, 203, 228, 229, 233, 243, 244, 245, 246, 247, 275, 278, 280, 281, 282, 303, 341, 352, 368, 394
rattlesnakes, 256
rayon gauze, 48, 139, 166
razors, 198
red clover, 287, 357
respiration, 95, 194, 299, 309, 372, 374
respiratory syncytial virus, 284, 301
restless leg syndrome, 76, 77
reverse osmosis, 37
Reyes syndrome, 97
rheumatoid arthritis, 97, 98, 234
Rhodiola, 270
riboflavin, 60, 61
rice, 55, 58, 60, 62, 64, 138, 265, 305, 346, 401
rickettsiosis, 246
RID, 238
Rocky Mountain spotted, 121, 245
rodents, 266, 271, 272
rosemary, 178, 231, 236, 241, 362, 402
rotavirus, 35
roundworms, 133
RSV, 301, 302, 400
rubella, 24
Rule of Nines, 218, 222
Rule of Threes, 26
RZ masks, 145
safety goggles, 149

safety pin, 373
saline, 85, 86, 90, 91, 97, 98, 141, 158, 159, 186, 259, 382, 384, 386
Salmonella, 35, 87, 112, 116, 130, 274, 304, 305, 306, 318, 319, 320
salmonellosis, 318
salt, 33, 72, 73, 74, 141, 152, 235, 236, 238, 348, 349, 353, 360, 387
SAM splint, 164, 167, 168, 180, 193, 382
Sanitary Control and Surveillance of Field Water Supplies, 29, 30
SARS, 41, 400
saturated fats, 53
sauerkraut, 74
Sawyer extractor, 257
Saxl, Eva, 357, 358
scabies, 42, 232, 233, 234, 235, 244
scalpels, 47, 324
schistosomiasis, 74
scissors, 32, 46, 48, 49, 86, 167, 198
sclera, 74
scrapes, 91, 151, 334
scurvy, 66, 67
sedative, 94
selenium, 362
sepsis, 299, 315, 319, 339
septicemia, 315
Septra, 338
sexually transmitted disease, 233
Sharpie, 32, 168, 257, 380, 386, 388
Shigella, 35, 112, 116, 120, 305, 306, 321
shigellosis, 321
shingles, 177, 227, 228, 229, 401
Shingrix, 228
shivering, 193, 345, 347
shoe repair, 181
shortness of breath, 59, 64, 66, 74, 127, 176, 267, 273, 356
shower cap, 178, 238
sida, 270
signs, 127, 308, 337, 368
silk, 162, 163, 344, 384
Silvadene, 107, 219, 411
silver sulfadiazine, 219
simethicone, 362
sinus infections, 109, 115
sinusitis, 113, 129, 203
skin grafts, 140
skunks, 262
slivers, 195, 199
slow heart rate, 53
slow wound healing, 54
smallpox, 41, 273, 399
smoking, 67, 73, 325, 330
snakebite, 173, 256, 258
sneezing, 38
soap, 39, 40, 41, 200, 249, 251, 262, 296, 318, 339
social distancing, 148
socks, 95, 242, 344
soda, 33, 76, 78, 95, 154, 173, 174, 250, 251, 305, 332, 352
SODIS, 26, 33, 34, 35, 37
sodium bicarbonate, 87
sodium hypochlorite, 29, 46
SOF-T, 169
SOFTT, 169
sore muscles, 157, 225
sore throat, 60, 125, 183, 247, 272, 274, 301, 302, 303, 392
South Carolina, 34
soy, 55
Spanish-American War, 274, 279
spasms, 69, 70, 80, 225, 226, 348
spearmint, 240, 241
sphygmomanometer, 192
spinach, 60, 64, 67, 80, 336
splinter, 174, 179, 198, 226, 379
splints, 167, 170, 180, 202
spoon nails, 75
sprains, 170, 202, 203, 394
sprouts, 319
squash, 58, 60, 61
St. John's wort, 229, 402
stabilized oxygen, 37
Staphylococcus, 90, 110, 130, 260, 305
Staphylococcus aureus, 130, 305, 320
staples, 83, 163, 164, 198
STDs, 42, 123, 203, 237, 340, 341, 395
sterile gown, 167, 324
sterile saline, 86
sterilization, 26, 45, 46, 47, 48, 49, 157, 162
sterilization indicator tape, 48
Steri-Strips, 163, 202
steroids, 249, 250, 289, 325, 356, 364
stethoscope, 46, 193, 300
stiff neck, 247, 315
stings, 83, 89, 90, 91, 115, 126, 174, 177, 248, 250, 392
stomach, 76, 88, 92, 93, 97, 98, 114, 175, 201, 202, 228, 247, 305, 306, 311, 319, 326, 327, 330, 331, 332, 333, 362
stomach acid, 313, 316, 331, 332
straws, 300, 387, 388
strep, 16, 120, 125, 202, 205, 284, 302, 303, 429
strep throat, 16, 113, 122, 125, 202, 203, 302, 303
Streptococcus mutans, 174
Streptococcus pneumoniae, 125
Streptococcus pyogenes, 125, 130
Streptococcus viridans, 260
streptomycin, 273
stress, 22, 54, 93, 159, 188, 190, 227, 228, 327
stunted growth, 54, 69, 70, 73
sucralfate, 362
Sudafed, 95, 283, 284, 292, 356, 411

sugar, 76, 101, 141, 174, 183, 184, 188, 189, 190, 286, 346, 359, 387, 396
sugardyne, 190, 191
suicide, 22
sulfa drugs, 127
sulfonamides, 107
sulfur, 234, 235, 314
sumatriptan, 98
sun, 33, 34, 47, 68, 69, 71, 217, 336, 349
sunburns, 91, 174, 216
sunscreen, 25, 68, 69, 71, 217, 240
superglue, 163
surgery, 53, 59, 65, 70, 78, 81, 152, 155, 162, 197, 198, 322, 324, 325, 327, 334, 369
Survival and Austere Medicine, 3rd Edition, 223, 324, 397, 405
suture, 47, 83, 159, 160, 161, 162, 164, 166, 167, 180, 185, 197, 202, 324, 386
SWAT-T, 169, 382
sweating, 79, 80, 252, 335, 345
swelling, 59, 65, 98, 127, 137, 157, 166, 249, 251, 255, 257, 280, 288, 289, 322, 340, 342, 343, 348, 368, 392
symptoms, 53, 58, 63, 69, 80, 228, 273, 274, 281, 290, 301, 306, 316, 317, 319, 320, 321, 340, 349, 368, 392
Synthroid, 361, 362, 363
syphilis, 120, 341
syringes, 21, 45, 48, 91, 166, 359
Tagamet, 65, 78
Tamiflu, 295
tape, 31, 49, 132, 163, 164, 165, 168, 179, 180, 181, 182, 198, 199, 201, 202, 220, 379, 380, 382
tapeworms, 133
tea, 16, 95, 178, 183, 220, 229, 236, 238, 242, 249, 259, 297, 332, 366, 388
tea tree, 178, 183, 236, 238, 242, 249
tea tree oil, 178, 183, 220, 236, 238, 242
tears, 57, 164
Telfa non-stick pads, 139
temperature, 34, 47, 49, 142, 154, 157, 158, 243, 274, 297, 310, 320, 345, 347, 348, 349, 350, 356, 364, 374, 375
tendinitis, 98, 99, 137, 325
Tennessee, 245, 247
tension headache, 98, 175
tetanus, 24, 185, 223, 224, 225, 226
tetracycline, 72, 87, 101, 102, 107, 119, 123, 127, 128, 130, 226, 246, 265, 266, 291, 298, 333, 341
Texas, 34, 276, 280, 282
thalassemia, 75
The Medical Letter, 128, 129
The Year Without a Summer, 277
thermometer, 46, 86, 346, 382
thiamine, 58, 59, 60
thirst, 74, 360
Thirty Years' War, 277
thrush, 114, 178, 340
thyme, 130, 241, 287, 357, 400
thyroid, 153, 345, 350, 351, 352, 360, 361, 362, 392
Thyromine, 363
thyroxine, 361
tick, 108, 114, 120, 129, 202, 242, 243, 244, 245, 247, 271, 272, 400
time-release tablets, 101
tincture, 157, 163, 229, 254, 258, 259, 270, 314, 357, 386, 401
tincture of benzoin, 163
tingling, 66, 70, 80, 127, 228, 255, 342
tinidazole, 340
TMP-SMZ, 107, 108, 110, 112, 123, 275, 312, 316, 323, 329, 337, 338, 339
tobacco, 133, 232, 366
tongue, 64, 65, 127, 130, 364, 372, 373
tonsillitis, 115, 272
toothaches, 202
tourniquet, 149, 151, 168, 169, 171, 203, 257
trachoma, 129
Tramadol, 336
transfusion, 247, 281, 359
trash, 38
trauma shears, 167, 198, 199
triage, 22, 23
triangle bandage, 170
trichobezoars, 326
trichomonas, 340
trichomoniasis, 124
trimethoprim-sulfamethoxazole, 107
triple antibiotic, 243, 387
TSH, 361
t-shirt, 32, 33, 220
tuberculosis, 41, 44, 268, 269, 270, 271
tubing, 47
tularemia, 271, 272, 273
Tums, 78, 86, 130, 332, 382
turmeric, 133, 297
tweezers, 49, 193, 198, 199, 243
Tylenol, 89, 95, 99, 100, 229, 280, 282, 286, 292, 325, 379
Tylenol-3, 95, 99, 286
type-1 diabetic, 15, 357
type-2 diabetes, 78
typhoid, 19, 87, 114, 274, 275
Typhoid Mary, 275
typhus, 120, 121, 129, 237, 276, 277, 278
ulcer, 189, 253, 330, 331, 333, 341
ulcerative colitis, 57, 67, 81
ulcers, 75, 76, 88, 92, 93, 98, 176, 185, 201, 272, 304, 328, 392
ultraviolet radiation, 33, 34
umbilical cord, 226
upper respiratory infections, 68, 99, 113, 115, 120, 121, 202, 356
urinalysis strips, 358

urinary tract infections, 108, 120, 129, 174, 203, 311, 337, 394
urine, 79, 223, 253, 334, 337, 338, 347, 349, 359
Uristat, 338
Usnea, 164, 271, 287, 297, 316, 386, 398, 402
uterine infections, 123
vaccines, 24, 228, 262, 264, 274, 366
Vagisil, 83
valacyclovir, 228
valium, 226
Vanquish, 98
Vaseline, 140
vector-borne diseases, 42, 397
vegan, 69, 73
vegetables, 51, 55, 56, 57, 61, 64, 65, 66, 67, 74, 76, 77, 78, 80, 138, 307, 316, 319, 336, 362
vegetarianism, 76, 81
vertigo, 90
vet wrap, 138
Vet-Bond, 163
Vibrio cholerae, 265
Vicks VapoRub, 95
Vicodin, 95, 100, 386
vigorous exercise, 356
vinegar, 156, 178, 220, 235, 238, 240, 241
viral hemorrhagic fever, 41, 279
viruses, 31, 32, 33, 36, 40, 45, 142, 144, 151, 155, 156, 157, 244, 247, 262, 301, 399
vital signs, 299, 374, 375
vitamin A, 56, 57, 58
vitamin B1, 58
vitamin B12, 65, 76, 93, 202, 229
vitamin B3, 61
vitamin B9, 63
vitamin C, 35, 66, 67, 76, 152, 336, 338
vitamin D, 67, 70
vomiting, 59, 79, 80, 93, 94, 97, 116, 123, 124, 127, 203, 245, 246, 247, 252, 253, 255, 265, 273, 274, 281, 299, 306, 312, 316, 317, 320, 322, 326, 327, 328, 329, 331, 335, 337, 339, 349, 394
walnuts, 63, 362
War of Grenada, 277
warfarin, 121, 362
warts, 179
water, 19, 24, 26, 27, 28, 29, 30, 31, 32, 33, 34, 35, 36, 37, 39, 40, 41, 45, 46, 61, 62, 64, 65, 66, 71, 81, 85, 90, 91, 105, 119, 122, 124, 132, 138, 141, 151, 152, 153, 154, 155, 156, 157, 170, 172, 173, 174, 179, 182, 183, 186, 216, 217, 218, 220, 221, 222, 231, 235, 236, 237, 241, 243, 244, 249, 251, 256, 258, 259, 263, 265, 271, 272, 273, 274, 277, 286, 289, 291, 296, 297, 298, 300, 305, 317, 318, 320, 335, 338, 343, 344, 345, 346, 347, 348, 349, 355, 357, 379, 390, 403
weight gain, 73, 361
weight loss, 59, 269, 326, 327, 360
West Nile virus, 281
wheat, 55, 58, 62, 67, 71
wheezing, 96, 127, 175, 287, 301, 356
Where There Is No Doctor, 341
whipworms, 74, 133
whole grains, 51, 55, 62, 63, 77, 78, 367
whooping cough, 285
witch hazel, 236, 238, 251
wool, 344, 356
World Health Organization, 35
World War I, 175, 185, 277
World War II, 185, 357, 358
worms, 120, 132, 133, 184
wormwood, 133
wound salve, 178
Xeroform, 140
yarrow, 297, 357, 402
yeast infection, 116
yellow fever, 41, 278, 279, 280
yogurt, 81
Yugoslavia, 277
Zantac, 65, 78, 88, 93, 204, 249, 332, 260, 364
Zika, 280, 281
zinc, 57, 80, 81, 130, 216, 362
Zipstitch, 163
Zithromax, 127, 129, 204, 265, 275, 291, 312, 319, 340, 341, 382, 384
Zofran, 94
Zostavax, 228
Zyrtec, 88, 95, 204, 356

Made in United States
Orlando, FL
10 October 2026

88905713R00252